Food Science and Technology

Fermented Foods and Beverages in a Global Age

Medicine & Health
New York

Food Science and Technology

Food Byproducts: Valorization Through Nutraceutical Production
Sandra Teresita Martín-del-Campo, PhD; Anaberta Cardador-Martínez, PhD; Jessica del Pilar Ramírez-Anaya, PhD
2023. ISBN: 979-8-88697-612-0 (Hardcover)
2023. ISBN: 979-8-88697-876-6 (eBook)

Bioprospecting of Natural Compounds in Food, Pharmaceutical and Biomedical Science
Siddhartha Pati, PhD; Tanmay Sarkar, PhD; Dibyait Lahiri, PhD
2022. ISBN: 979-8-88697-361-7 (Hardcover)
2022. ISBN: 979-8-88697-431-7 (eBook)

More information about this series can be found at https://novapublishers.com/product-category/series/food-science-and-technology-series/

Fermented Foods and Beverages in a Global Age

New Frontiers in Sparkling Wine Production
Rosanna Tofalo, Hervé Alexandre
2024. ISBN: 979-8-89113-562-8 (Hardcover)
2024. ISBN: 979-8-89113-642-7 (eBook)

Fermented and Distilled Alcoholic Beverages: A Technological, Chemical and Sensory Overview. Distilled Beverages
Maurício Bonatto Machado de Castilhos (Editor)
Vanildo Luiz Del Bianchi (Editor)
Vitor Manfroi (Editor)
2021. ISBN: 978-1-53619-026-7 (Softcover)
2021. ISBN: 978-1-53619-053-3 (eBook)

More information about this series can be found at https://novapublishers.com/product-category/series/fermented-foods-and-beverages-in-a-global-age/

Maria Simona Chiș
Adriana Paucean
Editors

Lactobacillus plantarum and Its Role in Human Health

nova
Medicine & Health
New York

DOI: https://doi.org/10.52305/VWNC0146

Library of Congress Cataloging-in-Publication Data

Names: Chiş, Maria Simona, editor. | Paucean, Adriana, editor.
Title: Lactobacillus plantarum and its role in human health / editors Maria Simona Chiş, PhD, Lecturer, Department of Food Technology, Faculty of Food Science and Technology, University of Agricultural Sciences and Veterinary Medicine Cluj-Napoca, Cluj-Napoca, Romania, Adriana Paucean, PhD, Faculty of Food Science and Technology, University of Agricultural Sciences and Veterinary Medicine Cluj-Napoca, Cluj-Napoca, Romania.
Description: New York : Nova Science Publishers, [2024] | Series: Fermented foods and beverages in a global age | Includes bibliographical references and index. |
Identifiers: LCCN 2024021203 (print) | LCCN 2024021204 (ebook) | ISBN 9798891136960 (hardcover) | ISBN 9798891138452 (adobe pdf)
Subjects: LCSH: Lactobacillus plantarum.
Classification: LCC QR82.L3 L335 2024 (print) | LCC QR82.L3 (ebook) | DDC 579.3/7--dc23/eng/20240521
LC record available at https://lccn.loc.gov/2024021203
LC ebook record available at https://lccn.loc.gov/2024021204

Published by Nova Science Publishers, Inc. † New York

Contents

Preface vii

Chapter 1 *Lactobacillus plantarum*: **History and Versatility** 1
Chirag Patel, Priya Shukla, Sonal Pande,
Jayesh Beladiya and Ketan Ranch

Chapter 2 **An Overview of** ***Lactobacillus plantarum*** **Strains with Probiotic Effect on Human Health** 23
Jiancun Zhao, and Zhenshang Xu

Chapter 3 **Macro, Micro and Nanoencapsulation as Delivery System of** ***Lactobacillus plantarum*** 45
Camila Cristina Avelar de Sousa,
Juliana Sant'Ana Falcão Leite,
Rafael Sepúlveda Fonsêca Trevisan Passos,
Thiago da Matta Pires Cruz,
Maurício Costa Alves da Silva
and Carlos Pasqualin Cavalheiro

Chapter 4 *Lactobacillus plantarum*: **Food Supplements and Pharmaceutical Uses** 75
Călina Ciont, Ramona Suharoschi,
Andreea Diana Kerezsi, Dan Cristian Vodnar
and Oana Lelia Pop

Chapter 5 *Lactobacillus plantarum* **in Bakery and Pastry Products**..115
Simona Maria Man, Adriana Păucean,
Anamaria Pop and Maria Simona Chiş

Chapter 6 ***Lactobacillus plantarum* and Its Role in Milk and Dairy Products Manufacturing** 157
Delia Michiu, Mirela Anamaria Jimborean, Cristina Anamaria Semeniuc, Elena Suzana Biriş-Dorhoi and Liana Claudia Salanţă

Chapter 7 ***Lactobacillus plantarum* and Its Role in Meat Products Manufacturing** 185
Rafael Sepúlveda Fonsêca Trevisan Passos, Camila Cristina Avelar de Sousa, Thiago da Matta Pires Cruz, Juliana Sant'Ana Falcão Leite, Maurício Costa Alves da Silva and Carlos Pasqualin Cavalheiro

Chapter 8 ***Lactobacillus plantarum* in Cereals, Fruits and Vegetables** 207
Elena Suzana Biriş-Dorhoi, Mihaela Mihai and Delia Michiu

Chapter 9 **The Use of *Lactobacillus plantarum* in Sugar Confectionery and Chocolate-Based Products** 237
Andreea Puşcaş, Alexandra Lazăr and Vlad Mureşan

Index 265

Preface

This book provides scientific information about fermentation processes with different *Lactobacillus plantarum* strains and their influence on human health. Various vegetable matrices such as cereals, fruits, vegetables, cocoa beans, bakery and pastry, chocolate-based products, and non-vegetables ones such as milk and meat are discussed, aiming to highlight the applicability of *Lactobacillus plantarum* on food technology. Moreover, the history, and versatility of *Lactobacillus plantarum* strain together with its uses as a probiotic, its applicability on food supplements and pharmaceutical uses are emphasized. Macro, micro, and nano encapsulation as delivery systems for *Lactobacillus plantarum* is another chapter that overviews the controlled release of the strain in the human gastrointestinal tract.

Chapter 1

Lactobacillus plantarum: History and Versatility

Chirag Patel[1,*]
Priya Shukla[2]
Sonal Pande[1]
Jayesh Beladiya[1]
and Ketan Ranch[3]
[1]Department of Pharmacology, L. M. College of Pharmacy, Ahmedabad, India
[2]Department of Pharmacology, SSR College of Pharmacy, Silvassa, India
[3]Department of Pharmaceutics, L. M. College of Pharmacy, Ahmedabad, India

Abstract

Recently, the importance of fermented foods has increased in terms of illness prevention and improving overall health. One of the essential abundant families of gram-positive, acid-tolerant, food-related bacteria is lactic acid bacteria (LAB). *Lactobacillus* has more than 200 species and a greater genetic diversity than any other family. *Lactobacillus plantarum*, one of the important Lactobacillus species, is well recognised for its probiotic uses and has several functional qualities, including immune modulation, bioprotection, antioxidant activity, and antibacterial activity. In terms of genome size, protein count, and variation in antibacterial encoding loci, different strains of L. plantarum exhibit genetic variability. This chapter encompasses the variety and adaptability of many *L. plantarum* strains isolated from various sources, along with their history, isolation, phenotypic, and genotypic characterization.

---

* Corresponding Author's Email: chiragapatel@lmcp.ac.in.

In: Lactobacillus plantarum and Its Role in Human Health
Editors: Maria Simona Chiş, Adriana Paucean
ISBN: 979-8-89113-696-0

Keywords: *Lactobacillus Plantarum,* genomic diversity, taxonomy, *L. plantarum* history

1. Introduction

One of the essential abundant fermented foods families of gram-positive, acid-tolerant, food-related bacteria is Lactic acid bacteria (LAB) [1]. The food, probiotic, dairy, and beverage industries all employ LAB extensively [2]. The importance of fermented foods has increased recently in terms of illness prevention and improving overall health [2]. The American Food and Drug Administration (FDA) has designated LAB as generally recognised as safe (GRAS) bacteria [3]. *Lactobacillus*, which has more than 200 species, is the LAB genus with the most diversity [3].

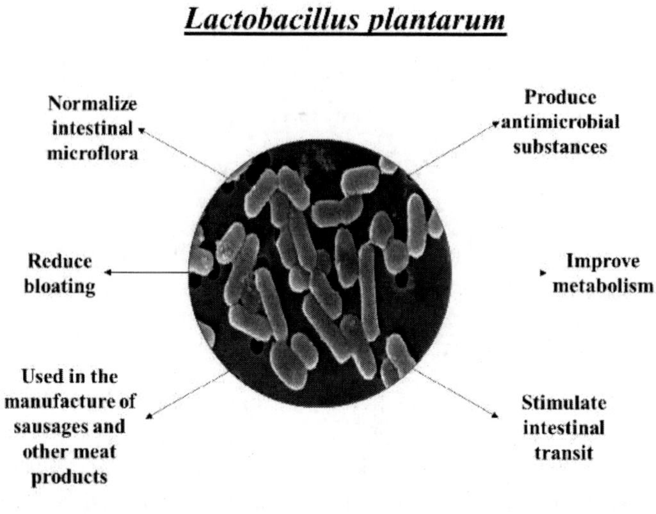

Figure 1. Modulatory potential of *L. plantarum.*

Despite being historically classified as a genus, *Lactobacillus* possesses a greater genetic diversity than the average family [4] *L. plantarum*, one of the numerous *Lactobacillus* species, is well recognised for its probiotic uses since it naturally lives in the human gastro intestinal tract [5]. It also has several functional qualities, including immune modulation, bio-protection, antioxidant activity, and antibacterial activity as shown in Figure 1 [6]. In terms of genome size, protein count, and variation in antibacterial encoding loci, different strains of *L. plantarum* exhibit genetic variability [6] Additionally, the molecular biology and genetics of *L. plantarum* directly influence its functional characteristics and traits [7]. Consequently, the chapter addresses the variety and adaptability of numerous *L. plantarum* strains isolated from various alongside their historical background, isolation, phenotypic and genotypic characterisation, and comparative genomics.

1.1. *L. plantarum* History

A kind of lactic acid bacterium called *L. plantarum* has been employed for many years in the fermentation of foods and drinks [8]. Its beginnings may be found in antiquity, when people became aware of how fermentation might be used to preserve and improve the flavour of food [9]. Traditional fermented foods are a great source of live, active microorganisms; in fact, it's assumed that lactic acid bacteria (LAB) is mostly obtained from traditional fermented foods [10]. When considering food fermentations, it is important to keep in mind that LAB is largely responsible for many of the bacterial changes seen in the more well-known fermented foods (as contrasted yeast-based alcoholic fermentations) [11]. This group, which frequently produces lactic acid as its principal by-product, consists of 261 species and families, including *Lactococcus, Lactobacillus, Enterococcus, Streptococcus, Leuconostoc, and Pediococcus* [12]. Human have ingested lactic acid bacteria, including *L. plantarum,* for a very long time before recorded history as shown in Figure 2. *L. plantarum* was initially employed to make sauerkraut in Germany in the 16th century, according to historical records [13]. Without the *Lactobacillus* genus is essential in the production of fermented milk products and has a long history of safe usage (particularly in the dairy sector) [14]. It is composed of Gram-positive, fermentative, facultatively anaerobic, and non-spore-forming bacteria, and Beijerinck first suggested the genus *Lactobacillus* in 1901 [15]. It has a wide range of applications and may be found in many environmental niches [15]. A rod-shaped, facultative hetero-fermentative group of lactobacilli belonging to the genus *Lactobacillus* is known as *L. plantarum* [16]. In 1919, OrlaJennsenand Holland first referred to *L. plantarum* as Streptobacterium plantarum [17]. In 1936, Pederson named *L. plantarum* after describing the species and noting various physical and biochemical characteristics [18]. *Lactobacillus pentosus, Lactobacillus arabinosus, Lactobacillus rudensis, and L. plantarum var. mobilis* were all wrongly thought to be members of the same species because of similarities in their phenotypic characteristics before the adoption of genetic techniques in the 1980s [19]. It belongs to the family of gramme-positive lactic acid bacteria (LAB) [19]. *L. plantarum* is commonly present in meals that have been soured by lactic acid bacteria, especially when the item is formed from a plant, such as brined olives, sauerkraut, etc. [20]. Individuals who consume food that has undergone fermentation by lactic acid bacteria, inadvertently consume a considerable amount of *L. plantarum* [21]. Researchers started looking into the health advantages of *L. plantarum* and other probiotic bacteria at the beginning of the 20th century [21]. These bacteria were shown to be capable of enhancing digestion, enhancing the immune system, and even preventing some illnesses [19].

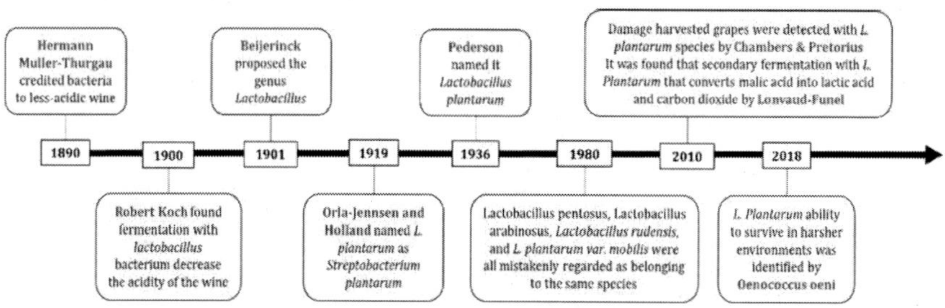

Figure 2. Timeline of *L. plantarum* in the history of probiotic.

Coincidentally, wine has been produced by fruit fermentation ever since civilization began [22]. When damaged grapes were harvested, they were put in a container and transformed into crude wine by local plants growing on the fruit skins [23]. It was discovered via farming that malolactic fermentation would make the wine less tart [24]. Less tart wine is produced through malolactic fermentation (MLF), a secondary fermentation that converts malic acid into lactic acid and carbon dioxide [25]. Hermann Muller-Thurgau attributed bacteria to less-acidic wine (malolactic fermentation) in 1891, and Robert Koch deliberately infected wine with bacteria to show that he could lessen the acidity of the beverage in 1900 [26].

A key player in malolactic fermentation has been identified as *Oenococcus oeni*; however, *L. plantarum* has also been used as a starter culture for MLF and has shown some advantages over O.oeni, including the capacity to thrive in more challenging environments and the capacity to produce more aromatic compounds [27]. In conclusion, *L. plantarum* DSM 33452 is safe for ingestion by humans, is effective in wine and must malolactic fermentation [26]. In the modern food business, *L. plantarum* is frequently utilised as a probiotic supplement and as a fermentation starter culture [28]. Additionally, probiotic drinks and nutritional supplements frequently include it. It is thought to be crucial in preserving a healthy gut flora, and studies into its health benefits are ongoing [28].

1.2. Taxonomy of *L. plantarum*

The taxonomic identity of *L. plantarum* was verified and registered by the German Collection of Microorganisms and Cell Cultures (Deutsche Sammlung von Mikroorganismen und Zellkulturen GmbH) on late February 2020 under the accession number DSM 33452, as shown in Table 1 [29]. During whole genome sequencing, identifying markers such the 16S rDNA and rpoA genes were employed to confirm the identity of the organism [30]. Although 16S cannot distinguish between all *Lactobacillus* species, it offers a standard for identifying bacteria. For further speciation analysis, the rpoA housekeeping gene was used [30]. The *L. plantarum* group has shown the applicability of the rpoA gene for precise species identification. Through the use of 16S rDNA and rpoA sequencing, the species of the strain has been identified [31].

Table 1. Taxonomical identification of *L. plantarum* [33]

Domain	*"Bacteria"*
Taxonomic Rank	Species
Synonym(s)	*L. plantarum; Lactobacillus arizonensis; Streptobacterium plantarum*
Full scientific name (PNU)	*Lactiplantibacillus plantarum*
Kingdom	Bacteria
Subkingdom	Posibacteria
Domain	*"Bacteria"*
Phylum	Firmicutes
Class	Bacilli
Order	Lactobacillales
Family	Lactobacillaceae
Genus	*Lactobacillus*
Species	*Lactiplantibacillus plantarum*
Subspecies	*L. plantarum* *L. plantarum argentoratensis*
Lineage	Cellular organisms > Bacteria (eubacteria) >Terrabacteria group >Firmicutes> Bacilli >Lactobacillales>Lactobacillaceae>Lactipantibacillus

Table 1. (Continued)

Domain	*"Bacteria"*
Strain	• DSM 4229 / 80 • C38 • LP80 • A-1 • L137 • KW30 • ATCC 8014 / DSM 20205 / CCM 1904 / CCUG 11253 / NCDO 82 / NCIMB 6376 / 17-5 (17-5, ATCC 8014 / DSM 20205 / CCM 1904 / NCDO 82 / NCIMB 6376, NCIMB 6376, NCIB 6376, CCUG 9289, BUCSAV 217, ICPB 2080, ATCC 8014, CCM 1904, ATCC 8014 / CCM 1904 / DSM 20205 / NCDO 82 / NCIB 6376) • NCDO 1088 • ATCC 14431 / CECT 221 / LMD 73.4 / T-1043-5 (ATCC 14431 / T-1043-5, CECT 221, T-1043-5) • C11

With names like *L. plantarum*, *Lactobacillus arizonensis*, and *Streptobacterium plantarum*, the domain of *L. plantarum* was found to be Bacteria [32]. It is also referred to as *Lactiplantibacillus plantarum*, a member of the bacterial kingdom. Its subkingdom is *Posibacteria* and are from the *Lactobacillaceae* family as shown in Table no. 1 [32].

1.3. Characterization of *L. Plantarum*

Gram-positive, nonmotile, nonspore-forming, microaerophilic, and mesophilic *L. plantarum* grows well between 10-15°C, but not at 45°C [34]. Straight rods with rounded ends that measure 0.9-1.2 X 3.0-8.0 mm make up cells, which can appear single, in pairs, or in short chains. It has been shown that under specific conditions, a few strains of *L. plantarum* have true catalase and pseudocatalase activity that contain manganese [35]. Moreover, it is a heterofermentative kind of lactobacilli that is acid-tolerant, non-respiring, and low in G + C. Furthermore, it can grow in the gastrointestinal tract despite having a low buffering capacity and demonstrating a high tolerance to repeated exposure to bile salts and HCL (pH 2.0) [36]. Some strains also display nitrate- and hematin-dependent nitrite reductases. Teichoic acid is either found in ribitol or glycerol in the cell wall, while certain strains have a different teichoic acid. The cell wall's peptididoglycan is of the meso-diaminopimelic acid (DAP) kind [37].

In addition to produce lactic acid as its principal metabolite by-product, *L. plantarum* needs a supply of fermentable saccharides for energ y [38]. Its adaptability to diverse ecological niches demonstrates *L. plantarum*'s astounding ability to ferment a variety of carbohydrates, including monosaccharides, disaccharides, and polysaccharides [39]. It may also ferment carbohydrates to produce significant metabolites like ethanol, carbon dioxide, and organic acids like acetic, succinic, and lactic acids under certain conditions and when using specific substrates [40]. These bacteria may switch between heterofermentative and homofermentative forms of metabolism depending on the carbon source [41].

To combat oxidative stress, *L. plantarum* has developed the P-type manganese translocation ATPase and a high intracellular concentration of manganese ions [Mn2+] to scavenge oxygen radicals [42]. The bacteria *L. plantarum* has tannase activity, which enables it to break down phenolic acids [43]. A flavan-3-ol-enriched grape seed extract was also metabolised by a strain of *L. plantarum* (IFPL935) using its galloylesterase, decarboxylase, and benzyl alcohol dehydrogenase activities [44].

The classic approach to identifying distinct *Lactobacillus* spp. focuses on patterns of carbohydrate fermentation responses, arginine hydrolysis, growth demands, growth at specified temperatures, and lactic acid configuration [45]. While more appropriate characterization techniques are being used, such as peptidoglycan structure, DNA base composition, electrophoretic mobility of L-lactate dehydrogenase, DNA homology, species-specific PCR (derived from rRNA sequences), RAPD-PCR (Random Amplified Polymorphic DNA-*polymerase chain reaction)*, PFGE (Pulse Field Gel Electrophoresis), and restriction enzyme analysis, these characteristics are still used as indicators [46]. Because many species are phenotypically quite similar yet genotypically varied, it is vital to define and categorise species using both phenotypic and genomic methodologies [47].

L. plantarum is a member of the *Lactobacillus* casei-Pediococcus group according to 16S rRNA-based phylogeny, which has recently received support from whole-genome DNA, DNA-RNA hybridization, and GC content studies. DNA-DNA hybridization studies have shown that *L. plantarum* forms two genomically related groups that are in turn divided by other streptobacteria and lactobacilli with DAP in the cell wall [48]. Although simple methods like the random amplified polymorphic DNA-polymerase chain reaction (RAPD-PCR) have been used for strain typing and differentiation from related *Lactobacillus* spp., accurate species identification requires a polyphasic strategy based on physiological tests and multiple molecular methods [49].

Due to their 99.7-99.9% sequence similarity, the closely related species *L. plantarum*, *Lactobacillus* pentosus, and *Lactobacillus paraplantarum* together known as the "*L. plantarum* group" cannot be separated from one another [50]. Moreover, the group's species display highly comparable fermentation processes. Repetitive element sequence-based polymerase chain reaction and species-specific PCR primers are two methods that may be used to distinguish between these species (Rep-PCR). Furthermore, utilising RFLP-PFGE, 16S ARDRA, AFLP employing restriction enzymes HindIII and MseI, ribotyping, and RAPD-PCR, strain separation between *L. plantarum* and *Lb. pentosus* could be accomplished. It could be useful to employ multilocus sequence typing (MLST) based on the housekeeping genes pgm, ddl, gyr B, purK1, gdh, and mutS to determine the genetic relatedness and distinguish between *L. plantarum* strains [51]. The direct identification of bacteria from a variety of matrices has recently been made possible thanks to the development of culture-independent methods. The most effective methods for this purpose are DGGE (Denaturing Gradient Gel Electrophoresis) and TGGE (Temperature Gradient Gel Electrophoresis), which were successfully used to find *L. plantarum* in cheese and other dairy products [49]. Table no. 2 displays some physiological and genetic properties of species.

Table 2. Characterization of *L. plantarum* [52]

Lactic Acid precursor	Arabinose, lactose, maltose, mannitol, mannose, melibiose, raffinose, sorbitol, salicin, ribose, galatose
Lactic acid are not formed from	Xylose, sorbose, inulin, inositol, starch, glycerol
Lactic acid isomer	D and L
Mol % G+C	44-46
Growth factor requirements	Calcium pentothenate, niacin, nicotinic acid
Growth with 4% taurocholate	+
Growth in presence of 10% NaCl	+
Hydrolysis of arginine	-
Production of dextran from saccharose	

'+', Present; '-' , absent.

1.4. Isolation of *L. plantarum*

The capacity of *L. plantarum* to tolerate the high salt and acidic content of fermented vegetables, especially cucumber, sauerkraut, and olive, accounts for the highest fraction of the species found in fermented vegetables [53]. Several investigations had proven the presence of *L. plantarum* in vegans, grains, meat, marine source and dairy products, plant-based diet, fermented food [54]. The above data shows different isolation source of *L. plantarum* species in Table 3.

Table 3. Isolation sources of *L. plantarum*

Product Isolation source	Sample	Genome	Reference
Breast milk	15 samples from their mother's milk	*L. plantarum* (210/29/24/*1)	[55]
Breast-fed infants	Fresh faecal samples were obtained from two healthy breast-fed infants	*L. plantarum* (P1) *L. plantarum* (P162) *L. plantarum* (P164) *L. plantarum* (P167) *L. plantarum* (P171) *L. plantarum* (P172) *L. plantarum* (P173) *L. plantarum* (P186)	[56]
Feces from young dairy calves	7-days of urine and fecal collection.	*L. plantarum* 27SC	[57]
Vagina	Vaginal swabs of 20 healthy women	*L. plantarum* 4B2	[58]
Human saliva	Saliva samples	*L. plantarum*	[59]
Human healthy rectal mucosa	42 healthy volunteers' biopsies were taken from the rectal mucosa during rectoscopy	*L. plantarum*, cluster 2 and cluster 16	[60]
Oral cavity	a cotton-tipped swab was pressed against the back of the tongue	*L. plantarum*	[61]
Ayurvedic medicine (Kutajarista)	Ayurvedic formulation prepared traditionally by fermentation of the decoction of Holarrhenaanti dysentrica	*L. plantarum* VR1	[62]
Amasi	Fermented milk food amasi	*L. plantarum* AMA-K	[63]
Dry fermented sausage	Argentinian dry-fermented sausage	*L. plantarum* LP 31	[64]
Fish	Gadusvirens	*L. plantarum*	[65]
Meat dry sausage	Dry sausage using MRS agar (Oxoid)	*L. plantarum* UG1	[66]
Olive products	Olives from Wageningen Centre for Food Sciences, NIZO Food Research	*L. plantarum* LPT57/1	[67]
Papaya	Papaya from Sao Paulo, SP, Brazil	*L. plantarum* ST16Pa	[68]

1.5. Genomic Diversity and Versatility of *L. Plantarum*

The versatile and adaptable species *L. plantarum* is found in a variety of environmental niches, including certain dairy, meat, and several vegetable or plant fermentations [69]. In addition, *L. plantarum* is commonly acknowledged as a natural resident of the human gastrointestinal tract. The considerable size of L. plantarum's genome, which surpasses many other lactic acid bacteria, indicates the species' remarkable ability for ecological adaptation [70]. Genetic tools have been developed for this species, including (controlled) gene expression systems and vectors that may be used to produce gene disruption or deletion variants, for several strains of *L. plantarum*. Here, we present *L. plantarum* WCFS1's whole genomic sequence [71].

Lactobacillus plantarum WCFS1, was first discovered in human saliva, has a single circular chromosome with a length of 3,308,274 base pairs, two small, cryptic plasmids (2,365 and 1,917 bp), and a larger plasmid (36,069 bp) that encodes genes for conjugal plasmid transfer and several other processes [72]. *L. plantarum* WCFS1 has 3,052 putative protein-encoding genes, of which 70% are anticipated to have biological functions [73]. As *L. plantarum* is a facultative heterofermentative lactic acid bacteria, its genome contains all the enzymes required for the glycolysis and phosphoketolase processes [73]. The genome of *L. plantarum* encodes every enzyme required for the glycolysis and phosphoketolase processes, supporting its classification as a facultative heterofermentative lactic acid bacterium [74]. In addition, *L. plantarum* additionally encodes 25 whole putative sugar transporter enzyme II complexes and a large number of pyruvate-dissipating enzymes that are involved in private metabolism [75]. Moreover, the chromosome codes for more than 200 extracellular proteins, many of which are believed to be associated with the cell membrane [75].

It was demonstrated that the *L. plantarum* group exhibits rather high levels of phenotypic heterogeneity even in the pre-genomic period [76]. The genetic diversity was originally recorded by employing molecular methods like AFLP (Amplified fragment length polymorphism) and RAPD (Randam Amplified polymorphic DNA) [77]. This work enabled the development of molecular markers that can distinguish *L. plantarum* from *L. paraplantarum* and *L. pentosus*. These two species have remarkably similar carbohydrate utilization traits and cannot be distinguished through 16S rRNA gene sequence analysis [78]. This research facilitated the creation of molecular markers that can distinguish L. plantarum from L. *paraplantarum* and L. *pentosus.*

Table 4. Characteristics of *L. plantarum* isolates ascertained through Multi-Locus Sequence Typing (MLST) analysis [87]

Strain no.	Strain	RT	ITS	ST	Allele no. at locus:						Source of isolate		
					pgm	Ddl	gyrB	purK1	gdh	mutS	Origin	Country	Year
1.	CECT 748T (ATCC 14917)	2	1	5	3	2	1	2	1	1	Pickled cabbage	Denmark	1919
2.	CECT 220 (ATCC 8014)	1	1	2	1	3	1	2	6	5	Corn silage	ND	1948
3.	CECT 749 (ATCC 10241)	2	1	6	3	2	1	2	3	1	Pickled cabbage	ND	1955
4.	WCFS1	ND	ND	1	1	1	1	1	1	1	Human Saliva	UK	1956
5.	CECT 4185 (NCBF 1193)	2	1	7	3	1	2	1	5	1	Silage	ND	1958
6.	CECT 4645 (NCBF 965)	4	1	8	2	4	7	8	10	4	Cheese	ND	1958
7.	CECT 221 (ATCC 14431)	2	1	3	1	1	6	3	8	1	Grass silage	ND	1960
8.	CECT 223	2	1	4	1	5	3	4	7	1	ND	Pamplona, Spain	1987
9.	CECT 224	2	1	4	1	5	3	4	7	1	ND	Pamplona, Spain	1987
10.	RM35	4	1	10	3	2	1	2	2	8	Wine	Toledo, Spain	1998
11.	RM38	2	1	11	3	1	4	2	4	2	Wine	Toledo, Spain	1998
12.	RM40	3	1	12	1	1	1	5	9	1	Wine	Toledo, Spain	1998
13.	RM28	2	1	9	1	2	1	7	7	3	Wine	Valladolid, Spain	2000

Table 4. (Continued)

Strain no.	Strain	RT	ITS	ST	Allele no. at locus:						Source of isolate		
Strain no.	Strain	RT	ITS	ST	Allele no. at locus:						Source of isolate		
					pgm	Ddl	gyrB	purK1	gdh	mutS	Origin	Country	Year
14.	RM73	2	1	14	3	2	1	2	1	7	Wine	Madrid, Spain	2000
15.	RM71	2	1	13	3	1	5	6	5	6	Wine	Valladolid, Spain	2001
16.	RM72	2	1	13	3	1	5	6	5	6	Wine	Valladolid, Spain	2001

RT, Ribotype; ITS, 16S–23S ISR type; ST, sequence type; ND, no data available.

The genetic diversity found in six loci of housekeeping genes is used in a multilocus sequence-typing (MLST) method for this organism, which may be used as a molecular tool for strain-level identification [79]. The utilization of these molecular techniques also brought to light the presence of a subspecies known as *L. plantarum* subsp. argentoratensis. This subspecies can be distinguished using nested PCR and is commonly found in fermented plant substrates [80]. Recent diversity studies have revealed that strains from the *L. plantarum* subsp. *argentoratensis* exhibit unique genomic characteristics. Notably, they lack two putative extracellular enzyme complexes that are believed to play a role in carbohydrate utilization. These investigations employed DNA microarrays based on the genome of L. plantarum WCFS1 and comparative genome hybridization methods [81]. Comparative genomics of different *L. plantarum* strains are presented in Table 4.

The chromosomes of the *L. plantarum* strains exhibit high conservation in gene order and in the sequence identity of orthologs. The chromosome does, however, include a few highly variable regions that deviate from this pattern. A few of these cases are discussed below [82].

Among the many strains of *L. plantarum*, there are significant differences in the chromosomal positions and gene contents of the cassettes encoding prophages and transposases [83]. The pln gene cluster of *L. plantarum*, comprising approximately 25 genes, is responsible for producing a range of class IIb bacteriocins. These bacteriocins exhibit full activity when two different peptides work together. Similar to other aspects of *L. plantarum*'s diversity, the pln gene cluster also demonstrates a significant level of variation [84]. Several strains of *L. plantarum* have a great deal of variation in CPS/EPS synthesis genes, which is likely what causes variations in the structure of capsular and exopolysaccharides. The large diversity of cassettes in the sugar lifestyle region, which was inferred from CGH studies, suggested that a lifestyle adaption island with a similar lifestyle would likely exist in many strains of *L. plantarum* [85]. Even the quantity of repeating motifs or domains varies between strains of the *L. plantarum* gene and protein, notably in extracellular proteins, suggesting that different strains interact with their environment differently [86].

Conclusion

The extensive phenotypic and genomic diversity, versatility, and flexibility of *L. plantarum* are the key of its success in diverse niches, including fermentation of vegetables, meat curing, dairy processing, Probiotic supplements, the gastro-intestinal tract health, and biotechnology industries. *L. plantarum is* most frequently tested for its probiotic properties as well as its in vivo efficacy on animals and human healthy volunteers for immune modulation, bio-protection, antioxidant activity, and antibacterial activity. Further investigation into the molecular mechanisms of *L. plantarum* in different diseases and its correlation with phenotypic and genomic diversity should be important for better therapeutic and industrial applications.

References

[1] Mokoena, M. P., Lactic Acid Bacteria and Their Bacteriocins: Classification, Biosynthesis and Applications against Uropathogens: A Mini-Review. *Molecules : A Journal of Synthetic Chemistry and Natural Product Chemistry.* 2017. 22, doi:10.3390/MOLECULES22081255.

[2] Shah, A. M.; Tarfeen, N.; Mohamed, H.; Song, Y., Fermented Foods: Their Health-Promoting Components and Potential Effects on Gut Microbiota. *Fermentation.* 2023. 9, 118, doi:10.3390/FERMENTATION9020118.

[3] Hill, C.; Guarner, F.; Reid, G.; Gibson, G. R.; Merenstein, D. J.; Pot, B.; Morelli, L.; Canani, R. B.; Flint, H. J.; Salminen, S.; Calder, P.C. The International Scientific Association for Probiotics and Prebiotics Consensus Statement on the Scope and Appropriate Use of the Term Probiotic. *Nature Reviews Gastroenterology & Hepatology* 2014. 11, 506–514, doi:10.1038/nrgastro.2014.66.

[4] Fessard, A.; Remize, F., Why Are Weissella Spp. Not Used as Commercial Starter Cultures for Food Fermentation? *Fermentation.* 2017. 3, 38, doi:10.3390/FERMENTATION3030038.

[5] Leroy, F.; De Vuyst, L., Lactic Acid Bacteria as Functional Starter Cultures for the Food Fermentation Industry. *Trends Food Sci Technol* 2004. *15*, 67–78, doi:10.1016/J.TIFS.2003.09.004.

[6] Stiles, M. E.; Holzapfel, W. H., Lactic Acid Bacteria of Foods and Their Current Taxonomy. *Int J Food Microbiol.* 1997, 36, 1–29, doi:10.1016/S0168-1605(96)01233-0.

[7] Buckenhüskes, H. J., Selection Criteria for Lactic Acid Bacteria to Be Used as Starter Cultures for Various Food Commodities. *FEMS Microbiol Rev.* 1993, *12*, 253–271, doi:10.1016/0168-6445(93)90067-J.

[8] Paul Ross, R.; Morgan, S.; Hill, C., Preservation and Fermentation: Past, Present and Future. *Int J Food Microbiol* 2002, *79*, 3–16, doi:10.1016/S0168-1605(02)00174-5.

[9] Terefe, N. S., Emerging Trends and Opportunities in Food Fermentation. *Reference Module in Food Science* 2016, doi:10.1016/B978-0-08-100596-5.21087-1.

[10] Lavefve, L.; Marasini, D.; Carbonero, F., Microbial Ecology of Fermented Vegetables and Non-Alcoholic Drinks and Current Knowledge on Their Impact on

Human Health. *Adv Food Nutr Res* 2019, 87, 147–185, doi:10.1016/bs.afnr.2018.09.001.

[11] Marullo, P.; Dubourdieu, D., Yeast Selection for Wine Flavour Modulation. *Managing Wine Quality* 2010, 293–345, doi:10.1533/9781845699987.2.293.

[12] Food Fermentation - an Overview | ScienceDirect Topics Available online: https://www.sciencedirect.com/topics/food-science/food-fermentation (accessed on 13 April 2023).

[13] Terefe, N. S., Food Fermentation. *Reference Module in Food Science* 2016, doi:10.1016/B978-0-08-100596-5.03420-X.

[14] McNeil, B.; Harvey, L.M.; Rowan, N.J.; Giavasis, I. Fermentation Monitoring and Control of Microbial Cultures for Food Ingredient Manufacture. *Microbial Production of Food Ingredients, Enzymes and Nutraceuticals* 2013, 125–143, doi:10.1533/9780857093547.1.125.

[15] Zheng, J.; Wittouck, S.; Salvetti, E.; Franz, C. M. A. P.; Harris, H. M. B.; Mattarelli, P.; O'toole, P. W.; Pot, B.; Vandamme, P.; Walter, J.; Watanabe, K. A., Taxonomic Note on the Genus *Lactobacillus:* Description of 23 Novel Genera, Emended Description of the Genus Lactobacillus Beijerinck 1901, and Union of Lactobacillaceae and Leuconostocaceae. *Int J Syst Evol Microbiol* 2020, 70, 2782–2858, doi:10.1099/IJSEM.0.004107.

[16] Ouwehand, A. C.; Röytiö, H., Probiotic Fermented Foods and Health Promotion. *Advances in Fermented Foods and Beverages: Improving Quality, Technologies and Health Benefits* 2015, 3–22, doi:10.1016/B978-1-78242-015-6.00001-3.

[17] Zheng, J.; Wittouck, S.; Salvetti, E.; Franz, C. M. A. P.; Harris, H. M. B.; Mattarelli, P.; O'toole, P. W.; Pot, B.; Vandamme, P.; Walter, J.; Watanabe, K. A., Taxonomic Note on the Genus Lactobacillus: Description of 23 Novel Genera, Emended Description of the Genus Lactobacillus Beijerinck 1901, and Union of *Lactobacillaceae* and Leuconostocaceae. *Int J Syst Evol Microbiol.* 2020, 70, 2782–2858, doi:10.1099/IJSEM.0.004107.

[18] Oren, A.; Garrity, G. M., Notification That New Names of Prokaryotes, New Combinations, and New Taxonomic Opinions Have Appeared in Volume 70, Part 4 of the Ijsem. *Int J Syst Evol Microbiol* 2020, 70, 4050–4060, doi:10.1099/IJSEM.0.004260.

[19] Kostinek, M.; Pukall, R.; Rooney, A. P.; Schillinger, U.; Hertel, C.; Holzapfel, W. H.; Franz, C. M. A. P., Lactobacillus Arizonensis Is a Letter Heterotypic Synonym of Lactobacillus Plantarum. *Int J Syst Evol Microbiol* 2005, 55, 2485–2489, doi:10.1099/IJS.0.63880-0.

[20] Tamang, J. P.; Watanabe, K.; Holzapfel, W. H., Review: Diversity of Microorganisms in Global Fermented Foods and Beverages. *Front Microbiol* 2016, 7, doi:10.3389/FMICB.2016.00377.

[21] Medina, E.; de Castro, A.; Romero, C.; Ramírez, E.M.; Brenes, M., Safety of Fermented Fruits and Vegetables. *Regulating Safety of Traditional and Ethnic Foods* 2016, 355–367, doi:10.1016/B978-0-12-800605-4.00018-9.

[22] Zhang, Z.; Dong, Y.; Xiang, F.; Wang, Y.; Hou, Q.; Ni, H.; Cai, W.; Liu, W.; Yang, S.; Guo, Z. Analysis of Bacterial Diversity and Genetic Evolution of

Lacticaseibacillus Paracasei Isolates in Fermentation Pit Mud. *J Appl Microbiol* 2022, *133*, 1821–1831, doi:10.1111/JAM.15672.

[23] Mele, M. A.; Kang, H. M.; Lee, Y. T.; Islam, M. Z., Grape Terpenoids: Flavor Importance, Genetic Regulation, and Future Potential. *Crit Rev Food Sci Nutr* 2021, *61*, 1429–1447, doi:10.1080/10408398.2020.1760203.

[24] Morata, A.; González, C.; Tesfaye, W.; Loira, I.; Suárez-Lepe, J.A. Maceration and Fermentation: New Technologies to Increase Extraction. *Red Wine Technology* 2018, 35–49, doi:10.1016/B978-0-12-814399-5.00003-7.

[25] Gil-Sánchez, I.; Bartolomé Suáldea, B.; Victoria Moreno-Arribas, M. Malolactic Fermentation. *Red Wine Technology* 2019, 85–98, doi:10.1016/B978-0-12-814399-5.00006-2.

[26] Takahashi, S.; Hudagula, H.; Minami, N.; Maeno, N.; Yoshida, K.; Onodera, S.; Takeda, Y.; Tobiyama, T.; Nakamura, T.; Hanai, J.; Tanaka, T. A., Model Study for Contributing Factors of the Fermentation of Qvevri Wine. *Food Control* 2023, *148*, doi:10.1016/j.foodcont.2023.109668.

[27] Pardo, I.; Ferrer, S. Yeast-Bacteria Coinoculation. *Red Wine Technology* 2018, 99–114, doi:10.1016/B978-0-12-814399-5.00007-4.

[28] Carpena, M.; Fraga-Corral, M.; Otero, P.; Nogueira, R. A.; Garcia-Oliveira, P.; Prieto, M. A.; Simal-Gandara, J. Secondary Aroma: Influence of Wine Microorganisms in Their Aroma Profile. *Foods* 2021, 10, doi:10.3390/FOODS 10010051.

[29] German Collection of Microorganisms and Cell Cultures GmbH: Welcome to the Leibniz Institute DSMZ Available online: https://www.dsmz.de/ (accessed on 13 April 2023).

[30] Saito, R.; Sato, N. *Characterization of Lactiplantibacillus Plantarum TO-A Growth Inhibition Activity against Pathogenic Bacteria*; 2021; Vol. 9;.

[31] Naser, S. M.; Thompson, F. L.; Hoste, B.; Gevers, D.; Dawyndt, P.; Vancanneyt, M.; Swings, J. Application of Multilocus Sequence Analysis (MLSA) for Rapid Identification of Enterococcus Species Based on RpoA and PheS Genes. *Microbiology (N Y)* 2005, 151, 2141–2150, doi:10.1099/MIC.0.27840-0.

[32] De Bruyne, K.; Camu, N.; De Vuyst, L.; Vandamme, P. Weissella Fabaria Sp. Nov., from a Ghanaian Cocoa Fermentation. *Int J Syst Evol Microbiol* 2010, 60, 1999–2005, doi:10.1099/IJS.0.019323-0.

[33] *Lactobacillus Plantarum* (Orla-Jensen, 1919) Bergey; Pederson, C. S., 1923 Available online: https://www.gbif.org/species/3227348 (accessed on 13 April 2023).

[34] Tamang, J. P.; Watanabe, K.; Holzapfel, W. H., Review: Diversity of Microorganisms in Global Fermented Foods and Beverages. *Front Microbiol* 2016, *7*, doi:10.3389/FMICB.2016.00377.

[35] Huang, C. H.; Chen, C.C.; Lin, Y. C.; Chen, C. H.; Lee, A. Y.; Liou, J. S.; Gu, C. T.; Huang, L., The Mutl Gene as a Genome-Wide Taxonomic Marker for High Resolution Discrimination of *Lactiplantibacillus Plantarum* and Its Closely Related Taxa. Microorganisms. 2021, *9*, doi:10.3390/MICROORGANISMS9081570/S1.

[36] Zheng, J.; Wittouck, S.; Salvetti, E.; Franz, C. M. A. P.; Harris, H. M. B.; Mattarelli, P.; O'toole, P. W.; Pot, B.; Vandamme, P.; Walter, J.; Watanabe, K. A Taxonomic

Note on the Genus Lactobacillus: Description of 23 Novel Genera, Emended Description of the Genus *Lactobacillus* Beijerinck 1901, and Union of Lactobacillaceae and Leuconostocaceae. *Int J Syst Evol Microbiol.* 2020, 70, 2782–2858, doi:10.1099/IJSEM.0.004107.

[37] De Bruyne, K.; Schillinger, U.; Caroline, L.; Boehringer, B.; Cleenwerck, I.; Vancanneyt, M.; De Vuyst, L.; Franz, C. M. A. P.; Vandamme, P. Leuconostoc Holzapfelii Sp. Nov., Isolated from Ethiopian Coffee Fermentation and Assessment of Sequence Analysis of Housekeeping Genes from Delineation of Leuconostoc Species. *Int J Syst Evol Microbiol* 2007, 57, 2952–2959, doi:10.1099/IJS.0.65292-0.

[38] Naser, S. M.; Dawyndt, P.; Hoste, B.; Gevers, D.; Vandemeulebroecke, K.; Cleenwerck, I.; Vancanneyt, M.; Swings, J. Identification of Lactobacilli by PheS and RpoA Gene Sequence Analyses. *Int J Syst Evol Microbiol.* 2007, 57, 2777–2789, doi:10.1099/IJS.0.64711-0.

[39] de Vries, M. C.; Vaughan, E. E.; Kleerebezem, M.; de Vos, W. M., *Lactobacillus Plantarum*-Survival, Functional and Potential Probiotic Properties in the Human Intestinal Tract. *Int Dairy J.* 2006, 16, 1018–1028, doi:10.1016/J.IDAIRYJ.2005.09.003.

[40] Koutsoumanis, K.; Allende, A.; Alvarez-Ordóñez, A.; Bolton, D.; Bover-Cid, S.; Chemaly, M.; Davies, R.; De Cesare, A.; Hilbert, F.; Lindqvist, R. Update of the List of QPS-Recommended Biological Agents Intentionally Added to Food or Feed as Notified to EFSA 12: Suitability of Taxonomic Units Notified to EFSA until March 2020. *EFSA Journal.* 2020, 18, doi:10.2903/J.EFSA.2020.6174.

[41] Oki, K.; Kudo, Y.; Watanabe, K., *Lactobacillus* Saniviri Sp. Nov. and *Lactobacillus Senioris* Sp. Nov., Isolated from Human Faeces. *Int J Syst Evol Microbiol* 2012, 62, 601–607, doi:10.1099/IJS.0.031658-0.

[42] Chao, S. H.; Sasamoto, M.; Kudo, Y.; Fujimoto, J.; Tsai, Y. C.; Watanabe, K. *Lactobacillus* Odoratitofui Sp. Nov., Isolated from Stinky Tofu Brine. *Int J Syst Evol Microbiol.* 2010, 60, 2903–2907, doi:10.1099/IJS.0.019307-0.

[43] Rosselló-Móra, R.; Amann, R., Past and Future Species Definitions for Bacteria and Archaea. *Syst Appl Microbiol* 2015, 38, 209–216, doi:10.1016/J.SYAPM.2015.02.001.

[44] Glaeser, S. P.; Kämpfer, P., Multilocus Sequence Analysis (MLSA) in Prokaryotic Taxonomy. *Syst Appl Microbiol.* 2015, 38, 237–245, doi:10.1016/J.SYAPM.2015.03.007.

[45] Goris, J.; Konstantinidis, K. cT.; Klappenbach, J. cA.; Coenye, T.; Vandamme, P.; Tiedje, J. M., DNA-DNA Hybridization Values and Their Relationship to Whole-Genome Sequence Similarities. *Int J Syst Evol Microbiol.* 2007, 57, 81–91, doi:10.1099/IJS.0.64483-0.

[46] Huang, C. H.; Liou, J. S.; Lee, A. Y.; Tseng, M.; Miyashita, M.; Huang, L.; Watanabe, K. Polyphasic Characterization of a Novel Species in the Lactobacillus Casei Group from Cow Manure of Taiwan: Description of L. Chiayiensis Sp. Nov. *Syst Appl Microbiol* . 2018, 41, 270–278, doi:10.1016/J.SYAPM.2018.01.008.

[47] Peter Jurtshuk, Jr., Bacterial Metabolism. *Medical Microbiology.* 1996.

[48] Ramamurthy, T.; Kumari, S.; Ghosh, A. Diarrheal Disease and Gut Microbiome., *Prog Mol Biol Transl Sci.* 2022, 192, 149–177, doi:10.1016/bs.pmbts.2022.08.002.

[49] Clifford, C. B.; Pritchett-Corning, K. R. Bacterial Infections of Laboratory Mice. *The Laboratory Mouse.* 2012, 481–501, doi:10.1016/B978-0-12-382008-2.00020-9.

[50] Zarour, K.; Vieco, N.; Pérez-Ramos, A.; Nácher-Vázquez, M.; Mohedano, M. L.; López, P. Food Ingredients Synthesized by Lactic Acid Bacteria. *Microbial Production of Food Ingredients and Additives.* 2017, 89–124, doi:10.1016/B978-0-12-811520-6.00004-0.

[51] Lonvaud-Funel, A. Leuconostocaceae Family. *Encyclopedia of Food Microbiology: Second Edition.* 2014, 455–465, doi:10.1016/B978-0-12-384730-0.00185-3.

[52] Feng, T.; Wang, J. Oxidative Stress Tolerance and Antioxidant Capacity of Lactic Acid Bacteria as Probiotic: A Systematic Review. *Gut Microbes.* 2020, *12*, doi:10.1080/19490976.2020.1801944.

[53] Archibald, F. Manganese: Its Acquisition by and Function in the Lactic Acid Bacteria. *Crit Rev Microbiol.* 1986, 13, 63–109, doi:10.3109/10408418609108735.

[54] Averina, O. V; Poluektova, E. U.; Marsova, M. V; Danilenko, V. N., Biomarkers and Utility of the Antioxidant Potential of Probiotic Lactobacilli and Bifidobacteria as Representatives of the Human Gut Microbiota. *Biomedicines.* 2021, 9, doi:10.3390/biomedicines9101340.

[55] Albesharat, R.; Ehrmann, M. A.; Korakli, M.; Yazaji, S.; Vogel, R. F., Phenotypic and Genotypic Analyses of Lactic Acid Bacteria in Local Fermented Food, Breast Milk and Faeces of Mothers and Their Babies. *Syst Appl Microbiol.* 2011, 34, 148–155, doi:10.1016/J.SYAPM.2010.12.001.

[56] Khalil, R.; Mahrous, H.; El-Halafawy, K.; Kamaly, K.; Frank, J.; Soda, M., El Evaluation of the Probiotic Potential of Lactic Acid Bacteria Isolated from Faeces of Breast-Fed Infants in Egypt. *Afr J Biotechnol* 2010, *6*, 939–949, doi:10.4314/ajb.v6i7.56977.

[57] Evaluation of Diet Containing Lactobacilli on Performance, Fecal Coliform, and Lactobacilli of Young Dairy Calves Available online: https://agris.fao.org/agris-search/search.do?recordID=NL9601253 (accessed on 13 April 2023).

[58] Kmet, V.; Lucchini, F., Aggregation-Promoting Factor in Human Vaginal Lactobacillus Strains. *FEMS Immunol Med Microbiol.* 1997, 19, 111–114, doi:10.1111/J.1574-695X.1997.TB01079.X.

[59] Kleerebezem, M.; Hugenholtz, J. Metabolic Pathway Engineering in Lactic Acid Bacteria. *Curr Opin Biotechnol.* 2003, 14, 232–237, doi:10.1016/S0958-1669(03)00033-8.

[60] Ahrné, S.; Nobaek, S.; Jeppsson, B.; Adlerberth, I.; Wold, A. E.; Molin, G., The Normal Lactobacillus Flora of Healthy Human Rectal and Oral Mucosa. *J Appl Microbiol.* 1998, 85, 88–94, doi:10.1046/J.1365-2672.1998.00480.X.

[61] Lönnermark, E.; Nowrouzinan, F.; Adlerberth, I.; Ahrné, S.; Wold, A.; Friman, V., Oral and Faecal Lactobacilli and Their Expression of Mannose-Specific Adhesins in Individuals with and without IgA Deficiency. *Int J Med Microbiol.* 2012, 302, 53–60, doi:10.1016/J.IJMM.2011.08.004.

[62] Kumar, H.; Rangrez, A.Y.; Dayananda, K. M.; Atre, A. N.; Patole, M. S.; Shouche, Y. S., *Lactobacillus Plantarum* (VR1) Isolated from an Ayurvedic Medicine (Kutajarista) Ameliorates in Vitro Cellular Damage Caused by Aeromonas Veronii. *BMC Microbiol* 2011, 11, 1–11, doi:10.1186/1471-2180-11-152/FIGURES/5.

[63] Todorov, S. D., Bacteriocin Production by Lactobacillus Plantarum AMA-K Isolated from Amasi, a Zimbabwean Fermented Milk Product and Study of the Adsorption of Bacteriocin AMA-K TO Listeria Sp. *Brazilian Journal of Microbiology*. 2008, 39, 178, doi:10.1590/S1517-83822008000100035.

[64] Müller, D. M.; Carrasco, M. S.; Tonarelli, G. G.; Simonetta, A. C., Characterization and Purification of a New Bacteriocin with a Broad Inhibitory Spectrum Produced by Lactobacillus Plantarum Lp 31 Strain Isolated from Dry-Fermented Sausage. *J Appl Microbiol*. 2009, 106, 2031–2040, doi:10.1111/J.1365-2672.2009.04173.X.

[65] Jónsson, S.; Clausen, E.; Raa, J. Amino Acid Degradation by a Lactobacillus Plantarum Strain from Fish. *Syst Appl Microbiol.* 1983, 4, 148–154, doi:10.1016/S0723-2020(83)80043-5.

[66] Enan, G.; El-Essawy, A. A.; Uyttendaele, M.; Debevere, J. Antibacterial Activity of *Lactobacillus Plantarum* UG1 Isolated from Dry Sausage: Characterization Production and Bactericidal Action of Plantaricin UG1. *Int J Food Microbiol*. 1996, 30, 189–215, doi:10.1016/0168-1605(96)00947-6.

[67] Piekarska-Radzik, L.; Klewicka, E. Mutual Influence of Polyphenols and Lactobacillus Spp. Bacteria in Food: A Review. *European Food Research and Technology* 2021, 247, 9–24, doi:10.1007/S00217-020-03603-Y.

[68] Todorov, S. D.; Prévost, H.; Lebois, M.; Dousset, X.; LeBlanc, J. G.; Franco, B. D. G. M. Bacteriocinogenic *Lactobacillus Plantarum* ST16Pa Isolated from Papaya (*Carica Papaya*) - From Isolation to Application: Characterization of a Bacteriocin. *Food Research International.* 2011, 44, 1351–1363, doi:10.1016/J.FOODRES.2011.01.027.

[69] Genner, M. J.; Turner, G. F., The Mbuna Cichlids of Lake Malawi: A Model for Rapid Speciation and Adaptive Radiation. *Fish and Fisheries*. 2005, 6, 1–34, doi:10.1111/J.1467-2679.2005.00173.X.

[70] Jeun, J.; Kim, S.; Cho, S. Y.; Jun, H. jin; Park, H. J.; Seo, J. G.; Chung, M. J.; Lee, S. J., Hypocholesterolemic Effects of Lactobacillus Plantarum KCTC3928 by Increased Bile Acid Excretion in C57BL/6 Mice. *Nutrition*. 2010, 26, 321–330, doi:10.1016/J.NUT.2009.04.011.

[71] Downs, E.; Bottrell, A. D.; Naylor, K., Identifying the Effects of Reactive Oxygen Species on Mitochondrial Dynamics and Cytoskeleton Stability in Dictyostelium Discoideum. *Cells*. 2021, 10, doi:10.3390/cells10082147.

[72] Paulino do Nascimento, L. C.; Lacerda, D. C.; Ferreira, D. J. S.; de Souza, E. L.; de Brito Alves, J. L., *Limosilactobacillus Fermentum*, Current Evidence on the Antioxidant Properties and Opportunities to Be Exploited as a Probiotic Microorganism. *Probiotics Antimicrob Proteins*. 2022, 14, 960–979, doi:10.1007/s12602-022-09943-3.

[73] Schallreuter, K. U.; Moore, J.; Wood, J. M.; Beazley, W. D.; Gaze, D. C.; Tobin, D. J.; Marshall, H. S.; Panske, A.; Panzig, E.; Hibberts, N. A., In Vivo and in Vitro Evidence for Hydrogen Peroxide (H2O2) Accumulation in the Epidermis of Patients

with Vitiligo and Its Successful Removal by a UVB-Activated Pseudocatalase. *Journal of Investigative Dermatology Symposium Proceedings*. 1999, 4, 91–96, doi:10.1038/sj.jidsp.5640189.

[74] Allgood, G. S.; Perry, J. J., Characterization of a Manganese-Containing Catalase from the Obligate Thermophile Thermoleophilum Album. *J Bacteriol.* 1986, 168, 563–567, doi:10.1128/jb.168.2.563-567.1986.

[75] Beyer, W. F.; Fridovich, I. Pseudocatalase from *Lactobacillus Plantarum*: Evidence for a Homopentameric Structure Containing Two Atoms of Manganese per Subunit. *Biochemistry.* 1985, 24, 6460–6467, doi:10.1021/bi00344a023.

[76] Fuhren, J.; Schwalbe, M.; Peralta-Marzal, L.; Rösch, C.; Schols, H. A.; Kleerebezem, M., Phenotypic and Genetic Characterization of Differential Galacto-Oligosaccharide Utilization in Lactobacillus Plantarum. *Sci Rep.* 2020, 10, doi:10.1038/S41598-020-78721-4.

[77] Van Leeuwen, S. S.; Kuipers, B. J. H.; Dijkhuizen, L.; Kamerling, J. P., Comparative Structural Characterization of 7 Commercial Galacto-Oligosaccharide (GOS) Products. *Carbohydr Res.* 2016, 425, 48–58, doi:10.1016/J.CARRES.2016.03.006.

[78] Martin, C. R.; Ling, P. R.; Blackburn, G. L. Review of Infant Feeding: Key Features of Breast Milk and Infant Formula. *Nutrients.* 2016, 8, doi:10.3390/NU8050279.

[79] Milani, C.; Duranti, S.; Bottacini, F.; Casey, E.; Turroni, F.; Mahony, J.; Belzer, C.; Delgado Palacio, S.; Arboleya Montes, S.; Mancabelli, L.; Lugli, G. A. The First Microbial Colonizers of the Human Gut: Composition, Activities, and Health Implications of the Infant Gut Microbiota. *Microbiology and Molecular Biology Reviews.* 2017, 81, doi:10.1128/MMBR.00036-17.

[80] Azcarate-Peril, M. A.; Ritter, A. J.; Savaiano, D.; Monteagudo-Mera, A.; Anderson, C.; Magness, S. T.; Klaenhammer, T. R. Impact of Short-Chain Galactooligosaccharides on the Gut Microbiome of Lactose-Intolerant Individuals. *Proc Natl Acad Sci U S A.* 2017, 114, E367–E375, doi:10.1073/PNAS.1606722113.

[81] Bakker-Zierikzee, A. M.; Alles, M. S.; Knol, J.; Kok, F. J.; Tolboom, J. J. M.; Bindels, J. G., Effects of Infant Formula Containing a Mixture of Galacto- and Fructo-Oligosaccharides or Viable Bifidobacterium Animalis on the Intestinal Microflora during the First 4 Months of Life. *British Journal of Nutrition.* 2005, 94, 783–790, doi:10.1079/BJN20051451.

[82] Zhang, Z.; Lv, J.; Pan, L.; Zhang, Y.. Roles and Applications of Probiotic Lactobacillus Strains. *Appl Microbiol Biotechnol.* 2018, 102, 8135–8143, doi:10.1007/S00253-018-9217-9.

[83] Fuhren, J.; Rösch, C.; ten Napel, M.; Schols, H. A.; Kleerebezem, M. Synbiotic Matchmaking in *Lactobacillus Plantarum:* Substrate Screening and Gene-Trait Matching to Characterize Strain-Specific Carbohydrate Utilization. *Appl Environ Microbiol.* 2020, 86, doi:10.1128/AEM.01081-20.

[84] Moro, G.; Minoli, I.; Mosca, M.; Fanaro, S.; Jelinek, J.; Stahl, B.; Boehm, G., Dosage-Related Bifidogenic Effects of Galacto- and Fructooligosaccharides in Formula-Fed Term Infants. *J Pediatr Gastroenterol Nutr.* 2002, 34, 291–295, doi:10.1097/00005176-200203000-00014.

[85] Thongaram, T.; Hoeflinger, J. L.; Chow, J. M.; Miller, M. J., Human Milk Oligosaccharide Consumption by Probiotic and Human-Associated Bifidobacteria and Lactobacilli. *J Dairy Sci*. 2017, 100, 7825–7833, doi:10.3168/JDS.2017-12753.

[86] Davis, L. M. G.; Martínez, I.; Walter, J.; Hutkins, R. A Dose Dependent Impact of Prebiotic Galactooligosaccharides on the Intestinal Microbiota of Healthy Adults. *Int J Food Microbiol*. 2010, 144, 285–292, doi:10.1016/J.IJFOODMICRO. 2010.10.007.

[87] Siezen, R. J.; van Hylckama Vlieg, J. E. T., Genomic Diversity and Versatility of *Lactobacillus Plantarum*, a Natural Metabolic Engineer. *Microb Cell Fact*. 2011, 10, doi:10.1186/1475-2859-10-S1-S3.

Chapter 2

An Overview of *Lactobacillus plantarum* Strains with Probiotic Effect on Human Health

Jiancun Zhao[1], PhD
and Zhenshang Xu[2,*], PhD

[1]Department of Pharmacy and Biotechnology, Zibo Vocational Institute, Zibo, Shandong Province, PR China
[2]State Key Laboratory of Biobased Material and Green Papermaking, Qilu University of Technology, Shandong Academy of Science, Jinan, Shandong Province, PR China

Abstract

Lactobacillus plantarum, belonging to the *Lactobacillus* genera, widely exists in natural niches, including pickles, silages, and various fermented milk products. Recent studies have shown that *L. plantarum* is also an important component of probiotics in the human gastrointestinal tract. Probiotics have good effects on regulating intestinal flora structure, improving intestinal microecological stability, and promoting health. Based on the excellent physiological characteristics and probiotic function, *L. plantarum* has become a hot topic in the field of probiotics. Different strains of *L. plantarum* have been proven to have diverse health effects, such as regulating immune function, antagonizing pathogenic bacteria infection, and improving chronic metabolic diseases and psychiatric diseases. This chapter mainly reviews the probiotic function and clinical application of different *L. plantarum* strains, and describes the possible mechanism of these effects, thus providing information for the research and application of *L. plantarum* in maintaining and improving human health.

---

* Corresponding Author's Email: xuzhenshang@126.com.

In: Lactobacillus plantarum and Its Role in Human Health
Editors: Maria Simona Chiş, Adriana Paucean
ISBN: 979-8-89113-696-0

Keywords: *Lactobacillus plantarum*, clinical application, human health

1. Introduction

Lactobacillus plantarum is a Gram-positive bacterium classified as *Firmicutes*, *Bacilli*, *Lactobacilliaceae*, and *Lactobacillus*. It is a facultative anaerobic organism, non-spore-producing, with straight rods and round ends. When grown on MRS Medium, their colonies are round and smooth, with colors ranging from white to light yellow and dark yellow. *L. plantarum* is capable of producing both D-type and L-type lactic acid, and its optimal growth temperature is 30-35°C, with an optimum pH of 6.5 (Goldstein et al., 2015). These bacteria can be found in a variety of food sources, such as vegetables, meat, dairy products, and wine, as well as in the gastrointestinal tract of humans and other animals, where it is a natural component of the important flora (Seddik et al., 2017). As of April 2023, a total of 887 strains of *L. plantarum* had completed whole genome sequencing in the NCBI (National Center for Biotechnology Information) database. The whole genome of this species is between 2.9-3.7 MB in length, making it the largest species within lactic acid bacteria. Its G+C (content of Guanine and Cytosine) percentage is roughly 45%. This sequencing of the genome has been highly beneficial in understanding the structure and composition of the genome, as well as the biological function and applications of *L. plantarum* on a molecular level (Siezen et al., 2011).

L. plantarum is widely utilized in industrial production, food fermentation, and other fields. Its metabolites include organic acids, bacteriocins, hydrogen peroxide, diacetyl, fatty acids, exopolysaccharides, and other functional substances. Such metabolites produced by *L. plantarum* are known to extend food shelf-life and add unique flavorings. In addition, *L. plantarum* can also absorb heavy metals, and plasticizers, degrade nitrites, and reduce other hazardous elements, thus increasing the safety of fermented food (Behera et al., 2018). In recent years, increasing evidence has highlighted the important role of *L. plantarum* in human health, such as regulating the stability and balance of gut microbes, inhibiting pathogens and harmful bacteria in the gut, modulating immune responses, improving nutrition, promoting growth, preventing chronic diseases, and reducing stress, which has attracted much attention in functional food and pharmaceutical industries (Fidanza et al., 2021). Based on the beneficial physiological characteristics and probiotic functions of *L. plantarum*, clinical research into its probiotic functions is gradually being carried out (Nordström et al., 2021). The present chapter reviews the prebiotic functions and clinical applications of *L. plantarum* strains and describes their possible mechanisms, providing references for the research and application of *L. plantarum* in the maintenance and improvement of human health.

1.1. Evidence-Based *L. Plantarum* Strains Related to Human Health

Probiotics are a group of active microorganisms that are beneficial to their host by colonizing the human body and altering the composition of the host flora (Azad et al., 2018). In the past, it was believed that *L. plantarum* was an important probiotic. However, modern science requires a more precise definition of probiotic application, such that it needs to be specified at the strain level (Cantero et al., 2022). Therefore, the scientific view is that one or more strains of *L. plantarum* can be considered probiotics, which involves a screening process. The selection of probiotics typically involves the evaluation of their growth characteristics, physiological and biochemical characteristics, metabolic characteristics, and their effect on nutrition and clinical pathology. The target strains are then selected from the samples and verified for safety, efficacy, and analysis (Shokryazdan et al., 2017). Table 1 lists all *L. plantarum* strains associated with human health that have undergone randomized, double-blind, placebo-controlled trials, which show that they all have positive effects on human health. By looking at these *L. plantarum* strains, they all have common traits such as tolerance, colonization, and microecology regulation, as well as some specific properties that lead to different effects.

1.2. Tolerance

The premise of *L. plantarum* as probiotic is that it can survive passage through the acidic and duodenal environment of the stomach to reach the small and large intestine, where it can then perform the function of micro-ecological adjustment. Therefore, tolerance to gastric acid and bile salt is an essential physiological characteristic for the screening of probiotic *L. plantarum* (Reuben et al., 2020). The mechanisms of *L. plantarum* against acid stress include ammonia production, decarboxylation, protection or repair of damaged macromolecules, and alteration of metabolic pathways.

Table 1. *L. plantarum* strains with definite efficacy verified by randomized, double-blind, placebo-controlled trials

Strain	Function	Intervention period	Participants	Dosage	Reference
DR7	alleviate stress and anxiety in adults	12 weeks	probiotic group, n=56, placebo group, n=55.	1×10^{9} cfu	Chong et al., 2019
P8	alleviate stress and anxiety and enhance memory and cognition in stressed adults	12 weeks	probiotic group, n=52, placebo group, n=51.	1×10^{10} cfu	Lew et al., 2019
299v	reduce cortisol levels in human saliva during examination-induced stress	14 days	probiotic group, n=21, placebo group, n=20.	1×10^{10} cfu	Andersson et al., 2016
PS128	improve the depressive symptoms and sleep quality of insomniacs	30 days	probiotic group, n=20 placebo group, n=20.	6×10^{10} cfu	Ho et al., 2021
PS128	ameliorate opposition/ defiance behaviors in Children with autism spectrum disorder	4 weeks	probiotic group, n=36, placebo group, n=35.	3×10^{10} cfu	Liu et al., 2019
OLL2712	protective effects against memory function decline in older adults	12 weeks	probiotic group, n=39, placebo group, n=39.	5×10^{9} cfu	Sakurai et al., 2022
299v	decrease kynurenine concentration and improve cognitive functions in patients with major depression	8 weeks	probiotic group, n=30, placebo group, n=30.	2×10^{10} cfu	Rudzki et al., 2019
TWK10	elevate exercise performance and improve fatigue-associated features in healthy humans	6 weeks	low probiotic group, n=9, high probiotic group, n=9, placebo group, n=9.	3×10^{10} or 9×10^{10} cfu	Huang et al., 2019
TWK10	improve muscle mass and functional performance in frail older adults	18 weeks	low probiotic group, n=12, high probiotic group, n=13, placebo group, n=17.	2×10^{10} or 6×10^{10} cfu	Lee et al., 2021
PS128	improve muscle damage, renal damage, and oxidative stress on exercise capacity recovery after a half-marathon	4 weeks	probiotic group, n=4, placebo group, n=4.	2×10^{10} cfu	Fu et al., 2021
Dad-13	modulate the moderate undernutrition in infants	50 days	probiotic group, n=15, placebo group, n=15.	8.96×10^{8}-1.16×10^{9} cfu	Kamil et al., 2022

Strain	Function	Intervention period	Participants	Dosage	Reference
299V	resolute the abdominal pain, normalization of stools frequency in patients with irritable bowel syndrome	4 weeks	probiotic group, n=20, placebo group, n=20.	3×10^{10} cfu	Niedzielin et al., 2001
DSM 9843	decrease pain and flatulence in patients with irritable bowel syndrome	4 weeks	probiotic group, n=25, placebo group, n=27.	2×10^{10} cfu	Nobaek et al., 2000
APsulloc 331261	enhance intestinal discomfort symptoms, defecation consistency, quality of life, beneficial microbiota, and overall intestinal health on diarrhea-predominant irritable bowel syndrome	4 weeks	probiotic group, n=18, placebo group, n=8.	1×10^{10} cfu	Jung et al., 2022
299v	improve symptoms including abdominal pain and bloating of irritable bowel syndrome	4 weeks	probiotic group, n=105, placebo group, n=99.	1×10^{10} cfu	Ducrotté et al., 2012
CCFM1143	alleviate chronic diarrhea	4 weeks	probiotic group, n=28, placebo group, n=27.	3.52×10^{9} cfu	Yang et al., 2021
CJLP243	improve the symptoms of diarrhea and reduce fecal calprotectin levels	2 months	probiotic group, n=10, placebo group, n=12.	1×10^{10} cfu	Jung et al., 2022
Lp3a	relieve features of constipation in adult functional constipation patients	7 days	probiotic group, n=59, placebo group, n=58.	2×10^{10} cfu	Zhang et al., 2022
299v	preventive effect on milder gastrointestinal symptoms during treatment with antibiotics	until a week after termination of antibiotic treatment	probiotic group, n=80, placebo group, n=83.	1×10^{10} cfu	Lönnermark et al., 2010
DSM 9843	increase the bacterial diversity in the gut, and affect the concentration of some short-chain fatty acids	4 weeks	probiotic group, n=9, placebo group, n=7.	1×10^{11} cfu	Karlsson et al., 2010
IS-10506	reduce scoring atopic dermatitis index in children with atopic dermatitis	12 weeks	probiotic group, n=12, placebo group, n=10.	1×10^{10} cfu	Prakoeswa et al., 2017

Table 1. (Continued)

Strain	Function	Intervention period	Participants	Dosage	Reference
CJLP133	beneficial in the treatment of pediatric atopic dermatitis	12 weeks	probiotic group, n=58, placebo group, n=60.	5×10^{9} cfu	Han et al., 2012
IS-10506	alleviate atopic dermatitis symptoms in adults owing to its immunomodulatory effects	8 weeks	probiotic group, n=15, placebo group, n=15.	2×10^{10} cfu	Prakoeswa et al., 2022
CJLP55	beneficial to clinical state, skin sebum, hydration, and urine bacterial extracellular vesicles phylum flora in patients with acne vulgaris	12 weeks	probiotic group, n=14, placebo group, n=14.	1×10^{10} cfu	Kim et al., 2021
HY7714	increase the skin water content in the face and hands, suppress the transepidermal water loss in the face and forearm, reduce wrinkle depth, improve skin gloss and elasticity	12 weeks	probiotic group, n=55, placebo group, n=55.	1×10^{10} cfu	Lee et al., 2015
PCS 26	alleviate urinary tract infections symptoms and in urinary tract infections prevention	6 months	probiotic group, n=14, placebo group, n=16.	1×10^{9} cfu	Meštrović Popovič et al., 2022
P17630	improve vagina colonization of acid lactic bacteria, prevent episodes of vulvovaginal candidiasis	3 treatment cycles (15 days/cycle) separated by 15-day wash-out intervals	probiotic group, n=46, placebo group, n=47.	5×10^{9} cfu	Vladareanu et al., 2018
DR7	improve upper respiratory tract infections via enhancing immune and inflammatory parameters	12 weeks	probiotic group, n=56, placebo group, n=53.	1×10^{9} cfu	Chong et al., 2019

Strain	Function	Intervention period	Participants	Dosage	Reference
LP14	improve the ocular symptom-medication score in seasonal allergic disease	6 weeks	Two studies. probiotic group, n=16, placebo group, n=17. probiotic group, n=10, placebo group, n=10.	8.7×10^{8} cfu	Nagata et al., 2010
299v	reduce the cardiovascular disease risk factors in smokers	6 weeks	probiotic group, n=18, placebo group, n=18.	2×10^{10} cfu	Naruszewicz et al., 2002
ECGC 13110402	reduce cardiovascular risk	12 weeks	probiotic group, n=23, placebo group, n=23.	4×10^{9} cfu	Costabile et al., 2017
299v	affect maternal and neonatal hematological and iron status	from 15-20 weeks of gestation through delivery	probiotic group, n=1, placebo group, n=8.	1×10^{10} cfu	OjiNjideka Hemphill et al., 2023
299v	modulate the gut barrier function in patients with obstructive jaundice	until 7 days after biliary drainage	probiotic group, n=8, placebo group, n=7.	1×10^{10} cfu	Jones et al., 2013
Lp-G18	immunomodulatory and hypolipidemic effect in nephrotic and dyslipidemic pediatric subjects	12 weeks	probiotic group, n=2, placebo group, n=2.	5×10^{9} cfu	Fortes et al., 2020
Q180	maintain healthy postprandial lipid levels by modulating the gut environment	12 weeks	probiotic group, n=35, placebo group, n=35.	8×10^{9} cfu	Park et al., 2020
K50	reduce the total cholesterol and triglyceride levels	12 weeks	probiotic group, n=35, placebo group, n=36.	4×10^{9} cfu	Sohn et al., 2022
299v	decrease in fibrinogen and LDL-cholesterol levels in subjects with moderately elevated cholesterol	6 weeks	probiotic group, n=15, placebo group, n=15.	1×10^{10} cfu	Bukowska et al., 1998
Dad-13	decrease in body weight and BMI in overweight adults	90 days	probiotic group, n=30, placebo group, n=30.	2×10^{9} cfu	Rahayu et al., 2021

Table 1. (Continued)

Strain	Function	Intervention period	Participants	Dosage	Reference
LMT1-48	decrease body weight, abdominal visceral fat area, insulin resistance, and leptin levels in overweight subjects	12 weeks	probiotic group, n=50, placebo group, n=49.	2×10^{10} cfu	Sohn et al., 2023
Dad-13	improve the HbA1c level, modulate some beneficial bacteria that promote metabolites in type 2 diabetic women	11 weeks	probiotic group, n=18, placebo group, n=18.	1×10^{10} cfu	Rustanti et al., 2022
HAC01	improve glycemic control in prediabetic subjects	8 weeks	probiotic group, n=20, placebo group, n=17.	4×10^{9} cfu	Oh et al., 2021
299v	increase in the serum albumin concentration, reduce the frequency of vomiting and flatulence in cancer patients	4 weeks	probiotic group, n=21, placebo group, n=14.	2×10^{10} cfu	Kaźmierczak-Siedlecka et al., 2020

Additionally, it can form biofilms in acidic environments, and upregulate the expression of related proteins, thus conferring a certain degree of tolerance to low pH (Heunis et al., 2014). Exopolysaccharides and surface proteins of *L. plantarum* interact with intestinal epithelial cells to form a protective barrier against high concentrations of bile salts. Moreover, bile salt hydrolase produced by *L. plantarum* can convert primary bile salts, which are more toxic to the organism, into secondary bile salts, which are less toxic (Wu et al., 2022). In addition to being resistant to acid, the strain also has tolerance to osmotic pressure, temperature, oxidation, and starvation stress, which gives it an enhanced competitive advantage (Ricciardi et al., 2012).

1.3. Colonization

In the gut, only resident bacteria have an essential role. Nonetheless, due to intestinal peristalsis and other factors, some well-tolerated strains, even though they can endure the gastrointestinal environment, are unable to stay in the body for a long enough period to be expelled. Therefore, strains with strong colonization capabilities have more potential to be used as probiotics (Han et al., 2021). The adhesion of *L. plantarum* to human intestinal epithelial cells and mucosal surfaces is one of the principal criteria for screening probiotic strains *in vitro*. The ability of *L. plantarum* to attach to the intestinal mucosa provides them with a competitive advantage. Specifically, adhesion is the particular process between microbes and intestinal epithelial cells. Numerous *in vitro* and *in vivo* experiments have demonstrated that certain *L. plantarum* strains have an affinity to intestinal cells, which contributes to the colonization of *L. plantarum* in the intestinal tract (Darmastuti et al., 2021). The mechanism of *L. plantarum* adhesion to intestinal epithelial cells is linked to mannose-specific lectin binding (Buntin et al., 2017). It is noteworthy that some *L. plantarum* strains have a special ability to colonize other parts of the body, such as the vagina and skin. This grants *L. plantarum* a varied niche and guides its functional development.

1.4. Regulation of Microecology

The gut microbiota plays an essential role in human health (Gomaa, 2020). *L. plantarum* is a probiotic bacteria in the human gut, which has a probiotic impact on the body. This is reflected by *L. plantarum* by influencing the structure and composition of the intestinal flora, thereby affecting intestinal metabolism and intestinal immunity to maintain the natural equilibrium of the gut microbiota. *L. plantarum* can colonize the adsorption sites of gastrointestinal epithelial cells, occupy the niche, and inhibit the adsorption of pathogenic bacteria, thus protecting the intestinal tract from the invasion of pathogens (Cui et al., 2021). *L. plantarum* and its metabolites can also suppress the growth of intestinal pathogenic bacteria, thus preserving the balance of the intestinal microecology. Moreover, bacteriocins, small peptides, proteases, hydrogen peroxide, organic acids, carbon dioxide, and diacetyl produced by *L. plantarum* are all antibacterial agents, killing foreign and pathogenic bacteria to better maintain the physiological function of the intestine (Zhao et al., 2020). These physiological characteristics of *L. plantarum* allow it to effectively regulate the intestinal microecological environment. Beyond regulating intestinal microecology, *L. plantarum* may also be involved in the regulation and improvement of other microecological environments.

1.5. Strain Specificity

Generally speaking, tolerance, colonization, and regulation of microecology are the essential characteristics for screening probiotic *L. plantarum* strains. Moreover, probiotics from different plants usually have strain-specificity, where each *L. plantarum* strain has a distinct genetic makeup, resulting in unique physiological processes, metabolites, and probiotic characteristics (Liu et al., 2022). To develop the probiotic functions of *L. plantarum*, targeted screening steps are usually conducted according to the desired outcome. As screening for strains that can reduce blood sugar, the activity of α-glucosidase, lipase, and so on is usually started by the strain and its fermentation products, and to screen the strain that can improve IBD (inflammatory bowel disease), the antioxidant capacity of the strain is first measured (Kim et al., 2018; Ren et al., 2022). These procedures lead to the selection of different *L. plantarum* strains with unique probiotic function characteristics.

1.6. Possible Mechanisms of Action

1.6.1. Treatment of Inflammatory Bowel Disease

Inflammatory bowel disease comprises Crohn's disease, ulcerative colitis, and some other forms that differ from the former two. Transmural inflammation, complications such as abscesses and fistulas, and the ability to affect any part of the gastrointestinal tract, primarily the distal ileum or perianal area, are common features of crohn's disease. In contrast, ulcerative colitis is limited to the colon and manifests as inflammation of the mucous membranes (Ducrotté et al., 2012). Initially discovered in the West, inflammatory bowel disease has, in recent decades, become a global phenomenon.

Probiotics have been found to ameliorate inflammation through their positive effect on the dysfunction of epithelial cells and the mucosal immune system that underlies inflammation. Consequently, the application of probiotics to alleviate or treat inflammatory bowel disease has become an area of extensive research. Studies have demonstrated that probiotics employ multiple mechanisms to relieve or treat inflammatory bowel disease, quickly making them one of the leading therapies for this condition (Jung et al., 2022). These mechanisms can be divided into (1) Regulation of the abundance and diversity of intestinal flora, thus improving immunity and enhancing intestinal barrier function. (2) Increasing antioxidant activity and regulating cytokine production, resulting in a reduction of clinical symptoms and histopathology damage. (3) Activation of the TLR-4/NF-KB signal pathway, regulation of Tlr-4, and suppression of inflammatory cytokines such as TNF-α, MPO (myeloperoxidase), and LPO (lipidperoxidation). (4) Decreased expression of p-selectin and leukocyte-platelet-endothelial interaction. (5) Inhibition of Th17 cells and reduction of Il-17 secretion. (6) Inhibition of apoptosis and promotion of proliferation and migration of epithelial cells. Overall, probiotics serve as an effective means to reduce the severity of inflammatory bowel disease and improve patient outcomes (Nobaek et al., 2020; Niedzielin et al., 2001; Wang et al., 2022).

1.6.2. Improvement of Diabetes

Type 2 diabetes is a metabolic disorder characterized by either inadequate insulin synthesis, insulin resistance, or both, leading to elevated levels of blood glucose. Diabetes and its associated effects have become a major global health problem. According to the International Diabetes Federation, in 2019, approximately 463 million (9.7%) adults aged 20-79 had diabetes, and this number is expected to increase to 700 million (10.9%) by 2045. Dysbiosis, which is the disruption of microbial homeostasis in the gut, can lead to the development of chronic diseases such as type 2 diabetes. Dysbiosis of the gut microbiota has a significant impact on the improvement of glucose metabolism (Iatcu et al., 2021).

The gut microbiota of patients with type 2 diabetes is altered, with a reduced *Bacteroides-Firmicutes* ratio and a reduced number of *Bifidobacteria*. In contrast, elevated levels of Gram-negative bacteria are observed. These bacteria produce endotoxin that disrupts the metabolic function of the host. Probiotics may help manage type 2 diabetes by altering the gut microbiota. When taken as food or supplements, probiotics can modulate beneficial metabolites of the gut microbiota, such as short-chain fatty acids including acetic acid, propionic acid, and butyric acid. According to a meta-analysis, probiotic therapy has been found to reduce HbA1c levels, fasting blood glucose levels, and insulin resistance in patients with type 2 diabetes. An 11-week intervention using *L. plantarum* Dad-13 powder was found to improve HbA1c levels in the probiotics group. Additionally, dietary supplementation with *L. plantarum* HAC01 significantly reduced 2-hour glucose levels and HbA1c levels in the group (Oh et al., 2021; Rustanti et al., 2022).

1.6.3. Reduction of Weight

Changes in lifestyle, diet, and physical activity have led to an increasing prevalence of obesity around the world. Many factors are thought to contribute to the development of this condition, including the gut microbiota. Studies have indicated that gut microbial ecology may influence nutrient absorption and energy regulation, thus impacting an individual's nutritional status (Green et al., 2020). Although excess calorie consumption is the primary cause of obesity, differences in gut microbial ecology between healthy and obese individuals may contribute to altered energy homeostasis. In other words, obese individuals may possess a gut microbial community that facilitates more efficient extraction and/or storage of energy from a given diet, as compared to lean individuals.

Probiotic consumption has been linked to the production of short-chain fatty acids such as acetic acid, propionic acid, butyric acid, and lactic acid. These metabolic byproducts have been associated with the regulation (inhibition or activation) of certain genes related to obesity and inflammation, providing a potential benefit to the host (Rahayu et al., 2021). Interestingly, it has been observed that in obese individuals, the number of probiotic bacteria is decreased, while the presence of certain pathogens, such as *Enterobacteriaceae* and *Staphylococcus*, is increased.Therefore, consuming probiotics that are alive and able to colonize the gut is beneficial for increasing the number of beneficial bacteria such as *Bifidobacterium* and *Lactobacillus*, and inhibiting the proliferation of harmful bacteria such as *Enterobacteriaceae* and *Staphylococcus*, thereby improving obesity (Sohn et al., 2023).

1.6.4. Treatment of Skin Diseases

In recent years, the establishment of the "Gut-Skin Axis" theory has provided a theoretical basis for the involvement of intestinal flora imbalance in the inflammatory response of skin diseases. Several studies have linked dysbacteriosis to inflammatory skin diseases such as psoriasis, acne, seborrheic dermatitis, atopic dermatitis, and alopecia areata, and probiotics have been demonstrated to have efficacy in the adjuvant treatment of these inflammatory skin diseases (Lee et al., 2015; Kim et al., 2021).

Atopic dermatitis is an inflammatory skin disorder that is characterized by recurrent dry skin, erythema, and pruritus. While the exact pathogenesis of this condition remains unclear, it is thought to be caused by an imbalance of Th2 and Th17 immune responses during both the acute and chronic phases (Prakoeswa et al., 2022). As such, modulating the immune response may be an effective way to relieve the symptoms associated with atopic dermatitis. Recent research has focused on the role of intestinal flora in the development of atopic dermatitis and other skin diseases. It has been demonstrated that an imbalance in gut flora can lead to an overproduction of TH2-type immune responses, which can increase the risk of developing atopic dermatitis (Han et al., 2012). A retrospective study also found that probiotics can improve the clinical performance of patients of all ages, from pregnant women to adults, in the treatment of atopic dermatitis, with significant efficacy (Prakoeswa et al., 2017).

1.6.5. Relief of Mental Illness

The gut-brain axis is a two-way communication channel between the intestinal flora and the brain. Composed of the autonomic nervous system, the hypothalamus-pituitary-adrenal axis, and the enteric nervous system, it is regulated by vagal and endocrine pathways, the intervention of neuronal structures and functions, and the immune response of central nervous system neurons and cerebral vessels, among others, to maintain the body's physiological stability. The intestinal flora affects the central nervous system in various ways (Ho et al., 2021).

The intestinal microbiota can influence the host's brain activity through the Vagus nerve. Moreover, gut bacteria can modify the structure and functioning of host neurons. These bacteria can secrete various neurotransmitters, such as GABA (γ-aminobutyric acid), noradrenaline, dopamine, acetylcholine, and 5-HT (5-hydroxytryptamine), that can permeate the intestinal mucosa of the host and thus reach the bloodstream, leading to alterations in the central nervous system (Liu et al., 2019; Chong et al., 2019). Furthermore, the short-chain fatty acids produced by the intestinal microbiota can boost the secretion of 5-HT by intestinal epithelial cells, which act on the brain through the circulatory system. Multiple studies have demonstrated that gut flora and its metabolites can induce an immune response in the host's nervous system, which consequently affects the functioning of the host's central nervous system (Andersson et al., 2016; Lew et al., 2019).

1.6.7. Prevention of Cardiovascular Diseases

Cardiovascular disease, also referred to as heart and cerebrovascular disease, is a collective term for all diseases involving the circulatory system. This includes the heart and the network of vessels that carry blood, such as arteries, veins, and microvessels, which can be further classified into acute and chronic conditions and are often linked to arteriosclerosis. Generally, the etiology, pathogenesis, and treatment strategies of cardiovascular diseases are similar (Naruszewicz et al., 2002). Some of the groups are more prone to developing such diseases. Elderly individuals should take particular note of any symptoms such as limb numbness or hearing loss. Overweight people are at risk due to the higher levels of fat and cholesterol in their bodies. Eating too much and irregularly can also increase the risk of cardiovascular disease. Smoking, drinking, and experiencing stress can lead to organ dysfunction and hinder blood circulation, thus increasing the chances of developing heart and cerebrovascular diseases.

The most severe type of arteriosclerosis heart disease is myocardial infarction. An important feature of patients with coronary atherosclerosis is an imbalance of cholesterol-metabolizing *Bifidobacteria*, *Lactobacillus*, *Bacteroides*, *Clostridium*, and other species. This is accompanied by stable or unstable gruel-like plaques, with identical or differential changes. Intestinal bacteria play a role in regulating inflammation and producing metabolites, which are highly effective in promoting arteriosclerosis (Costabile et al., 2017). Probiotics can act by regulating bile acid metabolism, which inhibits FXR/FGF15 and upregulates CYP7A1, thereby promoting bile acid synthesis in cholesterol and downregulating PCSK9/IDOL, leading to cholesterol reversal. In addition to regulating cholic acid metabolism, probiotics can also reduce TMAO (trimetlylamine oxide) levels, thus improving arteriosclerosis.

The relationship between hypertension and intestinal bacteria is also becoming clearer. Patients with hypertension have an altered abundance, breadth, and distribution of *Enterobacteriaceae*, and changes in some blood pressure-related hormones are determined by the gut-brain axis. Furthermore, gut bacteria are involved in the metabolism of tryptophan and GABA, affecting 5-HT, dopamine, epinephrine, and neurotransmitters such as noradrenaline, histamine, and gut-derived peptides, which are mostly related to the regulation of blood pressure (Sohn et al., 2022).

1.6.8. Improvement of Cognition

With the increasing age of individuals, cognitive function can decline in both quality and quantity, potentially resulting in dementia and negatively impacting the quality of life. Unfortunately, there is no specific treatment that can reverse such cognitive decline or dementia. Recent advances in microecology, however, have revealed a great deal of evidence indicating that intestinal flora can affect cognitive function in multiple ways, such as through the nervous, endocrine, metabolic, and immune systems. Probiotics may thus be a viable method for preventing or improving cognitive decline (Sakurai et al., 2022). Currently, the relationship between probiotics and cognitive function has been studied and found to be due to several possible mechanisms, including (1) reducing systemic inflammatory factors and alleviating chronic inflammation of the brain; (2) promoting the production of exogenous polyamines, such as putrescine, spermine, and spermidine, which can increase the secretion of intestinal mucus, protect the intestinal barrier function, suppress the production of inflammatory factors, and show anti-mutagenic and anti-oxidative properties that can delay aging; and (3) promoting the increase of serotonin precursor tryptophan and brain-derived neurotrophin, which can be beneficial in the prevention and early treatment of depression and cognitive dysfunction (Rudzki et al., 2019; Huang et al., 2019).

Conclusion

L. plantarum is a widely studied probiotic species that is known for its beneficial physiological characteristics and probiotic functions. In this chapter, the probiotic function and clinical application of *L. plantarum* strains were analyzed, and the potential mechanisms of its actions in maintaining and improving human health were described. It is important to note that this paper only considers studies using *L. plantarum* strains and does not take into account studies that use a combination of probiotic species containing *L. plantarum*, studies using inactivated *L. plantarum*, studies using *L. plantarum* in combination with other substances such as prebiotics, and studies using *L. plantarum* fermentation products such as yogurt. Nevertheless, these studies have also yielded encouraging results.

Through the above analysis, it is evident that the development process of *L. plantarum* probiotics involves three main steps. The first step consists of strain collection and screening. The second step involves the selection of probiotics using a high-throughput platform *in vitro*, which takes into account aspects such as safety, effectiveness, and stability. The third step involves the evaluation of the probiotics' function *in vivo*, mechanism of action, and safety to generate safety and effectiveness data. Currently, there is a great deal of research being conducted on *L. plantarum*, most of which remains in the animal experimentation stage. Many randomized, double-blind, placebo-controlled experiments have been conducted, and these research steps are worth studying in-depth to bring more *L. plantarum* into the human experimental stage. While the majority of clinical studies conducted thus far have had positive results, some have failed to meet expectations. Furthermore, even the results of different teams working on the same strain are inconsistent. As a result, large-scale, repeatable clinical research needs to be further developed.

References

Andersson H., Tullberg C., Ahrné S., Hamberg K., Lazou Ahrén I., Molin G., Sonesson M., Håkansson Å. Oral Administration of *Lactobacillus plantarum* 299v Reduces Cortisol Levels in Human Saliva during Examination Induced Stress: A Randomized, Double-Blind Controlled Trial. *Int J Microbiol.* 2016. 2016:8469018.

Azad M. A. K., Sarker M, Li T, Yin J. Probiotic Species in the Modulation of Gut Microbiota: An Overview. Biomed Res Int (2018) 2018:9478630.

Behera S. S, Ray R. C, Zdolec N. *Lactobacillus plantarum* with Functional Properties: An Approach to Increase Safety and Shelf-Life of Fermented Foods. *Biomed Res Int* (2018) 2018:9361614.

Bukowska H, Pieczul-Mróz J, Jastrzebska M, Chełstowski K, Naruszewicz M. Decrease in fibrinogen and LDL-cholesterol levels upon supplementation of diet with *Lactobacillus plantarum* in subjects with moderately elevated cholesterol. *Atherosclerosis* (1998) 137 (2):437-438.

Buntin N, de Vos WM, Hongpattarakere T. Variation of mucin adhesion, cell surface characteristics, and molecular mechanisms among *Lactobacillus plantarum* isolated from different habitats. *Appl Microbiol Biotechnol* (2017) 101 (20):7663-7674.

Cantero M. A, Guedes M. R. A., Fernandes R., Lollo P. C. B., Trimethylamine N-oxide reduction is related to probiotic strain specificity: A systematic review. *Nutr Res* (2022) 104:29-35.

Chong H. X., Yusoff N. A. A., Hor Y. Y., Lew L. C., Jaafar M. H., Choi S. B, Yusoff M. S. B., Wahid N., Abdullah M. F. I. L., Zakaria N, Ong K. L., Park Y. H., Liong M.T., *Lactobacillus plantarum* DR7 alleviates stress and anxiety in adults: a randomised, double-blind, placebo-controlled study. *Benef Microbes* (2019) 10(4):355-373.

Chong H. X., Yusoff N. A. A., Hor Y. Y, Lew L. C., Jaafar M. H., Choi S. B, Yusoff M. S. B, Wahid N., Abdullah M. F. I. L., Zakaria N, Ong K. L., Park Y.H., Liong M. T. *Lactobacillus plantarum* DR7 improved upper respiratory tract infections via enhancing immune and inflammatory parameters: A randomized, double-blind, placebo-controlled study. *J Dairy Sci* (2019) 102 (6):4783-4797.

Costabile A, Buttarazzi I, Kolida S, Quercia S, Baldini J, Swann JR, Brigidi P, Gibson G. R. An *in vivo* assessment of the cholesterol-lowering efficacy of *Lactobacillus plantarum* ECGC 13110402 in normal to mildly hypercholesterolaemic adults. *PLoS One* (2017) 12(12):e0187964.

Cui S, Chen C, Gu J, Mao B, Zhang H, Zhao J, Chen W. Tracing *Lactobacillus plantarum* within the intestinal tract of mice: green fluorescent protein-based fluorescent tagging. *J Sci Food Agric* (2021) 101(5):1758-1766.

Darmastuti A, Hasan P. N., Wikandari R, Utami T., Rahayu E.S, Suroto D. A. Adhesion Properties of *Lactobacillus plantarum* Dad-13 and *Lactobacillus plantarum* Mut-7 on Sprague Dawley Rat Intestine. *Microorganisms* (2021) 9(11):2336.

Ducrotté P, Sawant P, Jayanthi V. Clinical trial: *Lactobacillus plantarum* 299v (DSM 9843) improves symptoms of irritable bowel syndrome. *World J Gastroenterol* (2012) 18(30):4012-4018.

Fidanza M, Panigrahi P, Kollmann T. R. *Lactiplantibacillus plantarum*-Nomad and Ideal Probiotic. *Front Microbiol* (2021) 12:712236.

Fortes P. M, Teles Filho R.V, Azevêdo L. H. S, Queiroz V. C. J, Costa P. S. S. D. Inflammatory cytokines and lipid profile in children and adolescents with nephrotic syndrome receiving *L. Plantarum*: a randomized, controlled feasibility trial. *Rev Assoc Med Bras* (2020) 66 (11):1487-1492.

Fu S. K., Tseng W. C., Tseng K. W., Lai C. C, Tsai Y. C, Tai H. L, Hsu C. C. Effect of Daily Oral *Lactobacillus plantarum* PS128 on Exercise Capacity Recovery after a Half-Marathon. *Nutrients* (2021) 13(11):4023.

Goldstein E. J, Tyrrell K. L, Citron D. M. Lactobacillus species: taxonomic complexity and controversial susceptibilities. *Clin Infect Dis* (2015) 2:S98-107.

Gomaa E. Z. Human gut microbiota/microbiome in health and diseases: a review. Antonie Van Leeuwenhoek (2020) 113(12):2019-2040.

Green M, Arora K, Prakash S. Microbial Medicine: Prebiotic and Probiotic Functional Foods to Target Obesity and Metabolic Syndrome. *Int J Mol Sci* (2020) 21(8):2890.

Han S, Lu Y, Xie J, Fei Y, Zheng G, Wang Z, Liu J, Lv L, Ling Z, Berglund B, Yao M, Li L. Probiotic Gastrointestinal Transit and Colonization After Oral Administration: A Long Journey. *Front Cell Infect Microbiol* (2021) 11:609722.

Han Y, Kim B, Ban J, Lee J, Kim BJ, Choi BS, Hwang S, Ahn K, Kim J. A randomized trial of *Lactobacillus plantarum* CJLP133 for the treatment of atopic dermatitis. *Pediatr Allergy Immunol* (2012) 23(7):667-673.

Heunis T, Deane S, Smit S, Dicks L. M. Proteomic profiling of the acid stress response in *Lactobacillus plantarum* 423. *J Proteome Res* (2014) 13(9):4028-4039.

Ho Y. T, Tsai Y. C, Kuo T. B. J, Yang C. C. H. Effects of *Lactobacillus plantarum* PS128 on Depressive Symptoms and Sleep Quality in Self-Reported Insomniacs: A Randomized, Double-Blind, Placebo-Controlled Pilot Trial. *Nutrients* (2021) 13(8):2820.

Huang W. C, Lee M. C, Lee C. C, Ng K. S, Hsu Y. J, Tsai T. Y, Young S. L, Lin J. S, Huang C. C. Effect of *Lactobacillus plantarum* TWK10 on Exercise Physiological Adaptation, Performance, and Body Composition in Healthy Humans. *Nutrients* (2019) 11(11):2836.

Iatcu C. O, Steen A, Covasa M. Gut Microbiota and Complications of Type-2 Diabetes. *Nutrients* (2021) 14(1):166.

Jones C, Badger S. A, Regan M, Clements B. W, Diamond T, Parks R. W, Taylor M. A. Modulation of gut barrier function in patients with obstructive jaundice using probiotic LP299v. *Eur J Gastroenterol Hepatol* (2013) 25(12):1424-1430.

Jung K, Kim A, Lee J. H., Cho D, Seo J, Jung E. S, Kang H. J, Roh J, Kim W. Effect of Oral Intake of *Lactiplantibacillus plantarum* APsulloc 331261 (GTB1TM) on Diarrhea-Predominant Irritable Bowel Syndrome: A Randomized, Double-Blind, Placebo-Controlled Study. *Nutrients* (2022) 14(10):2015.

Jung M, Jung S, Kim N, Ahn H, Yun H, Kim K. N. A. Randomized, Double-Blind, Placebo-Controlled Trial to Assess the Efficacy and Safety of *Lactiplantibacillus plantarum* CJLP243 in Patients with Functional Diarrhea and High Fecal Calprotectin Levels. *Nutrients* (2022) 14(2):389.

Kamil RZ, Murdiati A, Juffrie M, Rahayu E. S. Gut Microbiota Modulation of Moderate Undernutrition in Infants through Gummy *Lactobacillus plantarum* Dad-13 Consumption: A Randomized Double-Blind Controlled Trial. *Nutrients* (2022) 14(5):1049.

Karlsson C, Ahrné S, Molin G, Berggren A, Palmquist I, Fredrikson GN, Jeppsson B. Probiotic therapy to men with incipient arteriosclerosis initiates increased bacterial diversity in colon: a randomized controlled trial. *Atherosclerosis* (2010) 208(1):228-233.

Kaźmierczak-Siedlecka K, Folwarski M, Ruszkowski J, Skonieczna-Żydecka K, Szafrański W, Makarewicz W. Effects of 4 weeks of *Lactobacillus plantarum* 299v supplementation on nutritional status, enteral nutrition tolerance, and quality of life in cancer patients receiving home enteral nutrition - a double-blind, randomized, and placebo-controlled trial. *Eur Rev Med Pharmacol Sci* (2020) 24 (18):9684-9694.

Kim M. J, Kim K. P, Choi E, Yim J. H, Choi C, Yun H. S, Ahn H. Y, Oh J. Y, Cho Y. Effects of *Lactobacillus plantarum* CJLP55 on Clinical Improvement, Skin Condition and Urine Bacterial Extracellular Vesicles in Patients with Acne Vulgaris: A Randomized, Double-Blind, Placebo-Controlled Study. *Nutrients* (2021) 13(4):1368.

Kim S, Huang E, Park S, Holzapfel W, Lim S. D. Physiological Characteristics and Anti-obesity Effect of *Lactobacillus plantarum* K10. *Korean J Food Sci Anim Resour* (2018) 38 (3):554-569.

Lee D. E, Huh C. S, Ra J, Choi I. D, Jeong J. W, Kim S. H, Ryu J. H, Seo Y. K, Koh J. S, Lee J. H, Sim J. H, Ahn Y. T. Clinical Evidence of Effects of *Lactobacillus plantarum* HY7714 on Skin Aging: A Randomized, Double Blind, Placebo-Controlled Study. *J Microbiol Biotechnol* (2015) 25(12):2160-2168.

Lee M. C, Tu Y. T, Lee C. C, Tsai S. C, Hsu H. Y, Tsai T. Y, Liu T. H, Young S. L, Lin J. S, Huang C. C. *Lactobacillus plantarum* TWK10 Improves Muscle Mass and Functional Performance in Frail Older Adults: A Randomized, Double-Blind Clinical Trial. *Microorganisms* (2021) 9 (7):1466.

Lew L. C, Hor Y. Y, Yusoff N. A. A, Choi S. B, Yusoff M. S. B, Roslan N. S, Ahmad A, Mohammad J. A. M, Abdullah M. F. I. L, Zakaria N, Wahid N, Sun Z, Kwok L. Y, Zhang H, Liong M. T. Probiotic *Lactobacillus plantarum* P8 alleviated stress and anxiety while enhancing memory and cognition in stressed adults: A randomised, double-blind, placebo-controlled study. *Clin Nutr* (2019) 38(5):2053-2064.

Liu Y, Liu Q, Zhao J, Zhang H, Zhai Q, Chen W. Strain-specific regulative effects of *Lactobacillus plantarum* on intestinal barrier dysfunction are associated with their capsular polysaccharides. *Int J Biol Macromol* (2022) 222(Pt A):1343-1352.

Liu Y. W, Liong M. T, Chung YE, Huang H. Y, Peng W. S, Cheng Y. F, Lin Y. S, Wu Y. Y, Tsai Y. C. Effects of *Lactobacillus plantarum* PS128 on Children with Autism Spectrum Disorder in Taiwan: A Randomized, Double-Blind, Placebo-Controlled Trial. *Nutrients* (2019) 11(4):820.

Lönnermark E, Friman V, Lappas G, Sandberg T, Berggren A, Adlerberth I. Intake of *Lactobacillus plantarum* reduces certain gastrointestinal symptoms during treatment with antibiotics. *J Clin Gastroenterol* (2010) 44(2):106-112.

Meštrović Popovič K, Povalej Bržan P, Langerholc T, Marčun Varda N. The Impact of *Lactobacillus Plantarum* PCS26 Supplementation on the Treatment and Recurrence of Urinary Tract Infections in Children-A Pilot Study. J Clin Med (2022) 11(23):7008.

Nagata Y, Yoshida M, Kitazawa H, Araki E, Gomyo T. Improvements in seasonal allergic disease with *Lactobacillus plantarum* No. 14. *Biosci Biotechnol Biochem* (2010) 74(9):1869-1877.

Naruszewicz M, Johansson M. L, Zapolska-Downar D, Bukowska H. Effect of *Lactobacillus plantarum* 299v on cardiovascular disease risk factors in smokers. *Am J Clin Nutr* (2002) 76 (6):1249-1255.

Niedzielin K, Kordecki H, Birkenfeld B. A controlled, double-blind, randomized study on the efficacy of *Lactobacillus plantarum* 299V in patients with irritable bowel syndrome. *Eur J Gastroenterol Hepatol* (2001) 13(10):1143-1147.

Nobaek S, Johansson M. L, Molin G, Ahrné S, Jeppsson B. Alteration of intestinal microflora is associated with reduction in abdominal bloating and pain in patients with irritable bowel syndrome. *Am J Gastroenterol* (2000) 95(5):1231-1238.

Nordström E. A, Teixeira C, Montelius C, Jeppsson B, Larsson N. *Lactiplantibacillus plantarum* 299v (LP299V®): three decades of research. *Benef Microbes* (2021) 12(5):441-465.

Oh M. R, Jang H. Y, Lee S. Y, Jung S. J, Chae S. W, Lee S. O, Park B. H. *Lactobacillus plantarum* HAC01 Supplementation Improves Glycemic Control in Prediabetic Subjects: A Randomized, Double-Blind, Placebo-Controlled Trial. *Nutrients* (2021) 13(7):2337.

OjiNjideka Hemphill N, Pezley L, Steffen A, Elam G, Kominiarek M. A, Odoms-Young A, Kessee N, Hamm A, Tussing-Humphreys L, Koenig MD. Feasibility Study of *Lactobacillus Plantarum* 299v Probiotic Supplementation in an Urban Academic Facility among Diverse Pregnant Individuals. *Nutrients* (2023) 15(4):875.

Park Y. E, Kim M. S, Shim K. W, Kim Y. I, Chu J, Kim B. K, Choi I. S, Kim J. Y. Effects of *Lactobacillus plantarum* Q180 on Postprandial Lipid Levels and Intestinal Environment: A Double-Blind, Randomized, Placebo-Controlled, Parallel Trial. *Nutrients* (2020) 12(1):255.

Prakoeswa C. R. S, Bonita L, Karim A, Herwanto N, Umborowati MA, Setyaningrum T, Hidayati AN, Surono I.S. Beneficial effect of *Lactobacillus plantarum* IS-10506 supplementation in adults with atopic dermatitis: a randomized controlled trial. *J Dermatolog Treat* (2022) 33(3):1491-1498.

Prakoeswa C. R. S, Herwanto N, Prameswari R, Astari L, Sawitri S, Hidayati A. N, Indramaya D. M, Kusumowidagdo E. R, Surono I. S. *Lactobacillus plantarum* IS-10506 supplementation reduced SCORAD in children with atopic dermatitis. *Benef Microbes* (2017) 8 (5):833-840.

Rahayu E. S, Mariyatun M, Putri Manurung NE, Hasan P. N, Therdtatha P, Mishima R, Komalasari H, Mahfuzah NA, Pamungkaningtyas F. H, Yoga W. K, Nurfiana D. A, Liwan S. Y, Juffrie M, Nugroho A. E, Utami T. Effect of probiotic *Lactobacillus plantarum* Dad-13 powder consumption on the gut microbiota and intestinal health of overweight adults. *World J Gastroenterol* (2021) 27(1):107-128.

Ren R, Zhao A. Q, Chen L, Wu S, Hung WL, Wang B. Therapeutic effect of *Lactobacillus plantarum* JS19 on mice with dextran sulfate sodium induced acute and chronic ulcerative colitis. *J Sci Food Agric* (2022).

Reuben R. C, Roy PC, Sarkar S. L, Rubayet Ul Alam A. S. M, Jahid I. K. Characterization and evaluation of lactic acid bacteria from indigenous raw milk for potential probiotic properties. *J Dairy Sci* (2020) 103(2):1223-1237.

Ricciardi A, Parente E, Guidone A, Ianniello R. G, Zotta T, Abu Sayem S. M, Varcamonti M. Genotypic diversity of stress response in *Lactobacillus plantarum*, *Lactobacillus paraplantarum* and *Lactobacillus pentosus*. *Int J Food Microbiol* (2012) 157(2):278-285.

Rudzki L, Ostrowska L, Pawlak D, Małus A, Pawlak K, Waszkiewicz N, Szulc A. Probiotic *Lactobacillus Plantarum* 299v decreases kynurenine concentration and improves cognitive functions in patients with major depression: A double-blind, randomized, placebo controlled study. P*sychoneuroendocrinology* (2019) 100:213-222.

Rustanti N, Murdiati A, Juffrie M, Rahayu ES. Effect of Probiotic *Lactobacillus plantarum* Dad-13 on Metabolic Profiles and Gut Microbiota in Type 2 Diabetic Women: A Randomized Double-Blind Controlled Trial. *Microorganisms* (2022) 10(9):1806.

Sakurai K, Toshimitsu T, Okada E, Anzai S, Shiraishi I, Inamura N, Kobayashi S, Sashihara T, Hisatsune T. Effects of *Lactiplantibacillus plantarum* OLL2712 on Memory

Function in Older Adults with Declining Memory: A Randomized Placebo-Controlled Trial. *Nutrients* (2022) 14 (20):4300.

Seddik H. A, Bendali F, Gancel F, Fliss I, Spano G, Drider D. Lactobacillus plantarum and Its Probiotic and Food Potentialities. Probiotics Antimicrob Proteins (2017) 9(2):111-122.

Shokryazdan P, Faseleh Jahromi M, Liang J. B, Ho Y. W. Probiotics: From Isolation to Application. *J Am Coll Nutr* (2017) 36(8):666-676.

Siezen R. J, van Hylckama Vlieg J. E. Genomic diversity and versatility of *Lactobacillus plantarum*, a natural metabolic engineer. *Microb Cell Fact* (2011) 10:S3.

Sohn M, Jung H, Lee W. S, Kim T. H, Lim S. Effect of *Lactobacillus plantarum* LMT1-48 on Body Fat in Overweight Subjects: A Randomized, Double-Blind, Placebo-Controlled Trial. *Diabetes Metab J* (2023) 47(1):92-103.

Sohn M, Na G. Y, Chu J, Joung H, Kim B. K, Lim S. Efficacy and Safety of *Lactobacillus plantarum* K50 on Lipids in Koreans With Obesity: A Randomized, Double-Blind Controlled Clinical Trial. *Front Endocrinol* (Lausanne) (2022) 12:790046.

Vladareanu R, Mihu D, Mitran M, Mehedintu C, Boiangiu A, Manolache M, Vladareanu S. New evidence on oral *L. plantarum* P17630 product in women with history of recurrent vulvovaginal candidiasis (RVVC): a randomized double-blind placebo-controlled study. *Eur Rev Med Pharmacol Sci* (2018) 22(1):262-267.

Wang Z, Li C, He X, Xu K, Xue Z, Wang T, Xu Z, Liu X. *Platycodon grandiflorum* root fermentation broth reduces inflammation in a mouse IBD model through the AMPK/NF-κB/NLRP3 pathway. *Food Funct* (2022) 13(7):3946-3956.

Wu Q, Zhang C, Wa Y, Qu H, Gu R, Chen D, Song Z, Chen X. Correlation between exopolysaccharide biosynthesis and gastrointestinal tolerance of *Lactiplantibacillus plantarum*. *J Appl Microbiol* (2022) 132(1):584-591.

Yang B, Yue Y, Chen Y, Ding M, Li B, Wang L, Wang Q, Stanton C, Ross RP, Zhao J, Zhang H, Chen W. *Lactobacillus plantarum* CCFM1143 Alleviates Chronic Diarrhea via Inflammation Regulation and Gut Microbiota Modulation: A Double-Blind, Randomized, Placebo-Controlled Study. *Front Immunol* (2021) 12:746585.

Zhang C, Zhang Y, Ma K, Wang G, Tang M, Wang R, Xia Z, Xu Z, Sun M, Bao X, Gui H, Wang H. *Lactobacillus plantarum* Lp3a improves functional constipation: evidence from a human randomized clinical trial and animal model. *Ann Transl Med* (2022) 10(6):316.

Zhao Z, Chen L, Zhao Y, Wang C, Duan C, Yang G, Niu C, Li S. *Lactobacillus plantarum* NA136 ameliorates nonalcoholic fatty liver disease by modulating gut microbiota, improving intestinal barrier integrity, and attenuating inflammation. *Appl Microbiol Biotechnol* (2020) 104 (12):5273-5282.

Chapter 3

Macro, Micro and Nanoencapsulation as Delivery System of *Lactobacillus plantarum*

Camila Cristina Avelar de Sousa
Juliana Sant'Ana Falcão Leite
Rafael Sepúlveda Fonsêca Trevisan Passos
Thiago da Matta Pires Cruz
Maurício Costa Alves da Silva
and Carlos Pasqualin Cavalheiro[*]
Laboratório de Inspeção e Tecnologia de Carnes e Derivados (LabCarne),
Universidade Federal da Bahia, Salvador, Brazil

Abstract

Over the last few years, the growing health concern has led the food industry to develop new products by incorporating probiotic strains, such as *Lactobacillus plantarum*. The colonization of the gut with *L. plantarum* prevents dysbiosis, inflammatory bowel disease, and irritable bowel syndrome, and controls chronic disorders such as obesity, hypertension, and type 2 diabetes. Despite food being an effective delivery system for probiotic strains, the processing and storage conditions and the passage through the human digestive tract can be deleterious to *L. plantarum* cells. In this context, encapsulation emerges as a useful tool since the incorporation of *L. plantarum* into a carrier matrix may offer protection to enhance its viability and enable the controlled release in specific sites of the human gastrointestinal tract. Studies have tested several encapsulation techniques like spray drying,

[*] Corresponding Author's Email: carlos.cavalheiro@ufba.br.

In: Lactobacillus plantarum and Its Role in Human Health
Editors: Maria Simona Chiş, Adriana Paucean
ISBN: 979-8-89113-696-0

freeze-drying, and extrusion combined with different wall materials aiming to evaluate the effects on the encapsulation efficiency and controlled release capacity. Among the wall materials, sodium alginate is the most used, but chitosan, pectin, and starch have also been tested. Besides, the size of the particles is also important, depending on the application. In this sense, different technologies can be applied, such as macro, micro, and nanoencapsulation. Then, we aim to analyze recent studies about the encapsulation of *L. plantarum*, focusing on the techniques, the wall materials, and their impacts on the viability and controlled release of these microorganisms in the human gastrointestinal tract.

Keywords: lactic acid bacteria, encapsulating agents, gastrointestinal viability, controlled release, encapsulation techniques

1. Introduction

Nowadays, the search for functional foods is increasing because they can help to promote health and well-being to the consumers and reduce the chances of occurrences diseases. In addition, there is their well-known nutritional value. In this context, probiotics, prebiotics, symbiotics, antioxidants and other bioactive compounds has increasingly been used in industry to incorporate in foods to improve their quality.

Probiotics are live microorganisms, such as bacteria, that can provide health benefits when consumed in adequate amounts (FAO/WHO, 2002). To promote health effects, the daily recommended consumption of probiotic bacteria is 10^9 CFU/g (Atraki and Azizkhani, 2021). Probiotics are typically found in fermented foods such as yoghurt, but can be also incorporated in other foods as meat products, juices, candies or in the form of dietary supplements. The main probiotic microorganisms pertaining to the *Lactobacillus* and *Bifidobacterium* genera (Douglas and Sanders, 2008). *Lactobacillus* spp., constituting the most extensive category within the *Lactobacillaceae* family, comprises Gram-positive, facultative anaerobic bacteria that are commonly encountered within the respiratory, gastrointestinal, and genital tracts of animals and humans. However, they also can be found in other environments that contains carbohydrates, such as dairy, meat, fruits and vegetables. *Lactobacillus* can ferment sugars, producing lactic acid as a metabolic byproduct. One of the main species studied as probiotics are *Lactobacillus plantarum*.

L. plantarum is a lactic acid bacterium (LAB), mesophilic, produces lactic acid from the fermentation of glucose, but also produces acetic and formic acids, and ethanol (Todorov and Franco, 2010). Lactic acid production lowers the pH and prevents the growth of pathogens. In addition, it produces bacteriocins, which are antimicrobial proteins that inhibit the growth of other bacteria. The *L. plantarum* can grow in several conditions, including high salt concentrations, low pH levels, and high temperatures, which allows them to survive in different environments, such as the human gastrointestinal tract.

The regular consumption of probiotics, with emphasis on the *L. plantarum* strains, is effective in the healthy gut balance of microorganisms. Improving digestion, boosting the immune system, and reducing inflammation are some of the benefits of *L. plantarum* regular consumption. To achieve these effects, the ingestion and colonization of the gut must be done adequately but the passage through the human digestive tract can be deleterious to the bacteria which reduces cell viability. In this context, the encapsulation of microorganisms acts as a protection against stress factors, providing a greater cell viability.

Encapsulation can be defined as the technique of entrapping a liquid, solid or gaseous substance within another one. The substance to be encapsulated can be called core material or active agent, while the encapsulating substance can be called coating, carrier, or wall material (Nedovic, 2011). Many encapsulation techniques can be applied in the food industry, with different wall materials, releasing systems, and capsules sizes.

Regarding the wall materials used, biopolymers are the most due to the physical barrier with high protection effectiveness against the stress factors. Some examples are alginate, chitosan, pectin, and milk proteins (De Prisco and Mauriello, 2016). The release of the core material from the capsules can be due to mechanical stress, changes in temperature or pH values. The size of the capsules is also an important characteristic because it is directly related to their properties, such as their stability under different conditions, the viability during the storage period, and the controlled release of substances. Smaller capsules tend to have a faster release, while larger capsules tend to have a slower and prolonged release. The encapsulation process can be classified as macroencapsulation, with capsules bigger than 5 mm, microencapsulation, with capsules sizes ranging from 1 μm to 5 mm, and nanoencapsulation, when the size is less than 1 μm (Chopde et al., 2020). Some of the techniques to encapsulate *L. plantarum* in different wall materials and size of capsules are shown in Table 1.

1.1. Macroencapsulation of *Lactobacillus plantarum*

Macroencapsulation of probiotic microorganisms are not commonly used in the food industry to encapsulate probiotic microorganisms. Low cell viability is the main reason why this technique is not performed, as nutrients and oxygen do not diffuse to the center of large capsules, which would lead to the cell death in a few hours (Rathore et al., 2013). However, Zhang et al. (2018) developed sodium alginate/cellulose nanofiber gel macrospheres for *L. plantarum* encapsulation and analyzed the probiotic viability in the macrospheres and after exposure to *in vitro* simulated gastrointestinal tract (Table 1). The macrospheres were obtained from extrusion technique and five formulations were done with different concentrations of sodium alginate and cellulose nanofiber. The macrospheres become smaller during when exposed to the acid simulated gastric fluid due to the carboxyl groups protonation of the wall materials in acid environment, which resulted in an electrostatic charge repulsion reduction and in the formation of hydrogen bonds. However, it is a good characteristic because results in low penetration of gastric fluid into the macrospheres. In this context, they also observed that higher levels of cellulose nanofiber offer better protection to the encapsulated *L. plantarum* during exposure to the simulated gastrointestinal tract.

1.2. Microencapsulation of *Lactobacillus plantarum*

Several methods can be used for microencapsulation of *L. plantarum*, such as extrusion, emulsion, spray drying, spray cooling/chilling, fluidized-bed coating, liposomal entrapment, lyophilization, coacervation, centrifugal suspension separation, cocrystallization, inclusion complexation and thermal gelation. Extrusion, emulsion, and spray-drying are the most effective techniques used for encapsulation of *L. plantarum* (Kavitake et al., 2018).

Table 1. *L. plantarum* encapsulated under different techniques and different wall materials

Encapsulation technique		Wall materials	Main results	Reference
Macroencapsulation	Extrusion	Sodium alginate and cellulose	Existence and uniform dispersion of *L. plantarum* cells in the macrospheres and protection against simulated gastric conditions.	Zhang et al. (2018)
Microencapsulation	Spray-drying	Maltodextrin, sweet potato flour, pectin, agar-agar, and gelatin	Microcapsules showed to be resistant to heat treatment, acidic pH conditions and in vitro simulated gastrointestinal conditions. Also maintained the viability of *Lactiplantibacillus plantarum* during storage under refrigeration and freezing.	Costa et al. (2023)
	Spray-drying	Gum arabic, trehalose and maltodextrin	Encapsulation efficiency of 75%. Microcapsules provided storage viability rates between 60.41% and 89.74% for 120 days at 8°C and -18°C. and counts near 4 log CFU/g-1 under gastrointestinal conditions.	De Deus et al. (2023)
	Extrusion	Alginate and gelatin	Microcapsules showed great potential in protection (storage and heat resistance) and delivery of probiotics in simulated intestinal conditions.	Ni et al. (2023)
	Complex coacervation	Sodium caseinate and chitosan	Microcapsules offered protection in simulated gastric and intestinal fluids and during storage, with an increase in cell viability. They also reach distal areas of the small intestine and colon.	Peñalva et al. (2023)
	Spray-drying	Whey protein isolate and dextran	Microcapsules showed protective effect against processing stress conditions (high temperatures) and *in vitro* digestion.	Guo et al. (2022)
	Extrusion	Sodium alginate, milk powder, green banana flour and xanthan gum	Microcapsules showed a protective effect, increasing cell viability in storage	Trevisan et al. (2022)
	Extrusion	Sodium alginate, skim milk, dextrin, chitosan, and denatured whey protein	Microcapsules were successful in protect *L. plantarum* against stress factors (heating temperatures, refrigerated storage, exposure to acid latic and gastrointestinal conditions)	Mahmoud et al. (2020)

Table 1. (Continued)

Encapsulation technique		Wall materials	Main results	Reference
	Emulsion	Skim-milk	Higher survival rate after simulated gastric conditions and greater storage stability for microencapsulated *L. plantarum*.	Ma et al. (2020)
	Spray-drying	Whey, whey permeates and retentate	Wall materials can protect microorganisms from high temperatures during spray drying. Microcapsules offer protection during storage at 4°C and 20°C and provide stability for microorganisms in simulated gastrointestinal tract.	Eckert et al. (2017)
	Extrusion	Alginate and chitosan	Microcapsules increases cell viability during storage and a has a protective effect on cells in simulated gastric conditions.	Nualkaekul et al. (2012)
Nanoencapsulation	Electrospinning	Gum arabic and pullulan	Nanofibers exhibited great thermal stability. Nanofibers provided probiotic survivability between 85.38–97.83%, and retained viability during 28 days storage at 4°C.	Ma et al. (2021)
	Nanoemulsion	Sodium acetate, fructooligosaccharides and skim milk	Encapsulation of *Lactobacillus plantarum* powder with the Pickering HIPEs was successful to enhance the viable cell count after 14 days storage and GIT digestion.	Qin, Gao & Luo (2021)
	Nanoemulsion	Cell-free supernatant	Iinhibitory effect against *Streptococcus mutans*	Karimi et al. (2020)
	Electrospinning	Polyethylene oxide, sucrose, and trehalose	Nanofibers provided up to 7.6×10^8 CFU/mg *L. plantarum* cells. The addition of trehalose provided large survival benefits during storage and minimal loss of the probiotic viability over 24 weeks of storage at 4°C. The nanofibers released almost all the *L. plantarum* cells over 30 minutes.	Škrlec et al. (2019)
	Electrospinning	Poly (vinyl alcohol) and fructooligosaccharides (FOS)	Electrospun nanofibers with FOS improved probiotic cells viability. *L. plantarum* count above 6 log CFU/mL at 70°C	Feng et al. (2018)

1.3. Extrusion

The extrusion technique is the oldest and most common for converting hydrocolloids into capsules due to handling ease, low cost, and efficiency. The technique consists of a core material completely mixed with the wall material which is projected into a nozzle in a hardening solution (Figure 1). The shape and size of the microcapsules are on dependance on the nozzle diameter and its distance to hardening solution (Krasaekoopt, Bhandari and Deeth, 2003).

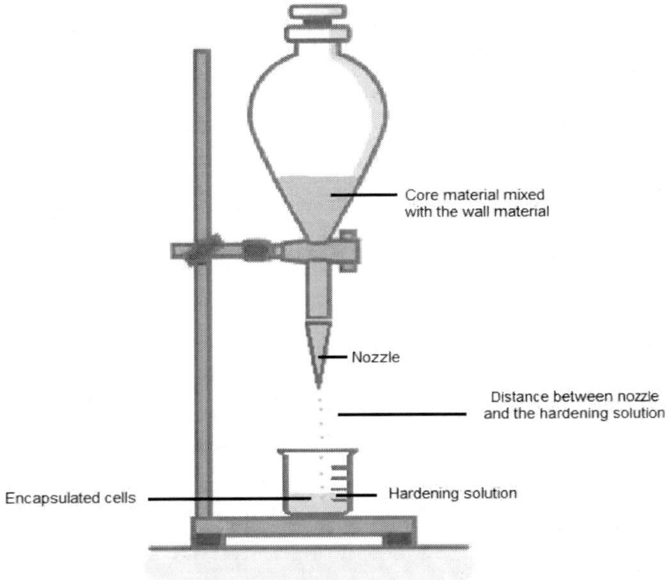

Figure 1. Schematization of extrusion method for *L. plantarum* encapsulation.

Generally, sizes between 300 μm to 3 mm can be achieved using the extrusion technique (Haffner et al., 2016). Several studies have been already conducted using the extrusion technique to encapsulate *L. plantarum* (Table 1), and the capsules sizes showed a large variety, which is associated with the wall material and the technique applications. Values of 180-300 μm, 80-220 μm and 200-1000 μm were found using alginate, alginate-psyllium and alginate-fenugreek as wall materials and extruded through a 21-gauge nozzle (Haghshenas et al., 2015). Using alginate and combining it with other substances such as gelatin, extruded through a syringe with a volume of 50 mL and an internal diameter of 2 cm, the sizes ranged from 4.0 to 4.9 mm (Ni et al., 2023). A syringe (25 G, 0.5 mm) used for extrusion resulted in capsules size from 501.54 to 800.739 μm in dry state, and from 1492 to 1635 μm in the wet state, using alginate associated with chitosan, dextrin, skim milk and whey protein as wall materials (Mahmoud et al., 2020).

Regarding the encapsulation efficiency (EE), using this technique the value is usually close to 100%. On Haghshenas et al. (2015) work, EE ranged from 98.7 to 99.8% using various alginate gel formulations. Similar results were obtained in other studies, values ranging from 98.11 to 94.94% (Mahmoud et al., 2020) and values of 97.1 and 97.7% (Ni et al., 2023). Although Trevisan et al. (2022) obtained a value of 86.17%, this can be explained by the temperature conditions (~25°C) without the use of organic solvent. These results show that the extrusion technique to encapsulate probiotics has high EE values and is suitable for application in living cells.

The encapsulation of probiotics shows the protective effect of the capsules during the storage period, increasing cell viability. According to Hagshenas et al. (2015), free cells showed a significant decrease in their viability, from 9.6 to 1.8 log CFU/mL. while encapsulated formulations had significantly higher viability. It was observed that treatments with higher concentrations of alginate resulted in better cell protection. Ni et al. (2023) showed that after the storage time of 6 days at 4°C, free cells had a significantly lower viable cell count (>2.1 log CFU) than encapsulated (alginate and alginate-gelatin capsules had a 1.5 log and 1.4 log CFU reduction, respectively). The protective effect was also demonstrated during 10 days of storage. The encapsulated treatment obtained higher *L. plantarum* counts when compared to the free treatment, 8.06 log CFU/g and 5.93 log CFU/g, respectively (Trevisan et al., 2022). An increase in cell viability during refrigerated storage was observed by Mahmoud et al. (2020). After 4 weeks, encapsulated *L. plantarum* counts increased by 1.40, 0.88, 0.84 and 0.19 log cycle using Sodium alginate-chitosan (Alg-Ch), Sodium alginate-dextrin (Alg-Dex), Sodium alginate-skim milk (Alg-Sm) and Sodium alginate-denatured whey protein (Alg-DWP) as wall materials. The protective effect can also be observed over long periods, after 3 months of freezing storage there was a reduction compared to the initial count (approximately 10^8 CFU/g sample) of approximately 1.66 and 1.48 log cycles for Alg-Sm and Alg-DWP, respectively.

Survival of microorganisms after contact with the gastrointestinal tract is important for bacteria to be effective as probiotics. The human stomach has a low pH and bacteria need to survive in this environment to reach the intestine and encapsulating it's a way to perform it. Free cells of *L. plantarum* were sensitive to exposure to low pH values, demonstrating loss of cell viability. Haghshenas et al. (2015) related that after the exposure, untreated *L.*

plantarum 15HN showed a survival rate around 37% while the encapsulated ones obtained high values, such as 84.63% and 86.41%. The decrease in the bacterial CFU counts for encapsulated cells ranged from 1.3 to 3.3 log. In Mahmoud et al. (2020) work, encapsulated microorganisms also showed similar decreases in counts, ranging from 1.24 to 1.71 log CFU. Higher values to the survival rates of cells after simulated gastric fluid were observed, 97.2% and 97.8% (Ni et al., 2023). Thus, encapsulation is adequate to protect microorganisms in adverse situations, such as low pH in the stomach environment.

In the intestinal tract, the microorganisms must remain viable, and the capsules must be able to release the probiotics into the environment. After exposure to simulated intestinal juice for 120 min, a reduction of only 0.68 log cycle for the cells encapsulated with sodium alginate-skim milk as wall material was observed, which indicates that encapsulation maintain good cell viability (Mahmoud et al., 2020). Regarding to the release of probiotics in simulated intestinal conditions, capsules of *L. plantarum* with low concentrations of alginate released the microorganisms completely after 1h. With increasing alginate concentration, complete release occurred in 2h. Alginate acts as a physical barrier that protects microorganisms, which results in a longer cell release time at higher concentrations (Haghshenas et al., 2015). In Ni et al. (2023) study, the release of probiotics occurred more intensely in the first hour and in the next two hours slowed down. At the end of the digestion, cell counts were above 9.0 log CFU, which indicates that most of the *L. plantarum* was released during the simulated intestinal digestion, site of action of probiotics. Capsules exposed to acidic environments remained viable. However, when exposed at pH 6-6.5 began to disintegrate, completely dissolving and releasing the bacteria over the incubation time. This indicates that the release of encapsulated probiotics is pH dependent and occurs in intestinal alkaline pH (Gbassi et al., 2011).

1.4. Emulsion

Emulsion is a technique based on dispersing the material to be encapsulated, such as probiotic cells (discontinuous phase) in an oily solution (continuous phase) (Figure 2A). The mixture is homogenized to form a water-in-oil (W/O) emulsion. When water-in-oil emulsion is formed, the water-soluble polymer must be insolubilized (cross-linked) so that the particles are formed in the oil phase. The emulsion can be broken by the addition of $CaCl_2$, and the microcapsules can be collected by centrifugation or filtration (Krasaekoopt, Bhandari and Deeth, 2003; Coghetto, Brinques and Ayub, 2016). When employing an oily solution as the discontinuous phase, to be dispersed within an aqueous solution (continuous phase), an oil-in-water (O/W) emulsion is generated (Figure 2B). It is also possible to prepare multiple emulsion formulations, such as water-in-oil (O/W/O) or water-in-oil-in-water (W/O/W) emulsions (McClements, Decker and Weiss, 2007). Capsule sizes vary from 200 μm-1 mm (Haffner et al., 2016) and are related to the emulsifier used and the agitation speed (Krasaekoopt, Bhandari and Deeth, 2003).

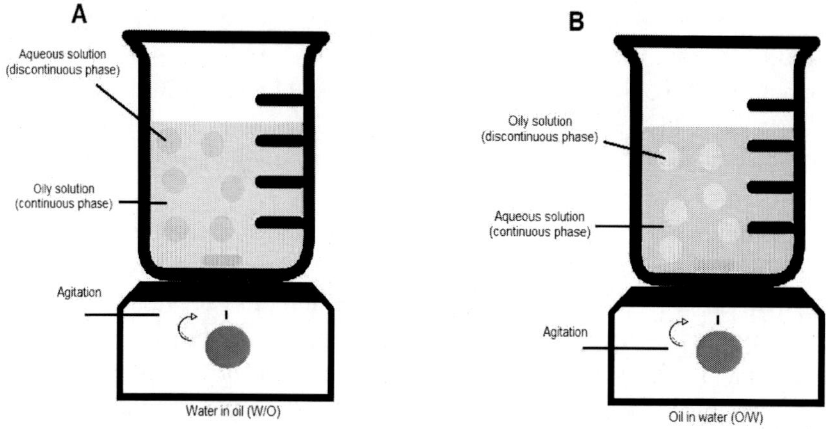

Figure 2. Encapsulation of *L. plantarum* in water-in-oil (A) and oil-in-water (B) emulsions.

To perform the technique, the substance most used in food industry as continuous phase is vegetable oils, but emulsifiers such as Tween 80 can be added to obtain a better emulsion. The addition of emulsifiers lowers the surface tension, resulting in smaller particles. For discontinuous phase, alginate, chitosan, and gelatin are commonly used. Emulsion proved to be viable to increase survival of probiotic microorganisms and it's easy to scale up (Krasaekoopt, Bhandari and Deeth, 2003).

The capsules sizes obtained from emulsion are usually smaller than that obtained from extrusion. However, a disadvantage of this technique is the formation of capsules with a wide variety of sizes and shapes (Burgain, Gaiani and Scher, 2011). Ma et al. (2020) described that the size of microcapsules ranged from 18.17–81.33 μm, with mean of 52.57 μm. Larger sizes were found ranged from 165 to 527 μm (Dong, Luan and Thuy, 2020; Pupa et al., 2021).

However, Luo et al. (2022) obtained larger variety in capsule sizes, ranging from 368.21 to 7896.67 nm.

Performing the emulsion encapsulation technique, high values for encapsulation efficiency (EE) are usually obtained. The encapsulation efficiency was 97.89 and 98%.05 for multilayer and conventional emulsion (Pour, Marhamatizadeh and Fattahi, 2022). High values for this parameter were also found in other studies, 93.50 and 89.25% (Dong, Luan & Thuy, 2020) and 92.66 to 94.10% (Pupa et al., 2021). Hassan et al. (2020) obtained a result for EE a little lower, 86.02% comparable to Ma et al. (2020), who obtained 86.59% but still great results.

Regarding to viability of the microorganisms, Pour, Marhamatizadeh and Fattahi (2022) evaluated the survival of encapsulated *L. plantarum* in yogurt for 3 weeks. The unencapsulated bacteria showed a significantly decreased during the storage time while the encapsulated ones showed a higher viability and higher counts at the end of storage. When the microorganisms were applied in soursop juice during storage for 4 weeks, it was observed a significant reduction in free cells counts, from 7.89 log CFU/mL to 4.90 log CFU/mL, while for encapsulated *L. plantarum* there was no statistical difference during storage, 7.87 log CFU/mL to 7.01 log CFU/mL (Hassan et al., 2020). In Ma et al. (2020) study, at day 0 of storage, counts of *L. plantarum* was 7.69 log units CFU/g, and after 21 days in storage at 4°C it decreased by 0.46 log units CFU/g. And after storage at 20°C for 21 days, the viable cells were 7.05 log units CFU/g. This indicates that microencapsulation by emulsification form a structure that protects *L. plantarum* from harsh environments.

Capsules obtained from emulsion are suitable for protecting bacteria under simulated gastric conditions. *L. plantarum* free and encapsulated were exposed to gastric juice and the results showed that encapsulated probiotics obtained higher viability than free cells. The initial count of free cells was 9.80 log CFU/g and after 60 min decreased to 1.036 log CFU/g. After 120 min, there were no viable free cells. At the same time of exposure, counts of encapsulated cells were 1.06 log CFU/g (Shah et al., 2016). Similar results were found by Ma et al. (2020), who observed a reduction in viable cell counts when exposed to acidic environments, but encapsulated cells had higher counts than free cells. This indicates an excellent protective capacity of microcapsules.

The release of probiotics from the microcapsules into the intestine must occur for the growth and colonization of bacteria in the host. Bacteria need to survive the intestinal environment to be able to colonize it. Shah et al. (2016)

showed that *L. plantarum* microencapsulated can survive in simulated intestinal juice for 6h, despite the decline in counts (initial counts decreased from 9.79 to 5.8 log CFU/g). Ma et al. (2020) related that after the 90 min release time in the SIF, the viable bacterial counts were close to the initial concentration. This result indicates that all bacteria were released from the microcapsules.

1.5. Spray-Drying

Spray-drying is a common technique in food industry and can be defined as a process that occur the dispersion of the core material, forming a dispersion or emulsion, followed by homogenization of the liquid, and atomization of the mixture in the drying chamber, which leads to the evaporation of the solvent and formation of microcapsules (Martín et al., 2014). In this method (Figure 3), liquid feeds are sprayed and directed into a flow of hot and dry air (usually 150 to 250°C).

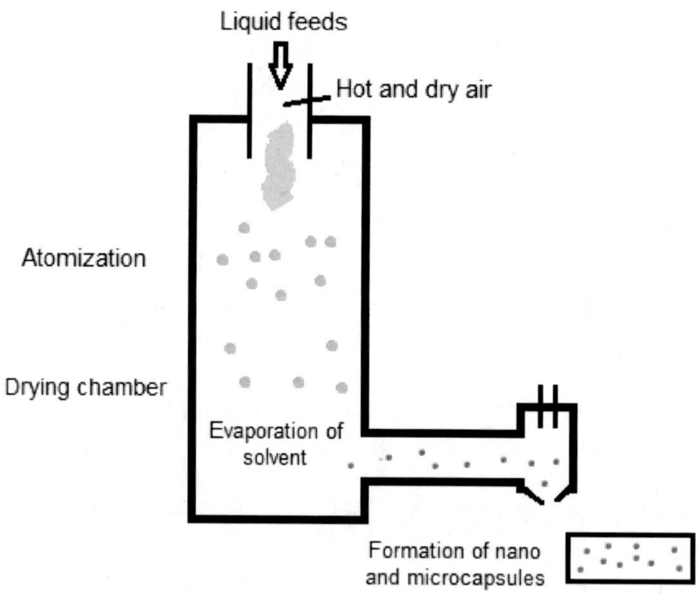

Figure 3. Representation of the spray-drying technique, performed on a spray-dryer to produce micro and nanocapsules of *L. plantarum*.

High temperatures can be deleterious for microorganisms, which suggests that use this technique in probiotics could be a challenge. Aiming to minimize cellular stress caused by spray drying, some protective agents have been used to enhance cellular protection, such as carbohydrates, maltodextrin with dextrose, inulin, and whey (Huang et al., 2017).

The particles size obtained from spray-drying is directly related to the wall materials used. According to Eckert et al. (2017) the mean size of microcapsules was 7.0 μm and whey, whey permeate and whey retentate were used as wall material. In the study performed by Guo et al. (2022) whey protein isolate (WPI) and dextran (DX) (WPI-DX) conjugates were used to develop microcapsules and the capsules sizes were in a range of 3–5 μm diameter. The sizes found are similar due to the similarity between the used wall materials. Marins et al. (2022) obtained slightly larger capsules, with sizes ranging from 10 to 12 μm, using alginate, β-cyclodextrin and xanthan gum. However, due to a variety of wall materials (maltodextrin, sweet potato flour, pectin, agar-agar, and gelatin), Costa et al., (2023) obtained capsule sizes ranging from 5.89 to 18.94 μm.

The wall materials and the temperature used during spray-drying are factors that can interfere with cell viability and encapsulation efficiency. In Eckert et al. (2017) study, the results showed that before spray drying the initial count was about 10.08-10.88 log CFU/g, and after spray drying, it was observed a reduction of 0.08-0.90 log cycles. The microencapsulation process was carried out at a temperature of 90°C to minimize the effects of high temperatures, and the cell counts remained high. Costa et al. (2023) obtained counts of *L. plantarum* before spray-drying of 10.14, 10.03, 9.56 and 10.09 log CFU/g, and after spray-drying of 9.60, 9.41, 8.17 and 8.69 log CFU/g, which represents an encapsulation efficiency of 94.67, 93.82, 85.46 and 86.12% respectively. Guo et al. (2022) obtained a percentage of 93.79% for encapsulation yield and Marins et al. (2022) an average of 90%. The values obtained in these studies (> 85%) demonstrate a high survival of bacteria after encapsulation by spray-drying.

It is important that the probiotic cells remain viable during storage. Costa et al. (2023) evaluated cell survivability at various temperatures. At 25 °C, microcapsules showed counts lower than 6 log CFU/g after 9 days and were unavailable after 27 days for microcapsule B (10% maltodextrin, 4% sweet potato flour and 2% gelatin) and 36 days for A (10% maltodextrin, 5% sweet potato flour and 1% pectin), indicating low survivability at room temperature. At 8 °C, *L. plantarum* were viable for 45 days with counts above 7 log CFU/g, highlighting microcapsule B with a count of 8.75 log CFU/g. Similar results were found on storage at -18°C for 45 days, with counts also above 7 log CFU/g. Survivability of *L. plantarum* was also evaluated in different temperatures of storage. After 56 days of incubation at 20 °C MW (microcapsule whey) and MP (microcapsule permeate) showed no reduction in cell viability and MWR (microcapsule whey retentate) showed a decrease of 1.11 log cycles ($p < 0.05$). But despite that, all showed *L. plantarum* counts above 6 log CFU/g. When incorporated into milk and stored for 42 days at 4°C, all counts remained stable and high (> 9 log CFU/g), which indicates that the capsules disintegrate slowly in storage (Eckert et al., 2017).

Regarding to exposure to simulated gastrointestinal tract, in gastric phase Costa et al. (2023) observed that free cells showed a reduction in viable counts of 6.04 log CFU/g meanwhile microcapsules A and B reduced 1.33 and 1.88 log CFU/g respectively. Guo et al. (2022) related that after exposure to pH 2.0 for 120 min, free cells showed a reduction of 1.73 log CFU/g and encapsulated 0.51 log CFU/g. These results showed that microcapsules can protect bacteria and maintain their viability under low pH conditions. When applied in milk it was observed that free and encapsulated cells did not showed differences in the results (8.76 and 9.19 log CFU/g, respectively), and after 28 remained similar (8.90 and 9.19 log CFU/g) (Eckert et al., 2017).

In the intestinal phase encapsulated cell showed greater resistance than free cells. At the end of the analysis, free cells obtained a decrease of 5.39 log CFU/g, meanwhile microcapsules A and B decreased 1.87 and 2.20 log CFU/g (Costa et al., 2023). Guo et al. (2022) observed that after 60 min in simulated intestinal conditions, free cells showed a decrease in viability of 2.97 log CFU/g and microcapsules decreased 1.22 log CFU/g. And after 2 hours, the results stayed similar. And in milk, all microcapsules showed counts above 8 log CFU/g (Eckert et al., 2017). These results indicates that capsules protect microorganisms so that they reach the intestine in adequate amounts to promote benefits as probiotics.

1.6. Nanoencapsulation of *Lactobacillus plantarum*

The use of nanotechnology includes the manufacturing, processing, and application of advanced materials to produce structures and devices with nanoscale dimensions. In this sense, the particle size influences the properties of materials since reducing dimensions to the nanoscale raises the surface-to-volume ratio, causing alterations in their physicochemical, biological, and functional properties. The nanoencapsulation allows the enhancement of the functional performance of active agents by improving their stability, bioactivity, and controlled release under specific conditions (Weisany et al., 2022). Although nanoencapsulation cannot be applied for probiotics since the cells have relatively large sizes (1–5 μm), the application of nanocoatings to protect probiotics has been studied recently (Assadpour and Jafari, 2019). Recent advanced approaches, such as single-cell encapsulation of probiotics, where individual cells are coated with nanomaterials, can improve bioavailability and mucoadhesion, provide resistance from enzymatic activity, pH, and antibiotic resistance, protection against chemicals, and help preventing and treating diseases at a cellular level (Centurion et al., 2021).

Nano-sized particles show greater adhesion and interaction with enzymes of the intestinal mucosa, as well as an easier penetration capacity through cell walls to achieve target cells. From a sensory point of view, nanocarriers cause less impact on the appearance of food products (Reque and Brandelli, 2021). Probiotics such as *L. plantarum* are among the most common encapsulated active agents (Dangi et al., 2023), and different nanotechnologies such as nanofibers, nano emulsions, nanoparticles, and nanoencapsulation show great potential in the food industry. Besides, nanostructures are reported to provide a larger contact area on the surface of the foods compared to micro or macro-size materials (Ceylan et al., 2019). Especially when using food as a delivery system for probiotics, from the sensory point of view, it is essential to decrease the matrix size from micrometers to nanometers, as well as develop new vehicles with improved delivery properties (López-Rubio and Lagaron, 2012). Probiotic agents with a size below 100 μm have the potential to mitigate adverse sensory effects in food. As a result, researching novel encapsulation technologies for probiotics becomes necessary (Xu et al., 2022).

1.7. Nanospray Drying

The conventional spray-drying technique produces microcapsules, which are considered to have lower solubility, absorption rate, controlled release capacity, imprecise targeting, and bioavailability of core compounds when compared to nanoparticles. Hence, there is an increased need for studies in new techniques, such as nanospray drying, which allows the production of particles with diameter up to 300 nm (Xu et al., 2022).

Despite studies using nanospray drying to encapsulate *L. plantarum* are still scarce, some studies using conventional spray drying technique (Figure 3) produced variable sizes of capsules of *L. plantarum* out of the nanoscale, achieving smaller sizes, ranging from 1 to 7.8 μm (Parlindungan, Dekiwadia, Maya and Jones, 2019), and bigger sizes, reaching between 23.89 μm and 27.30 μm (Rajam and Anandharamakrishnan, 2015; Guo et al., 2022; De Deus et al., 2023). Size variation depends, among other factors, on the core-to-wall ratio, since increasing the concentration of wall material and combining different wall materials can result in larger capsules (Rajam and Anandharamakrishnan, 2015).

The viability loss caused by the high temperatures is a disadvantage of spray drying. Hence, some studies reported low encapsulation efficiency, between 67.25% (Kalita, Saikia, Gautam, Mukhopadhyay and Mahanta, 2018) and 73.57% (De Deus et al., 2023). However, the encapsulation yield of *L. plantarum* encapsulated by spray drying can reach 93.79% (Guo et al., 2022). As well as the size, among other factors, the encapsulation efficiency when using the same technique may vary depending on the wall material, because each one of them show different properties that influence the protection of the core.

Regarding the survival of *L. plantarum* under storage, high survival indexes are reported on refrigeration (4°C) and freezing (-18°C) temperatures, reaching an average between 88.80% and 89.28%. Besides, the capsules produced by spray drying can maintain the viability of *L. plantarum* about 6 log CFU/g after 120 days of storage, which is the minimum limit required to provide benefits in the human gastrointestinal tract (De Deus et al., 2023). According to Romano, Mobili, Zuñiga-Hansen and Gómez-Zavaglia (2018), when stored at room temperatures (20°C), *L. plantarum* showed more susceptibility and lost 100% of the viability in 30 days. However, when reducing the water activity, *L. plantarum* maintained the viability of about 9 log CFU/g during the whole storage time, of 180 days, demonstrating the importance of the water activity for the long-term storage of *L. plantarum* at room temperature.

Different results on the viability of *L. plantarum* under gastrointestinal conditions are obtained depending on the initial count, encapsulation conditions, applied method, and the composition and concentration of the wall material. In this sense, showing no or low count in the simulated stomach stage, which is acid, represents a good ability of the capsule structure to protect *L. plantarum* from this adverse condition (De Deus et al., 2023), since the target of the controlled release is the bowel, an alkaline environment. Capsules produced by spray drying are told to provide final count of 5.80 log CFU/g (Kalita, Saikia, Gautam, Mukhopadhyay and Mahanta, 2018) for *L. plantarum*. However, according to De Deus et al. (2023), who reported a final count average of 3.73 log CFU/g to *L. plantarum* at the end of simulated gastrointestinal conditions, it is important to evaluate the controlled release capacity during the simulation of gastrointestinal conditions by observing the rupture of the capsules in the intestinal phase.

1.8. Nanoemulsion

Nanoemulsion is a technique to produce nanocapsules or nanoparticles of *L. plantarum*, usually applied to improve the effects against pathogenic microorganisms *in vitro* and *in vivo* (Karimi et al., 2020; Abdelhamid, Edris and Sadek, 2023).

The diameter of the particles in nanoemulsions can present a very wide range. Some studies report sizes smaller than 20 nm, which is very suitable for the addition in food, for example (Abdelhamid, Edris and Sadek, 2023), and particles with 92 nm (Karimi et al., 2018). However, nanoemulsion particles sizes can also reach bigger sizes, out of the nanoscale, ranging from 55 μm to 105 μm (Qin, Gao and Luo, 2021).

Nanoencapsulation and nanoemulsion of *L. plantarum* cell-free supernatant were reported as a delivery system for the development of candies to the inhibition of *Streptococcus mutans* in saliva. Despite the cell count on the nanoemulsion and the *L. plantarum* supernatant being very low, the treatment was successful against *S. mutans*. This might be due to the release of bioactive substances by the *L. plantarum* strains, which inhibit the growth of *S. mutans*. Therefore, nanoemulsions can serve as nanocarriers not just for probiotic cells, but also for bioactive compounds like bacteriocins, enzymes, and biosurfactants. They can be used to suppress the growth of pathogenic microorganisms (Karimi et al., 2020).

Nanoemulsion was reported by Qin, Gao and Luo (2021) as a suitable technique to encapsulate *L. plantarum*, since enhanced the viable cell count after 14 days of storage under 4°C for. Regarding the simulated gastrointestinal conditions, these authors reported the survival index of proximately 56%, with final count of 4.34×10^7 CFU/mL. Despite the loss in the viability of nanoencapsulated *L. plantarum*, this technique showed high efficiency against the acidic medium, bile salts, and digestive enzymes than the free probiotic cells. In this sense, nanoemulsion is considered a versatile and promising technique for encapsulating *L. plantarum*, but it remains underexplored and requires further studies to be enhanced.

1.9. Electrospinning

Recently, electrospinning has been gaining ground in the study of nanoencapsulation of probiotics in contrast to conventional techniques due to its efficiency and low cost. Electrospinning produces a nanofibre mat using a high-voltage electric field between two electrodes to create electrically charged jets from a polymeric aqueous solution, obtaining fibers or capsules after solvent's evaporation, without using temperature (Figure 4) (López-Rubio and Lagaron, 2012; Ma et al., 2021). This technique has been acknowledged as a workable method to protect dried and live probiotic bacteria because the execution does not include extreme temperature or pressure conditions (Sharma, Sharma, Bajwa, Chugh and Kumar, 2023).

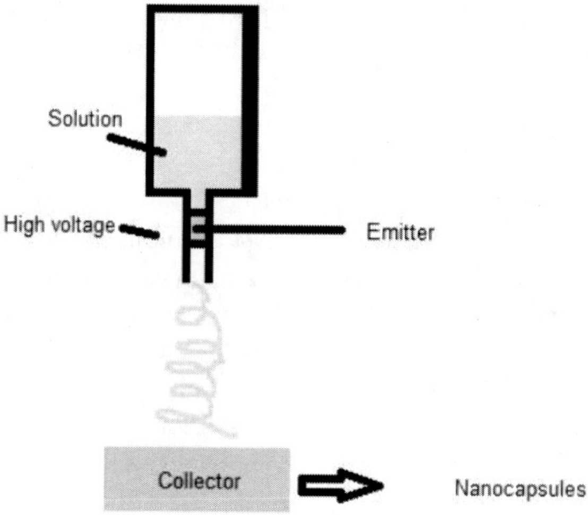

Figure 4. Representation of the electrospinning technique.

Although the *L. plantarum* cells have average diameter of 492 ± 35 nm, the electrospinning technique allows the entire coating with polymeric solution, enclosing the cells within the nanofibers as individual or dividing cells (Škrlec et al., 2019). Hence, the average diameter of electrospun nanofibers containing *L. plantarum* cells may reach lower values, between 676 ± 162 nm (Xu et al., 2020) and 815 ± 115 nm (Škrlec et al., 2019), but also higher values, up to 1.07 μm (Feng et al., 2018).

Regarding the encapsulation efficiency, Ma et al. (2021) reported a survival rate of 97.83% for *L. plantarum* encapsulated by electrospinning, which was the highest among other *Lactobacillus* strains tested, suggesting that electrospinning is a suitable technique to encapsulate *L. plantarum*. Electrospinning can be performed at room temperature, while other techniques and processes, such as spray drying and freeze drying, reaches extreme temperatures, causing damages to the cell membranes.

Ma et al. (2021) also reported that *L. plantarum* reached the highest storage viability rate (77.59%) among other *Lactobacillus* strains after 28 days at 4°C, suggesting that the encapsulation by electrospun nanofibers provided protection and thermal stability during the whole storage time, showing great potential to be used as a delivery system to *L. plantarum*. Regarding long-term storage, *L. plantarum* encapsulated by electrospinning can completely lose the viability when stored at room temperature (25 °C). Therefore, the association of lyoprotectants is an alternative to provide protection to *L. plantarum* cells from temperature and humidity during storage. At refrigeration storage temperature (4 °C), *L. plantarum* encapsulated by electrospinning shows better survival rates after long-term storage. Even so, the addition of the lyoprotectants provided better protection to *L. plantarum* (Škrlec et al., 2019).

In addition, electrospinning can provide a controlled release of *L. plantarum* cells over 30 minutes, which is sufficient time to attach to the surface of the intestinal mucosa, avoiding their rapid flushing with the body fluids and providing the quick removal of the delivery system from the gastrointestinal tract (Škrlec et al., 2019).

1.10. Wall Materials

The wall material selected for encapsulation directly reflects on the functional and morphological properties of the capsules, such as size, porosity, and texture (De Prisco and Mauriello, 2016). The ability to emulsify and stabilize the core material, low viscosity and hygroscopicity, insolubility, and non-reactivity with the core material, tasteless and protection against adverse conditions are some of the desired characteristics for wall materials (Aldana, Sandoval and Aponte, 2004). Biopolymers are the main substances used in cellular encapsulation, due to their high protection against stress factors, acting as a physical barrier, such as alginate, chitosan, and milk proteins (De Prisco and Mauriello, 2016).

To be used as a probiotic delivery system, nanomaterials must be generally recognized as safe (GRAS), biocompatible, bio tolerable, and biodegradable. These nanomaterials can be derived from natural sources, such as polysaccharides, proteins, and lipids, or artificially synthesized, such as metal-based polymers (Ashaolu, 2021).

Among the substances used for wall materials, sodium alginate is the most common. Alginate is a substance produced by algae and bacteria. The commercial alginates are mostly from algae, since that obtained from bacteria is not economically viable (Goh, Heng and Chan, 2012). Alginate is generally recognized as safe (GRAS) as it is non-antigenic, non-toxic, biocompatible, and biodegradable. These characteristics make it a popular option for encapsulating probiotics, as they protect microorganisms against adverse conditions, such as passage through the gastrointestinal tract, and improve viability during storage. Furthermore, alginate can form gels in the presence of calcium ions, which allows the production of microcapsules with high encapsulation efficiency (Lee and Mooney, 2012; Bennacef et al., 2021).

Alginate beads are quite used in a lab-scale, due to the easy preparation. However, the main disadvantage is that microcapsules obtained are very porous, which can compromise the viability of the encapsulated microorganisms. However, the porosity of the capsules can be solved by associating alginate with other compounds, such as chitosan and xanthan gum (Gouin, 2004; Etchepare et al., 2016; Chen et al., 2017). Other biopolymers can be added into alginate, such as skim milk, whey protein, dextrin, fenugreek, and psyllium to improve the structure stability of the capsule, and in some cases as prebiotics, to increase the microorganism viability (Haghshenas et al., 2015; Mahmoud et al., 2020; How and Pui, 2021). Recent studies have shown that the use of alginate for microencapsulation of probiotics can significantly improve the survival of microorganisms, in addition to promoting controlled release in the gastrointestinal tract (Trevisan et al., 2022; Ni et al., 2023).

Sodium alginate and starch are among the most used polysaccharides for nanoencapsulation of probiotics due to their low-cost and high availability (Atraki and Azizkhani, 2021). To enhance the survival of probiotic strains under gastrointestinal simulated conditions, Atraki and Azizkhani (2021) carried out the nanoencapsulation of *Lactobacillus acidophilus*, *Lactobacillus rhamnosus*, *Bifidobacterium bifidum*, and *Bifidobacterium animalis* using sodium alginate associated with starch as wall materials. Compared to the free cells, these authors obtained viability rates of 90% and 84.1% under simulated gastric conditions and 71.7% and 77.8% under simulated intestinal conditions for lactobacilli and bifidobacteria, respectively. Yilmaz et al. (2020) demonstrated that sodium alginate can maintain the survival rate of

Lactobacillus paracasei at 70.8%, demonstrating its viability as a wall material for maintaining the survival of microorganisms of this genus.

Regarding starch, the two most used nanostructures are starch nanoparticles (SNPs) and nanocrystals (SNCs). SNPs are amorphous structures generated from congealed starch, while SNCs are the crystalline portion of the starch granules that remain after hydrolysis of the amorphous structure. However, SNPs are not suitable for probiotics encapsulation, since the controlled release and thermal protection are not efficient, leading to cell death. In this sense, combining SNPs with other encapsulating materials improves their application in the encapsulation of probiotics (Razavi et al., 2021). On the other hand, the association of SNCs with sodium alginate was used for the encapsulation of *Lactobacillus brevis* ST-69 and showed a survival rate of 94.97% after 5 hours under gastrointestinal conditions, which was higher than the alginate survival rate, of 87.75%. Despite similar, the SNCs showed an enhancement of the protective function of alginate under the simulated gastrointestinal conditions (Thangrongthong et al., 2020).

Another common polysaccharide used for micro and nanoencapsulation is chitosan, a polysaccharide that has a rigid chemical structure, which is an important factor that makes it suitable for the formation of films, gels, and microcapsules. It has biocompatibility, biodegradability, and safety, which makes it a good option for encapsulating probiotics. This substance also has interesting biological activities, such as antimicrobial and antioxidant (Younes and Rinaudo, 2015). Chitosan is sensitive to pH variations, which allows for a controlled release of probiotics at specific sites, such as the gastrointestinal tract (Raza et al., 2020). This happens due to the amino group that becomes protonated at low pH, carrying a positive charge and deprotonates at neutral and basic pH, becoming neutral. In addition, chitosan structures have been applied as a vehicle due to their mucoadhesive properties, which allow prolonged residence time and enhanced absorption capacity by opening the tight junctions of the intestinal cells (Xiong et al., 2020).

Studies show that the microencapsulation of *L. plantarum* in chitosan capsules, chitosan associated with other materials, or as a coating material, increases cell viability during storage and has a protective effect on cells in simulated gastric conditions (Nualkaekul et al., 2012; Mahmoud et al., 2020). Peñalva et al. (2023) used sodium caseinate and chitosan by complex coacervation for the microencapsulation of *L. plantarum.* The microcapsules were cross-linked with substances such as vanillin, TPP (tripolyphosphate) e calcium salts. A significant increase in cell viability was observed during storage, especially in microcapsules cross-linked with vanillin. Greater protection was also observed in simulated gastric and intestinal fluids. The authors carried out biodistribution studies in rats and it was shown that microcapsules cross-linked with vanillin were able to reach distal areas of the small intestine and colon, the site where probiotics must be released and implanted to generate beneficial effects.

Shajahan et al. (2015) produced chitosan nanoparticles with average particle size ranging from 7 – 30 nm by ionic gelation and stability for 18 months at 4°C. In addition, the authors evaluated the adsorption of dyes and concluded that the nanoparticles can be used as adsorbents to treat commercial dye effluents. Considering these characteristics, these chitosan nanoparticles could be tested for other uses, such as a delivery system. Chitosan is among the most natural polymers used for the development of electrospun nanofibers, an efficient and promising nanomaterial due to the large surface area-to-volume ratios, flexibility, functionality, and superior mechanical properties for the building of nanomembranes (Panthi et al., 2015). Mojaveri, Hosseini and Garsallaoui (2020) nanoencapsulated *Bifidobacterium animalis* Bb 12 in nanofibers using chitosan associated with polyvinyl alcohol, inulin (as a prebiotic), and skimmed milk. The size distribution of nanofibers showed diameters between 117.51 ± 70.65 nm and 217.56 ± 62.74 nm. The initial count of *B. animalis* Bb 12 was 9.47 log CFU/mL and the loss after the electrospinning was minimal, of 1 log reduction, due to the rapid evaporation of the solvent and the osmotic change. The nanoencapsulated *B. animalis* viability was measured after the sequential incubation at 37°C in simulated gastric and intestinal fluids for 120 and 180 minutes, respectively. The exposure caused substantial damage to the free cells, which lost 4.5 log CFU/mL after the simulated gastric conditions and 1.0 log CFU/mL after simulated intestinal conditions, totalizing a loss of 5.5 log CFU/mL. The encapsulated cells instead showed satisfactory results: the final viability count ranged from 7.25 to 7.31 log CFU/mL. In this study, the chitosan nanofibers exhibited higher protection of encapsulated cells than the polyvinyl alcohol regardless of the use of inulin as a prebiotic. According to Hosseini et al. (2019), this might be due to the higher compacted chemical microstructure of the chitosan nanofibers compared to the pure polyvinyl alcohol nanofibers, which reduces the secretion of the core material.

Milk and milk proteins are also used as wall materials for encapsulation, such as skim milk, whey protein, caseins. Milk proteins can be used as carriers of ions and hydrophobic molecules and play an important role in the stabilization of emulsions containing hydrophobic bioactives. They can also trap different substances through the formation of hydrogels and emulsions

(Tavares et al., 2014). Mahmoud et al. (2020) performed microencapsulation by extrusion using alginate and skimmed milk, alginate and denatured whey protein and observed an increase in viability in frozen storage and survival of cells in gastrointestinal conditions. Ma et al. (2020) used skim milk to microencapsulate *L. plantarum* by emulsion and the cells showed greater storage stability and greater survival in harsh environments.

According to Dangi et al. (2023), other materials used to produce nanoparticles for the encapsulation of probiotics are cellulose, phthalyl pullulan, eudragit S100, magnesium oxide, silver, and titanium oxide. The field of nanotechnology for application in food technology is still underexplored.

Conclusion, Opportunities and Future Challenges

Encapsulation techniques have been shown to be effective for application in probiotic microorganisms. Macroencapsulation techniques are rarely reported for *L. plantarum*. However, more studies should be developed to improve these techniques, and possible adaptations to verify their viability or forms of application and consumption.

Microencapsulation of *L. plantarum* is a promising technique to increase survival during storage, exposure to adverse conditions such as high and low temperatures, and maintaining the stability of these microorganisms during passage through the gastrointestinal tract. The use of adequate encapsulating materials and the optimization of encapsulation conditions are crucial factors to obtain high-quality and effective microcapsules. Furthermore, microencapsulation of *L. plantarum* may be a viable alternative for delivering these probiotics in functional foods and nutritional supplements, contributing to health promotion and disease prevention. However, further research is still needed to study the biological activity of *L. plantarum* under different conditions, to develop techniques on an industrial scale, and to assess the feasibility of application in food and its acceptability. Constant research is also needed on wall materials that can be used to increase the effectiveness of the techniques.

Regarding the nanoencapsulation of *L. plantarum*, more studies on the characterization and application of nanomaterials to produce nanocapsules for the entrapment of probiotics and their bioactive compounds are needed. Given the superior characteristics of nanomaterials as delivery systems to bioactive compounds through the human gastrointestinal tract, further studies combining *in vitro* and *in vivo* experiments must be done to reveal the effects of the human gastrointestinal tract components on the stability and controlled release capacity of the nanoparticles. Moreover, studies about thermal stability and storage viability are also required, since the survival of *L. plantarum* under food processing conditions, such as temperature and storage time, is still a significant concern. Thus, the incorporation and commercialization of nanoparticles as vehicles for *L. plantarum* in the food industry would be achieved.

References

Abdelhamid, S. M., Edris, A. E., and Sadek, Z (2023). Novel approach for the inhibition of *Helicobacter pylori* contamination in yogurt using selected probiotics combined with eugenol and cinnamaldehyde nanoemulsions. *Food Chemistry*, 417, 135877, 1-8. http://doi.org/10.1016/j.foodchem.2023.135877.

Aldana, A. S., Sandoval, E. R., and Aponte, A. A. (2004). Encapsulación de Aditivos para la Industria de Alimentos. *Ingeniería y Competitividad*, v. 5, n. 2. http://doi.org/10.25100/iyc.v5i2.2298.

Ashaolu T. J., and Fernandez-Tomé, S. (2021). Gut mucosal and adipose tissues as health targets of the immunomodulatory mechanisms of probiotics. *Trends in Food Science & Technology*, 112, 764–779. https://doi.org/10.1016/j.tifs.2021.04.040.

Assadpour, E., and Jafari, S. M. (2019). Advances in spray-drying encapsulation of food bioactive ingredients: from microcapsules to nanocapsules. *Annual Review of Food Science and Technology*, 10, 103–131. https://doi.org/10.1146/annurev-food-032818-121641.

Atraki, R., and Azizkhani, M. (2021). Survival of probiotic bacteria nanoencapsulated within biopolymers in a simulated gastrointestinal model. *Innovative Food Science and Emerging Technologies*, 72, 102750. https://doi.org/10.1016/j.ifset.2021.102750.

Bennacef, C., Desobry-Banon, S., Probst, L., and Desobry, S. (2021). Advances on alginate use for spherification to encapsulate biomolecules. *Food Hydrocolloids*, 118, 106782. https://doi.org/10.1016/j.foodhyd.2021.106782.

Burgain, J., Gaiani, C., Linder, M., and Scher, J. (2011). Encapsulation of probiotic living cells: From laboratory scale to industrial applications. *Journal of Food Engineering,* 104(4), 467–483. doi:10.1016/j.jfoodeng.2010.12.031.

Centurion, F., Basit, A. W., Liu, J., Gaisford, S., Rahim, M. A., and Kalantar-Zadeh, K. (2021). Nanoencapsulation for probiotic delivery. *ACS Nano*, 15(12), 18653–18660. https://doi.org/10.1021/acsnano.1c09951.

Ceylan, Z., Uslu, E., İspirli, H., Meral, R., Gavgalı, M., 'Yilmaz, M. T., and Dertli, E. (2019). A novel perspective for *Lactobacillus reuteri*: Nanoencapsulation to obtain functional fish fillets. *LWT - Food Science and Technology*, 115, 108427. https://doi.org/10.1016/j.lwt.2019.108427.

Chen, L., Yang, T., Song, Y., Shu, G., and Chen, H. (2017). Effect of xanthan-chitosan-xanthan double layer encapsulation on survival of *Bifidobacterium* BB01 in simulated gastrointestinal conditions, bile salt solution and yogurt. *LWT - Food Science and Technology*, 81, 274 – 280. https://doi.org/10.1016/j.lwt.2017.04.005.

Chopde, S., Datir, R., Deshmukh, G., Anant Dhotre, A., and Patil, M. (2020). Nanoparticle formation by nanospray drying & its application in nanoencapsulation of food bioactive ingredients. *Journal of Agriculture and Food Research*, 2, 100085. https://doi.org/10.1016/j.jafr.2020.100085.

Coghetto, C. C., Brinques, G. B., and Ayub, M. A. Z. (2016). Probiotics production and alternative encapsulation methodologies to improve their viabilities under adverse environmental conditions. *International Journal of Food Sciences and Nutrition*, 67(8), 929–943. doi:10.1080/09637486.2016.1211995.

Costa, N. A., Silveira, L. R., Amaral, E. P., Pereira, G. C., Paula, D. A., Vieira, E. N. R., Martins, E. M. F., Stringheta, P. C., Júnior, B. R. C. L., and Ramos, A. M. (2023). Use of maltodextrin, sweet potato flour, pectin and gelatin as wall material for microencapsulating *Lactiplantibacillus plantarum* by spray drying: Thermal resistance, in vitro release behavior, storage stability and physicochemical properties. *Food Research International*, 164. https://doi.org/10.1016/j.foodres.2022.112367.

Dangi, P., Chaudhary, N., Chaudhary, V., Virdi, A. S., Kajla, P., Khanna, P., Jha, S. K., Jha, N. K., Alkhanani, M. F., Singh, V., and Haque, S. (2023). Nanotechnology impacting probiotics and prebiotics: a paradigm shift in nutraceuticals technology. *International Journal of Food Microbiology*, 388, 110083. https://doi.org/10.1016/j.ijfoodmicro.2022.110083.

De Prisco, A., and Mauriello, G. (2016). Probiotication of foods: A focus on microencapsulation tool. *Trends in Food Science & Technology*, 48, 27–39. https://doi.org/10.1016/j.tifs.2015.11.009.

Dong, L. M., Luan, N. T., and Thuy, D. T. K. (2020). The viability of encapsulated *Lactobacillus plantarum* during cupcake baking process, storage, and simulated gastric digestion. *Journal of Microbiology, Biotechnology and Food Sciences*, 9 (6), p. 1157-1161. doi: 10.15414/jmbfs.2020.9.6.1157-1161.

Douglas, L. C., and Sanders, M. E. (2008). Probiotics and prebiotics in dietetics practice. *Journal of the American Dietetic Association*, 108, p. 510–521. https://doi.org/10.1016/j.jada.2007.12.009.

Eckert, C., Serpa, V. G., Santos, A. C. F., Costa, S. M., Dalpubel, V., Lehn, D. N., and Souza, C. F. V. (2017). Microencapsulation of *Lactobacillus plantarum* ATCC 8014 through spray drying and using dairy whey as wall materials. *LWT - Food Science and Technology*, 82, 176–183. https://doi.org/10.1016/j.lwt.2017.04.045.

Etchepare, M. A., Raddatz, G. C., Flores, E. M. M., Zepka, L. Q., Jacob-Lopes, E., Barin, J. S., Grosso, C. R. F., and Menezes, C. R. (2016). Effect of resistant starch and chitosan on survival of *Lactobacillus acidophilus* microencapsulated with sodium alginate. *LWT – Food Science and Technology*, 65, 511–517. https://doi.org/10.1016/j.lwt.2015.08.039.

Feng, K., Zhai, M.-Y., Zhang, Y., Linhardt, R. J., Zong, M.-H., Li, L., and Wu, H. (2018). Improved viability and thermal stability of the probiotics encapsulated in a novel electrospun fiber mat. *Journal of Agricultural and Food Chemistry*, 66, 10890−10897. https://doi.org/10.1021/acs.jafc.8b02644.

Food and Agriculture Organization of the United Nations/World Health Organization FAO/WHO (2002). *Guidelines for the evaluation of probiotics in food. Joint FAO/WHO working group on drafting guidelines for the evaluation of probiotics in food*; London, Ontario, Canada.

Gbassi, G. K., Vandamme, T., Yolou, F. S., and Marchioni, E. (2011). In vitro effects of pH, bile salts and enzymes on the release and viability of encapsulated *Lactobacillus plantarum* strains in a gastrointestinal tract model. *International Dairy Journal*, 21(2), 97–102. doi:10.1016/j.idairyj.2010.09.006.

Goh, C. H., Heng, P. W. S., and Chan, L. W. (2012). Alginates as a useful natural polymer for microencapsulation and therapeutic applications. *Carbohydrate Polymers*, 88, 1–12, 2012. https://doi.org/10.1016/j.carbpol.2011.11.012.

Guo, Q., Li, S., Tang, J., Chang, S., Qiang, L., Du, G., Yue, T., and Yuan, Y. (2022). Microencapsulation of *Lactobacillus plantarum* by spray drying: Protective effects during simulated food processing, gastrointestinal conditions, and in kefir. *International Journal of Biological Macromolecules*, 194, 539-545. https://doi.org/10.1016/j.ijbiomac.2021.11.096.

Haghshenas, B., Abdullah, N., Nami, Y., Radiah, D., Rosli, R., and Yari Khosroushahi, A. (2015). Microencapsulation of probiotic bacteria *Lactobacillus plantarum* 15HN using alginate-psyllium-fenugreek polymeric blends. *Journal of Applied Microbiology*, 118(4), 1048–1057. https://doi:10.1111/jam.12762.

Hassan, S. S., Fadzil, I. N. A., Yazid, H. N. M., Yusoff, A., and Khalil, K. A. (2020). Effects of double emulsification on *Lactobacillus plantarum* NBRC 3070 stability and physicochemical properties of soursop juice during storage. *Asia-Pacific Journal of Molecular Biology and Biotechnology*, 28 (4), 11-25. doi:10.35118/apjmbb.2020.028.4.02.

Hosseini, S. F., Nahvi, Z., and Zandi, M. (2019). Antioxidant peptide-loaded electrospun chitosan/poly (vinyl alcohol) nanofibrous mat intended for food biopackaging purposes. *Food Hydrocolloids*, 89, 637–648. https://doi.org/10.1016/j.foodhyd.2018.11.033.

How, Y., and Pui, L. (2021). Efect of prebiotics encapsulated with probiotics on encapsulation efficiency, microbead size, and survivability: a review. *Journal of Food Measurement and Characterization*, 4899–4916. https://doi.org/10.1007/s11694-021-01059-6.

Huang, S., Vignolles, M.-L., Chen, X. D., Le Loir, Y., Jan, G., Schuck, P., and Jeantet, R. (2017). Spray drying of probiotics and other food-grade bacteria: A review. *Trends in Food Science & Technology*, 63, 1–17. https://doi.org/10.1016/j.tifs.2017.02.007.

Kalita, D., Saikia, S., Gautam, G., Mukhopadhyay, R., and Mahanta, C. L. (2018). Characteristics of synbiotic spray dried powder of litchi juice with *Lactobacillus plantarum* and different carrier materials. *LWT - Food Science and Technology*, 87, 351-360. http://dx.doi.org/10.1016/j.lwt.2017.08.092.

Karimi, N., Jabbari, V., Nazemi, A., Ganbarov, K., Karimi, N., Tanomand, A., Karimi, S., Abbasi, A., Yousefi, B., Khodadadi, E., and Kafil, H. S. (2020). Thymol, cardamom and *Lactobacillus plantarum* nanoparticles as a functional candy with high protection against *Streptococcus mutans* and tooth decay. *Microbial Pathogenesis*, 148, 104481. https://doi.org/10.1016/j.micpath.2020.104481.

Krasaekoopt, W., Bhandari, B., and Deeth, H. (2003). Evaluation of encapsulation techniques of probiotics for yoghurt. *International Dairy Journal*, 13, 3–13. https://doi.org/10.1016/S0958-6946(02)00155-3.

Lee, K. Y., and Mooney, D. J. (2012). Alginate: Properties and biomedical applications. *Progress in Polymer Science*, 37(1), 106–126. https://doi.org/10.1016/j.progpolymsci.2011.06.003.

López-Rubio, A., and Lagaron, J. M. (2012). Whey protein capsules obtained through electrospraying for the encapsulation of bioactives. Innovative Food Science and Emerging Technologies, 13, 200–206. https://doi.org/10.1016/j.ifset.2011.10.012.

Ma, J., Xu, C., Yu, H., Feng, Z., Yu, W., Liya Gu, L., Liu, Z., Chen , L., Jiang, Z. and Hou, J. (2021). Electro-encapsulation of probiotics in gum Arabic-pullulan blend nanofibres using electrospinning technology. *Food Hydrocolloids*, 111, 106381. https://doi.org/10.1016/j.foodhyd.2020.106381.

Ma, L., Shang, Y., Zhu, Y., Zhang, X., E, J., Zhao, L., and Wang, J. (2020). Study on microencapsulation of *Lactobacillus plantarum* LIP -1 by emulsification method. *Journal of Food Process Engineering*, 43(8), e13437. https://doi.org/10.1111/jfpe.13437.

Marins, A. R., Campos, T. A. F., Batista, A. F. P., Correa, V. G., Peralta, R. M., Mikcha, J. M. G., Gomes, R. G., and Feihrmann, A. C. (2022). Effect of the addition of encapsulated *Lactiplantibacillus plantarum* Lp-115, *Bifidobacterium animalis* spp. *lactis* Bb-12, and *Lactobacillus acidophilus* La-5 to cooked burger. *LWT - Food Science and Technology*, 155. https://doi.org/10.1016/j.lwt.2021.112946.

Martín, M. J., Lara-Villoslada, F., Ruiz, M. A., and Morales, M.E. (2014). Microencapsulation of bacteria: A review of different technologies and their impact on the probiotic effects. *Innovative Food Science and Emerging Technologies*, 27, 15-25. https://doi.org/10.1016/j.ifset.2014.09.010.

McClements, D. J., Decker, E. A. and Weiss, J. (2007). Emulsion-Based Delivery Systems for Lipophilic Bioactive Components. *Journal of Food Science*, 72(8), R109-R124. https://doi.org/10.1111/j.1750-3841.2007.00507.x.

Mojaveri, S. J., Hosseini, S. F., and Gharsallaoui, A. (2020). Viability improvement of *Bifidobacterium animalis* Bb12 by encapsulation in chitosan/poly(vinyl alcohol) hybrid electrospun fiber mats. *Carbohydrate Polymers*, 241, 116278. https://doi.org/10.1016/j.carbpol.2020.116278.

Nedovic, V., Kalusevic, A., Monojlovic, V., Levic, S., and Bugarski, B. (2011). An overview of encapsulation technologies for food applications. *Procedia Food Science*, 1, 1806 – 1815. http://doi:10.1016/j.profoo.2011.09.266.

Ni, F., Luo, X., Zhao, Z., Yuan, J., Song, Y., Liu, C., Huang, M., Dong, L., Xie, H., Cai, L., Ren, G., and Gu, Q. (2023). Enhancing viability of *Lactobacillus plantarum* encapsulated by alginate-gelatin hydrogel beads during gastrointestinal digestion, storage and in the mimic beverage systems. *International Journal of Biological Macromolecules*, 224, 94-104. https://doi.org/10.1016/j.ijbiomac.2022.10.106.

Nualkaekul, S., Lenton, D., Cook, M. T., Khutoryanskiy, V. V., and Charalampopoulos, D. (2012). Chitosan coated alginate beads for the survival of microencapsulated

Lactobacillus plantarum in pomegranate juice. *Carbohydrate Polymers*, 90(3), 1281–1287. http://dx.doi.org/10.1016/j.carbpol.2012.06.073.

Panthi, G., Park, M., Kim, H.-Y. and Park, S.-J. (2015). Electrospun polymeric nanofibers encapsulated with nanostructured materials and their applications: A review. *Journal of Industrial and Engineering Chemistry*, 24, 1–13. http://dx.doi.org/10.1016/j.jiec.2014.09.011.

Parlindungan, E., Dekiwadia, C., May, B. K., and Jones, O. A. H. (2019). Nutrient stress as a means to enhance the storage stability of spray dried microencapsulated *Lactobacillus plantarum* B21. *LWT - Food Science and Technology*, 111, 204–210. https://doi.org/10.1016/j.lwt.2019.05.010.

Peñalva, R., Martínez-López, A. L., Gamazo, C., Gonzalez-Navarro, C. J., González-Ferrero, C., Virto-Resano, R., Brotons-Canto, A., Vitas, A. I., Collantes, M., Peñuelas, I., and Irache, J. M. (2023). Encapsulation of *Lactobacillus plantarum* in casein-chitosan microparticles facilitates the arrival to the colon and develops an immunomodulatory effect. *Food Hydrocolloids*, 136, 108213. https://doi.org/10.1016/j.foodhyd.2022.108213.

Pour, H. M., Marhamatizadeh, M. H., and Fattahi, H. (2022). Encapsulation of Different Types of Probiotic Bacteria within Conventional/Multilayer Emulsion and Its Effect on the Properties of Probiotic Yogurt. *Journal of Food Quality*, 2022, 7923899. https://doi.org/10.1155/2022/7923899.

Pupa, P., Apiwatsiri, P., Sirichokchatchawan, W., Pirarat, N., Muangsin, N., Shah, A. A., and Prapasarakul, N. (2021). The efficacy of three double-microencapsulation methods for preservation of probiotic bacteria. *Scientific Reports*, 11(1). doi:10.1038/s41598-021-93263-z.

Qin, X.-S., Gao, Q.-Y., and Luo, Z.-G. (2021). Enhancing the storage and gastrointestinal passage viability of probiotic powder (*Lactobacillus plantarum*) through encapsulation with pickering high internal phase emulsions stabilized with WPI-EGCG covalent conjugate nanoparticles. *Food Hydrocolloids*, 116, 106658. https://doi.org/10.1016/j.foodhyd.2021.106658.

Rajam, R., and Anandharamakrishnan, C. (2015). Microencapsulation of *Lactobacillus plantarum* (MTCC 5422) with fructooligosaccharide as wall material by spray drying. *LWT - Food Science and Technology*, 60, 773-780. https://dx.doi.org/10.1016/j.lwt.2014.09.062.

Rathore, S., Desai, P. M., Liew, C. V., Chan, L. W., and Heng, P. W. (2013). Microencapsulation of microbial cells. *Journal of Food Engineering*, 116, 369-381. https://doi.org/10.1016/j.jfoodeng.2012.12.022.

Raza, Z. A., Khalil, S., Ayub, A., and Banat, I. M. (2020). Recent developments in chitosan encapsulation of various active ingredients for multifunctional applications. *Carbohydrate Research*, 492, 108004. https://doi.org/10.1016/j.carres.2020.108004.

Razavi, S., Janfaza, S., Tasnim, N., Gibson, D. L., and Hoorfar, M. (2021). Nanomaterial-based encapsulation for controlled gastrointestinal delivery of viable probiotic bacteria. *Nanoscale Advances*, 3, 2699–2709. https://doi.org/10.1039/d0na00952k.

Reque, P. M., and Brandelli, A. (2021). Encapsulation of probiotics and nutraceuticals: Applications in functional food industry. *Trends in Food Science & Technology*, 114, 1–10. https://doi.org/10.1016/j.tifs.2021.05.022.

Romano, N., Mobili, P., Zuñiga-Hansen, M. E., and Gómez-Zavaglia, A. (2018) Physico-chemical and structural properties of crystalline inulin explain the stability of *Lactobacillus plantarum* during spray-drying and storage. *Food Research International*, 113, 167–174. https://doi.org/10.1016/j.foodres.2018.07.007.

Shah, A., Gani, A., Ahmad, M., Ashwar, B. A., and Masoodi, F. A. (2016). β-Glucan as an encapsulating agent: Effect on probiotic survival in simulated gastrointestinal tract. *International Journal of Biological Macromolecules*, 82, 217–222. doi:10.1016/j.ijbiomac.2015.11.017.

Shajahan, A., Shankar, S., Sathiyaseelan, A., Narayan, K. S., Narayanan, V., Kaviyarasan, V. and Ignacimuthu, S. (2017). Comparative studies of chitosan and its nanoparticles for the adsorption efficiency of various dyes. *International Journal of Biological Macromolecules*, 104, 1449–1458. http://dx.doi.org/10.1016/j.ijbiomac.2017.05.128.

Sharma, H., Sharma, S., Bajwa, J., Chugh, R., and Kumar, D. (2023). Polymeric carriers in probiotic delivery system. *Carbohydrate Polymer Technologies and Applications*, 5, 100301. https://doi.org/10.1016/j.carpta.2023.100301.

Škrlec, K., Zupančič, Š., Mihevc, S. P., Kocbek, P., Kristl, J., and Berlec, A. (2019). Development of electrospun nanofibers that enable high loading and long-term viability of probiotics. *European Journal of Pharmaceutics and Biopharmaceutics*, 136, 108–119. https://doi.org/10.1016/j.ejpb.2019.01.013.

Tavares, G. M., Croguennec, T., Carvalho, A. F., and Bouhallab, S. (2014). Milk proteins as encapsulation devices and delivery vehicles: Applications and trends. *Trends in Food Science & Technology*, 37(1), 5–20. https://doi.org/10.1016/j.tifs.2014.02.008.

Thangrongthong, S., Narathip Puttarat, N., Ladda, B., Itthisoponkul, T., Pinket, W., Kasemwong, K., and Taweechotipatr, M. (2020). Microencapsulation of probiotic *Lactobacillus brevis* ST-69 producing GABA using alginate supplemented with nanocrystalline starch. *Food Science and Biotechnology*, 29(11), 1475–1482. https://doi.org/10.1007/s10068-020-00812-9.

Todorov, S. D., and Franco, B. D. G. M. (2010). *Lactobacillus plantarum*: Characterization of the Species and Application in Food Production. *Food Reviews International*, 26, 205-229. https://doi.org/10.1080/87559129.2010.484113.

Trevisan, A. B., dos Santos, M. C., Leite, J. S. F., Barreto, B. G., Passos, R. S. F. T., Franke, C. R., da Silva, M. C. A., and Cavalheiro, C. P. (2022). Encapsulation of probiotics and their application in beef patties. *Acta Scientarum Polonorum Technologia Alimentaria*, 21(3), 281-291. http://dx.doi.org/10.17306/J.AFS.2022.1038.

Weisany, W., Yousefi, S., Tahir, N.A., Golestanehzadeh, N., McClements, D.J., Adhikari, B., and Ghasemlou, M. (2022). Targeted delivery and controlled released of essential oils using nanoencapsulation: A review. *Advances in Colloid and Interface Science*, 303, 10265. https://doi.org/10.1016/j.cis.2022.102655.

Xiong, K., Zhou, L., Wang, J., Ma, A., Fang, D., Xiong, L., and Suna, Q. (2020). Construction of food-grade pH-sensitive nanoparticles for delivering functional food ingredients. *Trends in Food Science & Technology*, 96, 102–113. https://doi.org/10.1016/j.tifs.2019.12.019.

Xu, C., Ban, Q., Wang, W., Jou, J., and Jiang, Z. (2022). Novel nano-encapsulated probiotic agents: Encapsulate materials, delivery, and encapsulation systems. *Journal of Controlled Release*, 349, 184–205. https://doi.org/10.1016/j.jconrel.2022.06.061.

Yilmaz, M. T., Taylan, O., Karakas, C. Y., and Dertli, E. (2020). An alternative way to encapsulate probiotics within electrospun alginate nanofibers as monitored under simulated gastrointestinal conditions and in kefir. *Carbohydrate Polymers*, 244, 116447. https://doi.org/10.1016/j.carbpol.2020.116447.

Younes, I., and Rinaudo, M. (2015). Chitin and Chitosan Preparation from Marine Sources. Structure, Properties and Applications. *Marine Drugs*, 13(3), 1133–1174. https://doi.org/10.3390/md13031133.

Zaeim, D., Sarabi-Jamab, M., Ghorani, B. and Kadkhodaee, R. (2019). Double layer coencapsulation of probiotics and prebiotics by electro-hydrodynamic atomization, *LWT - Food Science and Technology*, 110, 102–109. https://doi.org/10.1016/j.lwt.2019.04.040.

Chapter 4

Lactobacillus plantarum: Food Supplements and Pharmaceutical Uses

Călina Ciont[1,2]
Ramona Suharoschi[1,2]
Andreea Diana Kerezsi[1,3]
Dan Cristian Vodnar[1]
and Oana Lelia Pop[1,2,*]
[1]Department of Food Science, University of Agricultural Sciences and Veterinary Medicine, Cluj-Napoca, Romania
[2]Molecular Nutrition and Proteomics Laboratory, Institute of Life Sciences, University of Agricultural Sciences and Veterinary Medicine, Cluj-Napoca, Romania
[3]Department of Food Science and Formulation, Gembloux Agro-Bio Tech, University of Liège, Gembloux, Belgium

Abstract

Due to their probiotic properties, which enhance the quality and functionality of both food and health-related products, *Lactobacillus plantarum* strains have found extensive applications in the fields of food processing and pharmaceuticals. However, for these probiotic bacteria to confer health benefits, they must endure the harsh conditions of the gastrointestinal tract and reach the colon in sufficient quantities. Additionally, they are susceptible to a rapid loss of vitality during various stages, such as preparation and storage, where they may be exposed to factors like heat or oxidative stress.

* Corresponding Author's Email: oana.pop@usamvcluj.ro.

In: Lactobacillus plantarum and Its Role in Human Health
Editors: Maria Simona Chiș, Adriana Paucean
ISBN: 979-8-89113-696-0

To address these challenges, encapsulation techniques have been proposed as a means to safeguard the viability of probiotic bacteria when subjected to digestive conditions. Current encapsulation technologies encompass a range of methods, including spray drying, freeze-drying, extrusion processes, emulsification, nanoencapsulation, and coacervation.
With a focus on incorporating probiotics, particularly *L. plantarum*, into food supplements and pharmaceuticals, numerous endeavors have been undertaken to employ encapsulation techniques that can maintain the viability of these beneficial microorganisms throughout the production process and up to the point of consumption.
This chapter aims to provide a comprehensive overview of the various encapsulation methods currently specifically in the context of *L. plantarum's* application in food supplements and pharmaceuticals.

Keywords: *L. plantarum* food supplements, pharmaceuticals, nutraceuticals, regulation, gut microbiota, therapy, encapsulation

1. Introduction

L. plantarum, a widely studied probiotic strain, has shown promising potential for various applications in functional foods, supplements, and pharmaceuticals [1, 2]. One of the critical challenges in using *L. plantarum* is maintaining its viability and stability during storage and distribution since temperature changes, moisture content, and oxygen exposure may all substantially influence the bacteria's survival and efficacy over time. Proper formulation, packaging, and preservation factors are crucial to sustaining the viability of bacteria in probiotics, functional foods, and other uses, ensuring that customers get the intended health benefits. To address this, encapsulation techniques have emerged as effective strategies for protecting and delivering *L. plantarum* in different products [3]. Microencapsulation involves enclosing *L. plantarum* within a protective matrix, enhancing resistance to environmental factors such as temperature, moisture, and pH. This approach enables the incorporation of *L. plantarum* in various functional foods, supplements, and pharmaceuticals while maintaining its viability and functionality [4]. Nanoencapsulation techniques have recently gained attention for their ability to enhance the stability and bioavailability of *L. plantarum*. Nano-sized carriers offer improved protection against harsh conditions and controlled release of *L. plantarum*, ensuring its viability and targeted delivery [5-7]. The therapeutic potential of *L. plantarum* extends beyond its role as a probiotic. Studies have demonstrated its antimicrobial and antifungal properties, making it a promising candidate for combating various pathogens. In addition, *L. plantarum* generates postbiotic metabolites that support its protective actions in the host, including organic acids, antimicrobial peptides, and bacteriocins [8-11]. Combining *L. plantarum* with prebiotics, such as fructooligosaccharides or inulin, can enhance its viability and promote its growth in the gastrointestinal tract. This symbiotic approach offers potential synergistic effects and improved health benefits for individuals consuming *L. plantarum*-based food supplements [12]. In symbiotic formulations, *L. plantarum* is combined with other probiotic strains, such as *Bifidobacterium* or different *Lactobacillus* strains, to create a synergistic effect. This approach aims to optimize the gut microbiota composition, supporting overall gut health and immune function [13, 14]. The nature and activity of the gut microbiota have been reported to be favorably impacted by *L. plantarum*-based dietary supplements. They have the potential to augment advantageous microbial populations, enhance the functionality of the gut barrier, regulate immunological responses, and promote overall gastrointestinal well-being. Using *L. plantarum* in pharmaceutical products requires adherence to stringent regulatory guidelines to ensure safety and efficacy [15]. Regulatory bodies establish criteria for quality control, safety assessment, and manufacturing practices to maintain the integrity and reliability of *L. plantarum*-based pharmaceuticals [16]. While *L. plantarum* is generally considered safe, assessing possible adverse effects is necessary, especially in vulnerable populations. Understanding the safety profile of *L. plantarum*-based pharmaceuticals is crucial for their responsible use in healthcare settings. Clinical studies investigating the benefits of *L. plantarum*-based pharmaceuticals have shown promising results in various therapeutic areas [17, 18]. However, limitations, such as study design, sample size, and heterogeneity, must be addressed to establish robust evidence and optimize the clinical application of *L. plantarum*.

This chapter explores the encapsulation methods for incorporating *L. plantarum* into food supplements and pharmaceuticals. The research includes the therapeutic properties of *L. plantarum*, its function in food supplements, and its possible applications in the pharmaceutical sector. Additionally, the investigation covers safety regulations, negative outcomes, methods for efficient administration, and the present state of clinical research involving *L. plantarum*. By examining these aspects, it was intended that a deeper understanding of *L. plantarum's* potential in dietary supplements and medications might be presented.

1.1. Encapsulation of *L. Plantarum* for Incorporation as a Food Supplement and in Pharmaceutical Items

L. plantarum is a strain of probiotic bacteria often used in various food and supplement items to enhance gastrointestinal health. Incorporating *L. plantarum* has gained significant attention as a food supplement and in pharmaceutical items. *L. plantarum*, a microorganism renowned for its resilience and advantageous characteristics, received acknowledgment for its prospective health advantages and medicinal properties [15].

As a food supplement, *L. plantarum* is often added to various products to enhance nutritional value and promote overall well-being. Among foods that contain *L. plantarum* are dairy products [19], vegetables [20, 21], cereals [22], wine, traditional fermented foods, or fodder [23]. *L. plantarum*'s presence in these food products aims to support digestive health, boost the immune system, and improve gut microbiota balance. It is also found throughout the gastrointestinal, vaginal, and urogenital systems [6].

In addition to its use as a food supplement, *L. plantarum* has also found relevance in pharmaceutical production. The organism's capacity to endure the challenging environment of the gastrointestinal system and its capability to attach to intestinal epithelial cells renders it a favorable contender for the advancement of probiotic treatments. Ongoing research is exploring the potential therapeutic uses of pharmaceuticals derived from *L. plantarum* in addressing gastrointestinal disorders such as inflammatory bowel disease, irritable bowel syndrome, and specific infections [2, 11, 24, 25].

Furthermore, *L. plantarum* exhibits genomic plasticity, allowing it to adapt and respond to various environmental conditions [15]. This characteristic makes it a versatile and adaptable probiotic strain, capable of exerting beneficial effects in different settings.

Incorporating *L. plantarum* as a food supplement and in pharmaceutical items showcases its versatility and potential to improve human health. Ongoing research and development efforts continue to explore its applications and unlock its full therapeutic potential.

It can be encapsulated in either micro or nano-sized particles for several reasons, including:

- Protection: Encapsulation can protect *L. plantarum* from harsh environmental conditions such as heat, moisture, and acidity. This helps maintain the bacteria's viability and activity during processing, storage, and digestion [19, 26].

- Controlled release: Encapsulation can provide an accurate dose of *L. plantarum* in the gastrointestinal tract, improving its effectiveness. The release rate can be adjusted by changing the size and composition of the encapsulation material [2, 3, 27, 28].
- Improved stability: Encapsulation can enhance the stability of *L. plantarum* during storage by preventing moisture and oxygen from reaching the bacteria. This can prolong the product's shelf life containing the bacteria [29, 30].
- Enhanced bioavailability: Nano-sized encapsulation can improve the bioavailability of *L. plantarum* by increasing its surface area and facilitating its absorption in the gut [31, 32].
- Improved sensory properties: Micro-encapsulation can improve the sensory properties of food products containing *L. plantarum* by masking the taste and odor of the bacteria [7, 33, 34].

Studies supporting *L. plantarum's* probiotic health benefits are multiplying. *L. plantarum* may be found in various ecological settings, drawing attention to its unique capacity for adaptation and its genome ability to undergo changes and modifications [1, 10, 35). The production of potent and varied bacteriocins by *L. plantarum* is another critical role. These peptide antibiotics have potential uses in both food preservation and as antibiotic supplements [11, 20, 36, 37]. These features establish *L. plantarum* as a reliable research model and a valuable bioactive agent with potential in dietary supplements and medicinal items innovation. *L. plantarum* formulations have advanced with microencapsulation and nanoencapsulation technologies, revolutionizing their applications in the food and pharmaceutical industries [38, 39]. Encapsulating *L. plantarum* at the micro or nanoscale can significantly enhance its viability and stability, ensuring the delivery of live probiotic cells to the desired target. In the food sector, microencapsulated or nano-encapsulated *L. plantarum* can be incorporated into various products, including functional foods, beverages, and supplements, offering improved shelf-life and controlled release [1, 38, 40]. In the pharmaceutical field, these advanced formulations showed promise for the targeted delivery of *L. plantarum* in treating gastrointestinal disorders and other therapeutic applications [8, 12, 41, 42].

1.2. Microencapsulation-for Enhanced Activity and Viability of *L. Plantarum*

Different materials and methods are being explored and researched for the encapsulation of *L. plantarum*. The carrier materials utilized for probiotics should fulfill two primary requirements: providing protection for the probiotics and ensuring safety for consumption, meeting the *Generally Recognized As Safe* (GRAS) standards. Moreover, considering cost-effectiveness is of critical significance, substantial cost would directly influence the overall value of the product. Economical carrier materials include starches, inulin, pectin, and other carbohydrates. Food-grade polymers such as alginate, chitosan, pectin, carrageenan, whey, gelatin, and lipids have undergone extensive testing to immobilize bacteria effectively [43]. Calcium alginate beads, produced using methods like extrusion and emulsion, generate a strong molecular network to capture cells efficiently. Although alginate hydrogel beads have shown promising results in protecting probiotics in gastrointestinal circumstances and during storage, it is essential to include other polymers to improve the stability of alginate microcapsules. The mechanical stability of alginate beads alone is limited, and probiotic retention remains uncertain in the presence of chelating agents [4, 44].

Newly introduced are functional beverages that offer enhanced bioactive compounds, providing ready-to-drink options [45]. These beverages benefit from incorporating bioactive elements, with lactic acid bacteria (LAB) being the food industry's most widely recognized and well-utilized probiotic cells [46, 47]. Probiotics are often included in various food and beverage products, such as fermented dairy products like sour milk and yogurt, fruit juices, fermented vegetables, and cereal [40, 45, 48].

Saniani et al. (2023) [39] gave an example, who obtained functional whey beverages containing encapsulated *L. plantarum* as a food supplement. A whey solution comprising 80% protein and 11% w/v milk powder was combined with 10.3% w/w sugar and homogenized at 10,000 rpm for 10 minutes. In the present study, the authors pasteurized the solution for 30 minutes at 75°C before being cooled to 40°C. The authors combined the pasteurized whey solution with 20 g/L of encapsulated *L. plantarum* (in alginate, inulin, and dextran) and free *L. plantarum* (10^8 CFU/mL), 0.3% v/v of fermentation starting culture including *L. acidophilus* and *Streptococcus thermophilus*. Overall, encapsulation improved *L. plantarum* survival during simulated gastric and biliary conditions and the sensory analysis attributes (taste, color, odor, concentration, and total acceptability). In another study, spray drying was used to co-encapsulate *L. plantarum and Bifidobacterium infantis.* Maltodextrin, chia, flax seed mucilage, and soluble protein were carriers for the probiotic bacteria with a significant survival (98%) rate. After 45 days of refrigeration, the encapsulated formula created the instant juice powder, proving> 9 log CFU/g [13]. These combinations of three ingredients provided protection to the probiotics and enhanced their ability to withstand bile and gastric simulated environment.

It is important to consider many aspects to achieve optimal encapsulation of a bioactive molecule. The factors included in this study are the selection of encapsulating material, encapsulation methodology, release mechanism, and processing parameters. This complexity may be addressed using various methods, including response surface analysis, genetic algorithms, and sequential quadratic programming (Table 1). The optimization process involves several key stages. Initially, diagnostic experiments are conducted to identify potentially promising factors for the enclosed material. Based on these findings, the encapsulation is designed according to an experimental plan. Response surface models are then constructed to analyze the data and identify optimal conditions. The optimization model is created and improved, followed by a validation of the optimal conditions. Research in this area should investigate encapsulation materials' physical and chemical properties. Additionally, conducting *in vivo* experiments to comprehensively understand the processes involved in the release process is essential. It is necessary to investigate the encapsulation of inexpensive materials with probiotic and prebiotic functions [4, 38, 43, 44].

Furthermore, ensuring stability, viability, and appropriate cellular concentration during storage is crucial to maintaining the efficiency of the encapsulated product for applications in the food industry. The optimization process can enhance bioactive molecule encapsulation's effectiveness and reliability by addressing these aspects [3, 6, 49].

Table 1. Diverse encapsulation approaches for *Lactobacillus plantarum*

Encapsulation material	Encapsulation technique	Effect of encapsulation	Final destination/ulilisation	Ref.
Sodium alginate inulin Dextran (0.5, 1, and 1.5 mg/l)	Cross-linking Gelation	• 93.55% ee for 0.5% of inulin and 0.5 mg/l of dextran • pH stabilization during storage • ↑ Survival during gastric and biliary conditions	Probiotic whey beverage	[39]
Maltodextrin MD:FM:FSP - 7.5:0.2:7.5%, w/w/w	Spray drying	• 9 x log CFU/g after 45 days storage at 4̊c • ↑ Survival during gastric and biliary conditions	Instant juice powder	[50]
Okara oil-caseinate1:2; 1:3 and 1:4 O/W ratios	Encapsulated by emulsion followed by freeze drying or spray drying	• ↓ Bacterial culturability is associated with ↑ oil content in emulsions • Spray drying showed ↑ viability (13.5 log CFU/g vs. 12.5 log CFU/g)	Freeze-dried or spray-dried capsules	[51]
Alginate/pectin, chitosan, bovine gelatin, or glucomannan coating	Cross-linking gelation Layer-by-layer coating	• 10^7 CFU/ml after 6 weeks of storage at 4̊c in the juice for the encapsulated form • Coating application improved survival in juice by at least 101 CFU/ml after 6 weeks of storage at 4̊c in the juice • ↑ Size of the single and double chitosan-coated alginate beads during storage in pomegranate juice • size unchanged of the single and double chitosan-coated alginate beads during storage in cranberry juice	Enriched pomegranate and cranberry juice	[38]
Native maize starch or partially hydrolyzed maize starches	Adhering -stirring and supernatant collection	• The modified starches, the initial cell numbers were approximately 9 log CFU/g, whereas the initial cell number for the native starch was 7.77 log CFU/g. • ↑ Acid resistance, with a significant reduction of viability • Significantly ↑ viable cell counts of the modified starches compared to unmodified maize starch after incubation at 60°C for 15 minutes.	Freeze-dried capsules	[52]

EE- encapsulation efficiency; ↑ - increased; ↓ - decreased; CFU- colony forming units.

1.3. Nanoencapsulation-Functional Foods, Supplements, and Pharmaceuticals Containing *L. plantarum*

Probiotics nanoencapsulation is an emerging field in probiotic research and technology. It involves encapsulating probiotic microorganisms within nanoscale (1 to 100 nms) structures, allowing for enhanced stability, targeted delivery, and improved viability of these beneficial bacteria [6, 7, 53]. The main objective of probiotic nanoencapsulation is to protect probiotic strains from several environmental variables, including moisture, heat, and acidity, which may reduce their viability and performance [26]. The enhancement of probiotic survival across several stages, including preparation, storage, and transit through the gastrointestinal tract, may be achieved by encapsulating them inside nano-scale carriers, such as liposomes, nanoparticles, or microcapsules [53, 54].

Nanoencapsulation techniques offer several advantages for probiotics. The small size of the carriers allows for better protection and controlled release of the probiotic strains at specific locations within the body, such as the intestines. This targeted delivery ensures a higher concentration of viable probiotics reaching the desired site, enhancing their efficacy [7, 26, 53, 54].

Furthermore, nanoencapsulation provides a means to enhance the stability of probiotics in various food products and dietary supplements. Encapsulated probiotics exhibit improved resistance to adverse conditions, prolonging their shelf life and maintaining their viability during storage.

Research in probiotics nanoencapsulation is focused on optimizing the encapsulation process, exploring different materials and techniques, and evaluating the impact of encapsulation on the survival and functionality of probiotic strains. Additionally, studies are being conducted to assess the potential health benefits of nanoencapsulated probiotics, such as improved immune function, gastrointestinal health, and prevention of certain diseases [55].

Although still early, probiotics nanoencapsulation holds significant promise for advancing probiotic research and commercial applications. It can potentially revolutionize how probiotics are formulated, delivered, and integrated into various products, ultimately enhancing their efficacy and improving consumer health outcomes.

An interesting study showed that nano encapsulated fish oil incorporated into yogurt containing *L. plantarum* helped maintain viability at 8.41 log CFU/mL during yougurt shelf life [56].

Another study incorporated nanoencapsulated *L. plantarum* in candy containing thymol and cardamom, which have been discovered to offer an excellent defense against tooth decay, especially *Streptococcus mutans* [5]. The electrostatic interaction between the cationic charge of nanoparticles and the anionic charge on the bacterium's membrane results to the disruption of the lipid bilayers in the membrane and subsequently enhances cellular permeability. This effect forms the fundamental mechanism behind the antibacterial efficacy of nanoemulsions [5, 25, 57].

Nanoencapsulation is a technique used to encapsulate probiotic bacteria into nanoparticles, which are smaller than microcapsules. This technique offers several advantages, including better protection against environmental stressors, improved bioavailability, higher stability, and solubility [26]. These advantages make nanoencapsulation of *L. plantarum* a better option for specific applications than microencapsulation.

1.4. *L. plantarum* Therapy

Dietary supplements regularly contain biological constituents, including probiotics, prebiotics, and other compounds with antioxidant properties and other beneficial impacts on consumers' well-being. Different scientists design novel nutraceutical formulations aiming to unlock the potential of probiotics in combination with these biological compounds. For example, *L. plantarum* and *L. paracasei* can generate a biosurfactant with proven antimicrobial and antiadhesive properties against different pathogens [42]. *L. plantarum* could be considered a natural antimicrobial agent, producing acetic and lactic acids, antimicrobial peptides, and hydrogen peroxide [25]. Besides *L. salivarius* and *L. rhamnosus*, *L. plantarum,* and *L. paracasei* exhibit the highest bioactivity among *Lactobacillus* species [58].

Using probiotics demonstrated clinical efficacy compared to a placebo for managing chronic diarrhea. For instance, *L. plantarum* CCFM1143 showed significant benefits by reducing bowel frequency and improving the Bristol stool score. It also played a role in inhibiting the rise of interleukin-6 and the decrease of motilin while positively influencing the gut microbiota by decreasing harmful bacteria and increasing the good ones. These findings offer valuable insights that can contribute to developing functional probiotic products for people with chronic diarrhea problems [59]. The same strain, *L. plantarum* CCFM1143 was used, but this time its efficiency was tested against *Escherichia coli.* The findings indicated that *L. plantarum* CCFM1143 exhibited the most pronounced protective impact against *Escherichia coli* - induced diarrhea [60].

Another similar study was conducted to check the ability of *L. plantarum* 299v on one of the most digestive problems encountered, irritable bowel syndrome (IBS). The test was done on two hundred and fourteen patients, and after 4 weeks of treatment with *L. plantarum* 299v, the bloating and abdominal pain were decreased [28].

Interestingly, the results on *L. plantarum* BPL207, *L. rhamnosus* PBL205 and *L. crispatus* BPL209 revealed that these strains help restore the vaginal environment for unhealthy women, positively impacting fertility and creating a favorable environment. Additionally, there is an observed improvement in inflammatory conditions for patients who encountered chronic endometritis [61]. Moreover, regarding food that impacts human health, a group of researchers has developed a gummy– supplement, which includes *L. plantarum* LUHS135, *L. paracasei* LUHS244 (probiotics), psyllium husk (prebiotics), and apple pomace as a pectin source. The researchers investigated the antibacterial activity of the LAB strains, the total phenolic compound content, texture, and color of the supplement. Related to the antimicrobial activity against *Escherichia coli*, *Enterococcus faecalis*, *Pseudomonas aeruginosa*, *Proteus mirabilis*, *Salmonella enterica*, *Staphylococcus aureus*, and *Streptococcus mutans*, these were all inhibited by *L. paracasei*. Additionally, pure strain *L. plantarum* inhibited 4 microorganisms out of 7. More interestingly, the mix of probiotics (*L. plantarum* and *L. paracasei*) inhibited all the pathogenic strains [62].

In addition, *L. plantarum* presents an antifungal capacity due to the active metabolites included, such as organic acids (lactic acid and its derivatives, fatty acids), proteinaceous substances (linear and cyclic peptide), and volatile organic compounds. The molecules mentioned are responsible for fungal inhibition and mycotoxin removal [31, 63, 64].

The presence of fungal contamination in food causes detrimental effects on both the quality of the food and human well-being. Moreover, compared with 2011, the number of publications about the antifungal and anti-mycotoxin of *L. plantarum* is increasing. *L. plantarum,* an antifungal agent, will replace conventional and chemical treatments [11].

Researchers have conducted various investigations to show the significance of the antimycoic effect of *L. plantarum*. The use of *L. plantarum* S61 and its cell-free supernatant has a beneficial impact on the prevention of *P. digitatum* rotting in apple and orange fruits. Moreover, the cell-free supernatant reduced *Salmonella enterica* (ATCC 14,028) in apple juice [8].

For example, *L. plantarum* MiLAB14 synthesizes two cyclic peptides (cyclo(L-Phe-trans-4-OH-L-Pro) and cyclo(L-Phe-L-Pro)) and one protein, all of which exhibit antifungal activity at a concentration in the milligram per milliliter. Other essential compounds, phenyllactic acid (PLA) and 4-hydroxyphenyllactic acid (OH-PLA), produced by the same strain inhibited *Penicillium* spp., *Aspergillus* niger, and *Fusarium* spp. [2].

Furthermore, it is also important to consider the postbiotic metabolites, which are less studied, and the mechanisms are not entirely known. These compounds are secreted by live bacteria or after lysis and can be considered by-products of the probiotic. They are known for their antimicrobial, antioxidant, anti-inflammatory, and anti-proliferative activity [17].

A study showed the effect of the postbiotic derived from *L. plantarum* M.2 and *L. curvatus* B.67 against *Listeria monocytogenes* in motility, biofilm state, and planktonic cells. They concluded that *L. plantarum* M.2 has a higher inhibition effect than the postbiotic isolated from *L. curvatus* B.67 (Hossain et al., 2021). Similarly, postbiotics isolated from *L. plantarum* (RG11, RG14, RI11, UL4, TL1, and RS5) in combination with inulin exhibited antimicrobial activity against different pathogens among *Listeria monocytogenes, E.coli, and S. enterica* [65].

Besides the antimicrobial and antioxidant effect, the postbiotic metabolites from *L. plantarum* can increase broiler chickens' body weight. More interestingly, a significant increase in daily egg production in hens was reported when the diet was supplemented with a postbiotic mix isolated from *L. plantarum* strains (RI11, RG14, and RG11). On the other hand, the postweaning piglets fed with postbiotics isolated from *L. plantarum* (TL1, RG14, and RS5) showed better protein digestibility and a decrease in diarrhea incidence [12, 65]. Additionally, future studies should be addressed to further understand the activity in vitro and in vivo to explore the potential of postbiotic metabolites [17].

Overall, *L. plantarum* exhibits remarkable antimicrobial, antifungal, and postbiotic activity. Its versatility makes it suitable for developing various nutraceuticals and beyond.

1.5. *L. plantarum* in Food Supplements

The world is becoming more aware of the association between nutrition and wellness. This has prompted further researchers to find foods and dietary components with particular health advantages for people. *L. plantarum,* with probiotic properties, has been proposed as a natural preservative for synthetic additives. According to the US Dietary Supplement and Health Education Act and Supplements of 2003, the term "dietary supplement" refers to a non-tobacco product designed to enhance the diet, which includes one or more of the subsequent dietary ingredients: concentrates, metabolites, constituents, extracts, and mixtures thereof [66]. The question comes from whether a nutrient used to treat an illness is medicine, functional food, or dietary supplements. Many European nations have implemented robust CODEX dietary supplement guidelines, making it impossible for consumers to buy supplements in therapeutic or relevant preventative quantities. The European Union is the first in a series of nations throughout the globe that have signed the United Nations' planned Codex Alimentarius (Latin for "Food Code"), a set of worldwide norms for nutritional supplements, food processing, manufacturing, and commerce [67]. On the contrary, in the United States, there are fewer restrictions on the types and dosages of nutritional supplements that may be sold than in other developed nations [67, 68]. Without authorization from the United States Food and Drug Administration (FDA), makers of dietary supplements are prohibited from making claims for the prevention or treatment of illness. And just a few of the supplements' disease-related claims have been authorized by the FDA [68]. In the case of probiotics, any probiotic listed as a food supplement that doesn't have scientific proof of a positive effect on the human body is not permitted to make any health claim. The key objectives of this legislation include evidence-based physiological efficacy and safety, safeguarding consumer interests, ensuring fair competition within the food sector, encouraging and protecting innovation, and effectively implementing Europe's internal framework [34]. When *L. plantarum* is incorporated into food supplements, it is generally used as freeze-dried or spray-dried cells, which remain inactive until reconstituted and released in the gastrointestinal system. These supplements may be found in various formats, including capsules, pills, and powders.

1.5.1. Role of Prebiotics in L. plantarum Food Supplements

The oldest definition of prebiotics described them as "non-metabolized food ingredients that increase probiotic bacteria" activity in the intestinal tract, stimulating their development and/or motility" [69, 70]. In 2017, a collective of specialists at the International Scientific Association for Probiotics and Prebiotics agreed to modify the definition of prebiotics. The revised report now characterizes prebiotics as a substrate used explicitly by microorganisms residing inside the host, conferring a positive efect after ingestion [70].

Essentially, the term "prebiotic" relates to inert dietary products, namely galactooligosaccharides, fructooligosaccharides, inulin, digestion-resistant starch, xylooligosaccharides, and lactulose. These substances can selectively sustain a limited population of advantageous bacteria within the colon, improving cardiometabolic and skeletal health [69, 71]. The selection criteria for a prebiotic include the following: (i) it should not undergo hydrolysis or absorption in the upper gastrointestinal tract; (ii) it should serve as a specific substrate for one or more beneficial colonic bacteria, thereby promoting their proliferation and metabolic stimulation; (iii) it should have the ability to alter the composition of the intestinal flora to the benefit of a healthier alternative; and (iv) it should induce positive changes either in the luminal environment or systemically [72]. The gut microbiota's composition, particularly the species present, is primarily influenced by diet, which has a significant and prompt impact on the microbial profile [69].

In the case of *L. plantarum*, various types of prebiotics have been reported with beneficial effects [69-75]. For example, two-color microarrays were employed to investigate genes expressed differently in *L. plantarum* WCFS1 cultured with short-chain fructooligosaccharides [75]. The study found that multiple genes (8- to 60-fold) were overexpressed, including sucrose phosphoenolpyruvate transport system, β-fructofuranosidase, fructokinase, α-glucosidase, and sucrose operon repressor. This study was the first example of β-fructofuranosidase associated with lactobacilli with the potential to degrade short-chain fructooligosaccharides [75]. Also, the prebiotic effects of resistant starch nanoparticles (0.5% w/v) were tested on the survival of *L. plantarum* through the fermenting process [73]. Hydrophobicity and β-sheet content of *L. plantarum* surface layer proteins were enhanced after starch nanoparticles addition, which may have contributed to improved intestine adherence. Also, the viability was maintained at 9.5 log CFU/mL, and the short-chain fatty acids (butyric acid) increased, which confirms the favorable activity [73].

Furthermore, to differentiate between strains in their consumption of prebiotic fibers, the growth efficiency of 77 *L. plantarum* strains on isomaltose- and galactooligosaccharides was examined [76]. Only one strain (*L. plantarum* Lp 900) showed similar growth efficiency on fructooligosaccharides- or inulin-containing media to its growth on its preferred substrate, glucose. Neither arabinoxylooligosaccharides nor sulfated fucoidan were metabolized by any bacteria in their testing panel. The establishment of genotype-phenotype correlations may be achieved by the identification and monitoring of gene clusters that are hypothesized to be involved in the use of isomaltose and other oligosaccharides, which are not yet identified as substrates for isomaltooligosaccharide metabolism [76]. In addition to the aforementioned factors, prebiotics have garnered significant attention in the fields of pharmacology and nutraceuticals owing to their favorable attributes of biocompatibility, non-toxicity, and biodegradability. The bioactive compounds possess the capacity to serve as antioxidants, agents that reduce cholesterol levels, and agents that combat microbial activity [74].

1.6. *L. plantarum* In Symbiotic Formulations

"Symbiotic" commonly describes the beneficial relationship between prebiotics and probiotics [69]. In May 2019, the definition of symbiotics was revised by a consortium of nutritionists, physiologists, and microbiologists affiliated with the International Scientific Association for Probiotics and Prebiotics. The fixed purpose of symbiotics, as agreed upon by the group, is as follows: "Symbiotics refer to a combination of live microorganisms and specific substrates that are selectively utilized by microorganisms residing within the host, resulting in a beneficial effect on the host's health." The underlying justification for the emergence of symbiotics is rooted in the susceptibility of probiotics to variations in growing conditions, including pH, oxygen levels, and temperature. Furthermore, probiotics are unable to survive inside the gastrointestinal tract of humans without the presence of prebiotics [73, 75, 77]. In their most recent paper, Jia et al. sustain the development of a symbiotic milk powder, prepared by combining the three (iso-malto-oligosaccharide, *L. plantarum* JJBYG12, and milk powder) and the impact of calcium supplementation on osteogenic activity [78]. The levels of L. *plantarum* activity and C-terminal telopeptide of type 1 collagen were reduced, whereas increases in serum calcium and phosphorus were seen after supplementation with symbiotic. The symbiotic effectively supplements calcium in the diet and rebuilds bones without adverse effects on other vital body systems [78]. Also, intestinal dysbiosis has a detrimental influence on the expression of metabolic and biochemical indicators throughout the course of chronic diseases that have a broad effect on overall health [79]. Of them, cardiovascular disease represents the highest mortality cause [80]. The capacity of *L. plantarum* has been reported to lower blood cholesterol levels through various mechanisms effectively. These mechanisms encompass the utilization of cholesterol for enhancing membrane stability, the attachment of cholesterol to the intestinal cell walls of bacteria, the conversion of cholesterol into coprostanol using bile salt hydrolase catalysis, and the restriction of hepatic cholesterol and triglyceride synthesis by short-chain fatty acids such as propionate [79, 81]. A research by Hijova et al. highlights the symbiotic effect of *L. plantarum* LS/07 and inulin (8% w/w) in modifying chronic disease risk factors [79]. The findings suggest a significant decrease in the concentrations of total cholesterol (1.8 mmol/L,) oxidized low-density lipoprotein (28 ng/m/L), and total bile acids (13 μmol/L) in comparison with control. In contrast, an increase of short-chain fatty acid synthesis was observed [79].

In interpreting the efficiency data of dietary administration of *L. plantarum* symbiotics, the researchers observe that it can be an ideal alternative to antibiotics [82]. *L. plantarum* has been proposed as a substitute for antibiotics in dietary because of its purported positive effects on intestinal microbiota issues, pathogenic intestinal bacteria, growth, and feed efficiency [82]. The previously mentioned consequences arise from the following mechanisms: (i) the prevention of gut colonization by harmful bacteria, (ii) the production of bacteriocins, (iii) the reduction of intestinal pH, and (iv) the modulation of immune function. Wang et al. data confirm the beneficial impact of microencapsulated *L. plantarum* ACCC 11016 (1.6×10^9 CFU/kg) with fructooligosaccharide (1.5 g/kg) affects weaned pigs' gut microbiota, blood immunological markers, and growth performance. After four weeks, the group fed with symbiotic showed higher plasma IgA (181.33 μg/mL) and IgG (3381.07 μg/mL) concentrations and colon lactic acid bacteria ($p < 0.05$) than the control group (99.99 μg/mL, respectively 1641.53 μg/mL) [82]. Furthermore, an assessment was conducted on the combined symbiotic blend derived from king oyster mushroom, *Pleurotus eryngii*, and *L. plantarum* 7-40, focusing on the growth and health of white shrimp [83]. Immune responses, such as phenoloxidase, respiratory burst, and lysozyme activity, as well as gene expression of pexn and pen4 in the haemocytes, and lgbp, sp, propoii, pexn, pen3a, pen4, and gpx in the haepatopancreas of shrimps, were significantly increased ($p < 0.05$) in the symbiotic group compared to the control, leading to lower cumulative mortality. Consequently, the proposed synbiotic has been suggested to increase growth performance, lower the danger of infectious disorders caused by *Vibrio*, and make a substantial contribution to the circular economy [83]. On the other hand, some probiotic strains' tolerance to antibiotics may help individuals whose gut imbalance directly results from antibiotic treatment [84]. A new functional beverage was developed by the fermentation of red seaweed (prebiotic) utilizing the probiotic bacteria *L. plantarum* DW12 as a starting culture. The results of the antibiotic testing indicated that strain DW12 exhibited susceptibility to just four antibiotics, namely ampicillin, cephalothin, ceftazidime, and chloramphenicol. Conversely, this strain showed resistance to seven additional antibiotics: vancomycin, bacitracin, gentamycin, kanamycin, streptomycin, norfloxacin, and polymyxin. Therefore, after antibiotic therapy, the functional beverage might be considered a synergistic dietary supplement [84].

Moreover, the antioxidant enzymes from *L. plantarum* play an essential role in neutralizing and destroying the reactive oxygen species that develop naturally, negatively impacting the body's many physiological systems [29, 85]. Hosseinifard et al. examined the oral supplementation of *L. plantarum* ATCC 8014 (10^7 CFU/ mL) with inulin (5% of daily food weight) to improve lipid profile and hypothalamic oxidative markers [29]. A statistically significant change ($p < 0.05$) was observed in the blood lipid profile (including low-density lipoprotein cholesterol, high-density lipoprotein cholesterol, very low-density lipoprotein cholesterol, triglyceride, and total cholesterol) between the group receiving symbiotic treatment and the control group. For oxidative stress indicators, the symbiotic increased superoxide dismutase and malondialdehyde levels in the hypothalamus [29]. Similar results were obtained in another experiment that utilized *L. plantarum* X1 (2×10^9 CFU/mL) and *L. plantarum* CCFM30 (2×10^9 CFU/mL) to improve antioxidant capacity in diabetic mice [85]. Superoxide dismutase (431.21 U/mgprot) was enhanced by bacteria supplementation. It has been proposed that *L. plantarum* might generate bioactive molecules (like glutathione) that can absorb free radicals, therefore protecting cells from oxidative damage [85]. Overall, *L. plantarum* is an effective medicine that might be regarded as a complementing alternative for preventing metabolic conditions [29, 82, 85].

1.7. Impact of *L. plantarum* Food Supplements on the Gut Microbiota

There has been a growing interest in the intricate nature of the human microbiota and its profound implications for human health [49]. Numerous researchers have shown connections between the diversity of a person's gut microbiota and their risk of contracting an infection, developing an illness, or experiencing a particular clinical state, opening up the possibility of innovative diagnostic procedures based on a patient's bacterial fingerprints [59, 71, 86-88]. For instance, a high-sugar diet leads to glucose intolerance, while a high-fat diet lowers microbiota diversity [89]. From a nutritional perspective, the inclusion of fibers, fermented dairy products, and polyphenols in the Mediterranean diet has been shown topositively impact the gut microbiota. This is achieved by a reduction in the ratio of *Firmicutes* to *Bacteroidetes* and an increase in the amounts of short-chain fatty acids [71]. Fermentation is the most common technique for increasing the presence of probiotics in food. When probiotics are added directly to meals like fruit drinks or cereals, the bacterial count may reach a billion CFU per serving [90].

The positive impacts of the administration of *L. plantarum* on gut microbiota are widely recognized by several studies [59, 71, 87]. However, there are barriers to modifying the gut microbiota for therapeutic research [27]. How gut health affects the onset and progression of illness may be investigated by changing the gut microbiota [27, 28]. One example is Ducrotte et al.'s clinical trial assessing the effectiveness of *L. plantarum* 299v DSM 9843 in relieving abdominal symptoms in a large group of patients (240) with irritable bowel syndrome who matched the Rome III criteria [28]. The dietary capsules were made from potato starch and magnesium stearate, each containing 10 billion CFU. After 4 weeks, the symptomatic impact of *L. plantarum* 299v was rated as excellent or good by 78.1% of patients, compared to 8.1% for placebo (p <0.01) [28]. Moreover, another research examined the alterations in the microbiome of triathletes by *L. plantarum* PS128 supplementation (100 mg cellulose with 3×10^{10} CFU/capsule) for exercise performance and possible physiological adaptation [91]. Athletes in the PS128 group had an endurance boost of roughly 130% compared to those in the placebo group; however, there was no change in maximal oxygen consumption between the two groups. Also, PS128 supplementation significantly decreased the abundance of *Anaerotruncus*, *Caproiciproducens*, *Coprobacillus*, *Desulfovibrio*, *Dielma*, *Family_XIII*, *Holdemania*, and *Oxalobacter* in the athlete's gut microbiota while simultaneously increasing the quantity of *Akkermansia*, *Bifidobacterium*, *Butyricimonas*, and *Lactobacillus* [91].

On the other hand, some studies have related the composition of an individual's gut microbiota to their dietary intake and energy balance [92, 93]. Although an imbalance between caloric intake and energy expenditure is primarily responsible for obesity, the gut microbiome of healthy and obese persons differs in ways that may influence energy homeostasis [92, 93]. Gut microbiota affects weight and obesity in particular [92]. Consequently, an Indonesian study aimed to evaluate the effects of the probiotic *L. plantarum* Dad-13 powder on overweight adults in Yogyakarta. The research's material was 1 g of skimmed milk powder containing 2×109 CFU of the probiotic *L. plantarum* Dad-13 in sachet form. The lipid profile, including cholesterol and triglyceride, high-density lipoprotein, and low-density lipoprotein, showed no significant changes between the probiotic and placebo groups before and after intake. Weight and body mass index were found to drop significantly ($p < 0.05$) in the therapy group from 84.54 ± 17.64 kg to 83.14 ± 14.71 kg and 33.10 ± 6.15 kg/m2 to 32.57 ± 5.01 kg/m2, respectively. Genetic study reveals that the introduction of *L. plantarum* Dad-13 reduced the number of Firmicutes and increased the number of Bacteroidetes, particularly *Prevotella* [92]. However, the results of Huang et al. indicate positive modifications in the investigated biomarkers point to *L. plantarum* KC28 having a weight-reduction effect similar to that of the two well-researched probiotic strains, *L. rhamnosus* GG and *L. plantarum* 299v. This was certainly caused by either probiotic strain modulating the cecal microbiota of the intermediate high-fat diet group distinctly since only the group receiving *L. plantarum* KC28 showed a significant increase in the *Desulfovibrionaceae* (0.78 ± 0.46% for high-fat diet group and 2.77 ± 1.22% for KC28) and *Lactobacillaceae* (12.0 ± 3.50% respectively, 25.6 ± 4.95%) families [93]. Thus, *L. plantarum* is a candidate probiotic for preventing and alleviating obesity.

1.8. *L. plantarum* in Pharmaceuticals

The human digestive tract has more than 1000 bacterial species, ranging in abundance. A limited number of probiotics, including *L. acidophilus*, *L. pentosus*, *L. brevis*, *L. lactis*, *L. amylovorus*, *L. casei*, *L. bulgaricus*, *L. fermentum*, *L. plantarum*, and *L. rhamnosus*, possess the ability to produce and release proteins, exopolysaccharides, bacteriocins, and lipoteichoic acids, which have significant implications for the host's overall health and physiological processes. The literature has shown that *L. plantarum* has been seen to have a beneficial influence on the immunological responses of other *Lactobacillus* strains.

1.8.1. Regulations on the Safety of L. plantarum

Lactobacilli have a history of safe use in human nutrition. Nevertheless, the introduction of any new strain, regardless of its prior safe use, necessitates a thorough evaluation of its safety and toxicity in compliance with existing regulations [36]. The predominant benefits of lactobacilli are often linked to the well-being of the urogenital, immunological, and gastrointestinal systems. Furthermore, current research indicates that lactobacilli have the potential to regulate lifestyle illnesses such as metabolic syndrome (which encompasses obesity, diabetes, cardiovascular disease, and related conditions), exert psychotropic effects *via* the gut-brain axis, and exhibit anti-mutagenic or anti-cancer properties. Nonetheless, lactobacilli might still result in opportunistic infections in those with weakened immune systems and defenses.

Consequently, *L. plantarum* has been studied extensively to understand its safety and probiotic properties [94-96]. Pradhan et al. studied the safety of *L. plantarum* MTCC 5690 using *in vitro* approaches and an *in vivo* murine model. For this purpose, mucin degradation, hemolytic activity, biogenic amine production, and platelet aggregation assay were used *in vitro*, applying a usual dosage (10^6 and 10^7 CFU/mL). The results of the toxicological risk evaluation indicated that the test strain lacked any hazardous metabolic or cytotoxic activity. Also, oral toxicity tests on mice showed that the probiotic strain's short-term and long-term feeding (10^{12} CFU/mL) did not change any hematological, general health, or organ-specific parameters [95]. Another safety study of *L. plantarum* ST8Sh, a strain isolated from fermented Bulgarian salami "Shpek," evaluated the total DNA isolated from bacteria for more than 50 genes associated with the production of biogenic amines and virulence factors [97]. The presence of virulence genes was minimal in *L. plantarum* ST8Sh. Only 13 genes (affiliated with sex pheromones, aggregating material, collagen adhesion, tetracycline, gentamicin, chloramphenicol, and erythromycin) were found, which may indicate safety for fermented food items [97]. Thus, *L. plantarum* received a qualified presumption of safety status from the European Food Safety Authority (EFSA) and GRAS classification by the US Food and Drug Administration [94, 96].

Another significant characteristic of lactobacilli is their capacity for synthesizing biogenic amines, particularly in protein-rich diets [32, 95, 98]. Biogenic amines cause migraines, headaches, stomach and intestinal ulcers, and allergic reactions, which might harm human health [32, 95]. For this reason, Ye et al. assessed the occurrence of biogenic amines and their correlations with the microbial community in sauerkraut made from cabbage (Dongbei Suancai) inoculated with *L. plantarum* SC-5 or spontaneously fermented after 60 days of fermentation [99]. Inoculated Dongbei Suancai showed a significantly lower total biogenic amine concentration (216.72-237.33 mg/kg) than spontaneously fermented (234.62-266.81 mg/kg) ($p < 0.05$). Accordingly, these results suggest that total biogenic amines in Dongbei Suancai can be controlled using the proper starter, like *L. plantarum* SC-5 [99]. Moreover, the malolactic fermentation of Cabernet Gernishct wine was investigated for the accumulation of biogenic amines by using *Oenococcus oeni* (Viniflora®® Oenos and CiNe) and *L. plantarum* strains (Lp39,

CICC6240 and C8-1, CICC23138) [100]. Before fermentation, Cabernet Gernischt wine had 7.29 mg/L of total biogenic amines, which decreased after fermentation only for *L. plantarum* C8-1 (6.94 mg/L) fermented wine. Concerning specific biogenic amines, histamine and putrescine were the predominant ones both before and after malolactic fermentation [100]. Based on limited available data, the following biogenic amines amounts in food (per person per meal) did not cause health problems: a) 50 mg histamine for healthy people but below detectable levels for those with histamine intolerance; b) 600 mg tyramine for healthy people not using monoamine oxidase inhibitor (MAOI) medicines, or 50 mg or 6 mg for those taking third-generation or traditional MAOIs [95, 101]. Monitoring biogenic amine concentrations in fermented foods might be helpful for quality control and scientific advancement. Further investigations on biogenic amine levels in fermented foods are required, especially on toxicity and concentrations, production process-based control strategies, process sanitation and/or food safety standards improvement, and validation of analytical methodologies.

1.8.2. Adverse Effects of L. plantarum Ingestion

The functions of *L. plantarum* are assumed to be a direct result of enzymatic actions or a modification of endogenous bacteria or the immune system. Some theoretical concerns have been expressed about using probiotics in humans [102]. These risks include transmigration and *L. plantarum* colonization, which might have unfavorable metabolic and physiological effects on the patient's digestive system [102]. Michail et al. reported that viable *L. plantarum* (10^9 CFU/mL) decreased neutrophil migration induced by enteropathogenic *Escherichia coli* and binding to monolayers when preincubated with host epithelia [103]. Also, *L. plantarum* CLP-0611 was evaluated for its inhibitory effect on 2,4,6-trinitrobenzene sulfonic acid (TNBS)-induced colitis in mice. The results indicate a significant reduction in TNBS-induced body weight loss, colon shortening (a measure of colon inflammation and damage), myeloperoxidase activity (an enzyme associated with inflammatory response), IRAK-1 phosphorylation (a key immune signaling event), NF-κB activation (a transcription factor involved in regulating immune and inflammatory genes), and MAP kinase activation (p38, ERK, JNK - signaling proteins in inflammatory pathways). Additionally, there is a decrease in iNOS (inducible Nitric Oxide Synthase) and COX-2 (Cyclooxygenase-2) expression, both of which are enzymes associated with inflammation, as influenced by the presence of bacteria [104]. Thus, *L.*

plantarum reduces the transmigration of pathogens during their use [87, 102, 103].

Concerning the possibility of toxicity from transmigration, there is no confirmation that *L. plantarum* has more binding characteristics than other bacterial isolates [33, 104]. Most *L. plantarum* species have generally been approved as safe status (GRAS), so the US Food and Drug Administration considers their bacteriocins safe [105]. Bacteriocins are antimicrobial peptides that bacteria, including *L. plantarum*, generate to prevent the development of competing pathogens. However, bacteriocin migration across gastrointestinal epithelial and vascular endothelial cells remains unclear. Although some research has shown that certain bacteriocins may be able to translocate across gastrointestinal epithelial cells, the exact nature of this migration is still limited and may be bacteriocin- or condition-specific [106, 107]. Dreyer et al. demonstrated the capacity of the probiotic strain, *L. plantarum* 423, to produce the bacteriocin (plantaricin 423) that, after 3 h, migrated across the Caco-2 (85%) and HUVEC (93%) cell monolayer [108]. These peptides may have been delivered paracellularly since they crossed the cell membrane without producing a cytotoxic effect.

Nevertheless, transcytosis (transcellular migration) of cationic peptides cannot be excluded and may represent the mechanism by which bigger bacteriocins (7 kDa) traverse the gastrointestinal epithelial [86, 108]. *In vivo,* bioluminescence investigations on mice have shown that *L. plantarum* 423 colonizes the gastrointestinal tract and inhibits *Listeria monocytogenes* EGDe from generating chronic infections [106]. Plantaricin 423 is a class IIa bacteriocin that inhibits Gram-positive bacteria, including pathogenic species like *L. monocytogenes* and *Enterococcus faecalis* [107]. In contrast, the ability of *L. plantarum* bacteriocins to pass through vascular endothelial cells is considerably more limited compared to gastrointestinal epithelial cells. Vascular endothelial cells play a crucial role in controlling the uptake of water, electrolytes, and nutrients from the gut cavity to ensure balance in the blood and gastrointestinal tract [88]. Due to the concentration of bacteriocin needed to induce noticeable cytotoxicity, it becomes challenging for these levels to be reached by bacteriocins crossing the gut-blood barrier. Nevertheless, this does not rule out the potential for bacteriocins to accumulate in organs like the liver and potentially cause membrane damage [86].

Another significant aspect reported for *L. plantarum* is the potential to produce bacteremia and endocarditis [109, 110]. In its most basic definition, bacteremia is the presence of living bacteria in the blood. Asymptomatic bacteremia may develop during everyday activities like oral hygiene or after receiving routine medical treatment. These infections are harmless to a healthy human host and will subside independently. However, bacteremia develops into a bloodstream infection, recognized as septicemia, when the immune response systems fail or become overwhelmed. Untreated, clinically significant bacteremia leads to systemic inflammatory response syndrome, sepsis, septic shock, and multiple organ degeneration syndromes [111]. In one case, bacteremia had been connected to a localized infection termed meningoencephalitis, which caused atrial fibrillation, left atrium swelling, and an indication of valve regurgitation. Still, there was no evidence of active endocarditis. The origin of the infectious agent was investigated by Biesiada et al., who observed one case of bacteremia caused by *L. plantarum* in a 63-year-old man with newly diagnosed metastatic planoepitheliale lung cancer. During antibiotic therapy, the condition of the patient improved [109].

Infectious endocarditis is an infection of the heart's endocardial surface, most often caused by bacteria, that may affect several body systems [57]. Less than 0.5% of all incidences of endocarditis are caused by *Lactobacillus* species, which was correlated with immunodeficiency, probiotics and antibiotics, recent surgery, and structural heart disorders [56]. On the other hand, endocarditis due to *L. plantarum* is extremely rare [110]. However, a rare instance of bioprosthetic aortic valve endocarditis was reported, caused by *L. plantarum,* that improved after the standard medical and surgical intervention. This example illustrates the value of transesophageal echocardiography in monitoring the whole course of endocarditis and improves our knowledge of the disease process caused by *L. plantarum* [110].

Future studies should perform population-based monitoring for *L. plantarum* bacteria isolated from infected patients to assess probiotic safety as they are introduced and utilized worldwide. The strain's susceptibility profile should be known before it is employed in a clinical experiment.

1.8.3. Formulations for the Effective Delivery

Prior to formulation design, it is essential to comprehend the many physicochemical and biological parameters that impact the stability and *in vivo* performance of *L. plantarum* [112]. These parameters considerably affect probiotic viability under environmental conditions (oxidation, humidity, temperature, pH change), stability in biological fluids, and enzymatic deterioration. Nevertheless, considering bacteria have different defensive mechanisms to combat internal damage and adapt to adverse external settings, the biological and pharmacological barriers should be evaluated with diverse defense mechanisms that let probiotics survive varied stress circumstances.

Table 2 shows the most used formulation approaches for *L. plantarum* with therapeutic applications.

Several dosage forms, such as tablets, capsules, oral films, and hydrogels, are available for the oral administration of probiotics. Hence, formulation options depend on probiotic strains, ways of delivery, and therapeutic locations. A randomized, double-blind, and placebo-controlled cross-over human experiment was performed to determine how *L. plantarum* (WCFS, CIP104448, TIFN101) may affect assessing the activity of the human mucosal and systemic immune systems in real-life scenarios with moderate mucosal stress through oral administration. The results indicate that some *L. plantarum* strains (TIFN101, WCFS) may mitigate the detrimental effects of immunological stress from regularly used medicines (NSAIDs) and even positively impact consumers' immunity by promoting antigen presentation (tetanus toxoid (TT)-antigen) and memory responses [112]. Also, another study conducted by Wang et al. chose *L. plantarum* WCFS1 as the oral administration method using genetically engineered tools to regulate the production of a modified, protease-resistant form of glucagon-like peptide-1 (mGLP-1) for treating type 2 diabetes mellitus [113]. The combination of bacteria (10^{10} CFU/mL) and mGLP-1 efficiently alleviated diabetes symptoms within 14 days after daily administration and might reverse diabetic kidney problems in male C57BL/KsJ-db/db rats. There was a correlation between these modifications and the reduction of pancreatic glucagon, the rise in the number of pancreatic cells, and the enhancement of insulin sensitivity [113].

In terms of doses, the use of multiple *L. plantarum* strains and the many doses, dosing patterns, strain variations, differences in the consumer, and the health endpoint being tested render it challenging to generalize. Most therapeutic studies applied daily dosages of 10^6–10^9 CFU [101, 114-117]. For example, the potential effect of dosage (1×10^{10} or 5×10^{10} CFU/capsule) from two species of *L. plantarum* (HEAL9, 299) against radiation therapy-induced comorbidities was investigated [118]. Study participants were women older than 18 with gynecologic cancer who were scheduled to receive external beam radiation treatment to the pelvis at a minimum dosage of 40 Gy. The significant improvement in the intensity of stomach discomfort was prominent two weeks after the end of radiation treatment for the probiotic and placebo groups. However, there were no noteworthy differences observed between the doses [118]. In another study, Cianci et al. investigated the effect of *L. plantarum* P17630 in preventing vaginal infections [119].

Table 2. Most used formulation approaches for *L. plantarum* with therapeutic applications

Bacterial strains	Dosage forms	Coatings	Dosage	Cell line/*in vivo* model	Disorder	Reported clinical effects	Ref.
L. plantarum CECT 220	Microencapsulated - spray-drying	Casein-chitosan	9.89- 10.98 Log CFU/g for 3 weeks		Immunology	• Potential to reach the distal ileum and colon in 4 h after treatment • An immunomodulatory impact that increased cytokine levels (TH1 and TH17 responses)	[30]
L. plantarum PBS067	Microencapsulated - cross-linking gelation	Alginated-glucose pleuran hydrogel (β-1,3-d-glucan)	3.9×10^{8}-1.3×10^{9} CFU/g for 24 h	Human intestinal cell line HT-29	Immunology	• Antioxidant effect of the cell line • The capacity to modulate the release of the interleukins (IL-4 and IL-10) and the TNF-α *in vitro*	[120]
L. plantarum YML009	Non-encapsulated	-	2.67×10^{9} CFU/ml for 72 h	MDCK cells	Virus H1N1	• High survival after gastric juice incubation 1.5×10^{8} CFU/ml, respectively bile juice incubation 6.9×10^{8} CFU/ml • Novel probiotic candidate for anti-influenza prevention and infection (hemagglutination assay)	[116]
L. plantarum HAC01	Capsules	-	4×10^{9} CFU/capsule for eight weeks	Human patients (n = 40)	Diabetes	• Significant reduction in 2 h postprandial glucose (170.30 mg/dl) and glycosylated hemoglobin (5.84%) levels compared to the placebo group (182.24 mg/dl, respectively 5.98%)	[114]

Table 2. (Continued)

Bacterial strains	Dosage forms	Coatings	Dosage	Cell line/*in vivo* model	Disorder	Reported clinical effects	Ref.
L. plantarum NCC1107	Intranasal- aerosol inhalation	-	10^9 CFU/ml for 20 min daily (30 days)	BALB/C mice (n=12)	Allergic airway inflammation	• Decreased pulmonary inflammation but enhanced neutrophilia (influx 4.8-fold) and macrophages	[115]
L. plantarum P17630	Capsules	-	5×10^9CFU/ capsule for 15 days intake and 15 days washout (90 days)	Caucasian women (n=93)	Recurrent vulvovaginal candidiasis	• Improves vagina colonization of lactic acid bacteria (41.94%) • Reduced vaginal mucosa redness	[117]
L. plantarum CCFM1143	Not mentioned	-	3.52×10^9 daily (30 days)	Human patients (n = 90)	Chronic Diarrhea	• Mitigate the apparent clinical symptoms • Reducing the accumulation of *Bacteroides* and *Eggerthella* • Enriching the abundance of *Akkermansia*, *Anaerostipes*, and *Terrisporobacter* • Inhibit the increase in interleukin 6 (IL-6) and the decrease in motilin	[59]
L. plantarum 299 v	Capsules	-	5×10^9 CFU/capsule 2 capsules daily for 8 weeks	Human patients (n = 92)	Irritable bowel syndrome	• No significant stomach pain alleviation difference between the trial and placebo groups • No difference in IBS-QOL scores between the groups	[121]

Bacterial strains	Dosage forms	Coatings	Dosage	Cell line/*in vivo* model	Disorder	Reported clinical effects	Ref.
L. plantarum CCFM8610	Powder	-	5×10^9/g 2 g·pack^{-1}daily for 8 weeks	Human patients (n = 75)	Irritable bowel syndrome	• Significantly decreased the IBS-SSS and IBS-QOL scores, reduced IBS-D symptom severity • Increased the relative abundance of butyric acid-producing by *Anaerostipes*, *Anaerotruncus*, • *Bifidobacterium*, *Butyricimonas,* and *Odoribacter*	[87]
Mixture *L. plantarum* CECT 7527, CECT 7528, and CECT 7529	Capsules	-	1.2×10^9/capsule daily for 12 weeks	Human patients (n = 60)	Cholesterol-lowering	• A significant reduction of 13.6% in plasma total cholesterol levels compared with the placebo group • No significant changes between the treatments in terms of weight, BMI, fat-free fat mass, and fat mass after 12 weeks of probiotic use	[122]

IBS-QOL- Irritable bowel syndrome- quality of life scale;
IBS-SSS-Irritable bowel syndrome -symptom severity scale;
IBS-D-Irritable bowel syndrome with diarrhea;
BMI- Body mass index

Eighty-five eligible women were selected with a diagnosis of bacterial vaginosis (more than 15 days) and documented history of recurrent vaginal infections. After 16 weeks of *L. plantarum* P17630 (10^8 CFU/g) vaginal treatment, the risk of recurrent disease was lowered (95%CI 0.7-9.4), although this reduction was not statistically significant. This may be because the incidence of infection in the community was lower than predicted, reducing the study's power [119]. Also, there was a significant variation between the indicated and actual probiotic content of commercially available formulations of probiotics. Consequently, suppliers of probiotic products often include substantial overages to compensate for this, which drives up manufacturing costs and results in a dosage of the probiotic that can differ considerably [94].

Regarding the mode of administration, oral delivery has been considered the most effective method of administering therapeutic live cells to human patients [112-114, 117, 120]. Accordingly, oral preparations (tablets, capsules, oral films, and hydrogels) are most frequent for therapeutic *L. plantarum* delivery, especially for treating gastrointestinal disorders such as Crohn's disease, ulcerative colitis, and irritable bowel syndrome; preserving intestinal microbiota following antibiotic therapy; and the inhibition of tumor development [59, 87, 104, 120, 121]. The target location is the colon in the gastrointestinal system [94]. Other ways of delivery consist of nasal, topical skin, vaginal and rectal administration [30, 115, 116, 119].

Since each formulation has benefits and drawbacks, the chosen method is determined by the probiotic species, the quantity of the dosage forms, the way of administration, and the size of the manufacturing process. *L. plantarum* efficacy might be improved by combining formulation tactics with bioengineered probiotic strains or cutting-edge medicinal devices.

1.9. Benefits and Limitations of *L. plantarum* Clinical Studies

Numerous research conducted in recent years have provided evidence that the indigenous gut microbiota has a significant role in regulating several physiological systems and behavioral patterns in humans [59, 71, 86, 87]. Clinical studies are fundamental to expanding medical knowledge and enhancing the quality of treatment for patients [27, 28]. Some of the benefits of *L. plantarum* clinical studies consist of evaluating treatment efficiency, safety profile, advancement of medical knowledge (the mechanisms of the diseases), regulatory approval, and manufacturing of new medicines [69, 96, 97, 121, 123]. In addition, evidence-based recommendations for healthcare providers may be strengthened using clinical research data [121]. By prescribing the most effective and safe therapies based on extensive scientific research, these recommendations could help direct clinical practice and improve patient outcomes. Equally, information on patients' backgrounds, physical attributes, biomarkers, and recessive genes is frequently collected from clinical research. This information contributes to the advancement of customized medicine, enabling doctors to create treatment plans that would allow doctors to develop treatment plans specifically for each patient.

On the other hand, more clinical trials are needed, especially comparing probiotic products or the current medical standard. This will allow for identifying *L. plantarum's* positive and negative effects. Documentation of proven clinical efficacy, known mechanisms of action, and clearly stated dosage, length of use, and safety parameters will make it easier for medical professionals to recommend products and for consumers to buy probiotic foods and over-the-counter products confidently. Also, more attention should be allocated to the individual variation. Factors such as age, genetics, nutrition, lifestyle, and the preexisting gut microbiota influence *L. plantarum* therapy. Probiotic interventions could generate varying degrees of receptivity from different people, making it difficult to generalize about their effects for diagnostic or therapeutic purposes.

In the same way, the study methodology's variability and quality are limited. Extreme caution must be exercised in interpreting clinical study data, such as sample sizes, follow-up periods, and other methodological aspects for clinical trials. Some studies have shortcomings, including limited sample size, lack of placebo controls, or a short follow-up time. These fluctuations may impact the accuracy and applicability of the results. Although more clinical data on the short-term effects of *L. plantarum* is accumulating, additional long-term trials are needed to evaluate its long-term benefits, safety, and possible adverse reactions. Thus, before beginning any probiotic supplementation or therapy, it is recommended to consult with a healthcare professional or medical specialist, who may provide individualized recommendations based on the patient's unique needs and medical history.

Conclusion

In conclusion, the book chapter highlights the versatile applications *of L. plantarum* in food supplements and pharmaceuticals.

Firstly, the encapsulation of *L. plantarum* has emerged as a promising technique for incorporating it into food supplements and pharmaceutical items. The encapsulation ensures the viability and stability of *L. plantarum* during storage and delivery, thereby enhancing its potential health benefits. Furthermore, nanoencapsulation offers exciting opportunities for developing functional foods, supplements, and pharmaceuticals containing *L. plantarum* with improved bioavailability and targeted delivery.

Secondly, *L. plantarum* has demonstrated significant therapeutic potential. Its antimicrobial properties make it a valuable candidate for combating various pathogens. Additionally, it shows detoxification properties, aiding in removing harmful substances from the body. Moreover, *L. plantarum* exhibits antidiabetic effects, making it a potential adjunct in managing diabetes. However, it is essential to consider the regulatory aspects and legislation surrounding the use of *L. plantarum* in therapy.

Thirdly, *L. plantarum* holds excellent promise as a component of food supplements. Its probiotic properties contribute to gut health and immune modulation, improving overall well-being. Incorporating L. plantarum into food supplements provides an accessible and convenient way to benefit from its therapeutic effects.

Fourthly, *L. plantarum* has shown potential for pharmaceutical applications. Its interaction with the human body's systems opens avenues for developing novel pharmaceutical products. However, further research and clinical studies must fully explore and harness its benefits in this context.

Overall, using *L. plantarum* in food supplements and pharmaceuticals offers numerous advantages. It possesses diverse therapeutic properties and can be effectively delivered through encapsulation techniques. However, it is crucial to acknowledge the limitations and challenges of conducting clinical studies on L. plantarum to ensure its safe and effective use.

In conclusion, *L. plantarum* shows immense potential as a valuable ingredient in food supplements and pharmaceuticals. Further research and development in this area will undoubtedly contribute to the expanding field of probiotics and their therapeutic applications in improving human health.

References

[1] Behera S. S., Ray R. C., Zdolec N. *Lactobacillus plantarum* with Functional Properties: An Approach to Increase Safety and Shelf-Life of Fermented Foods. *Biomed Res Int*. 2018; 2018:9361614.

[2] Mayo B., Flórez A. B. Lactic Acid Bacteria: *Lactobacillus plantarum. Encyclopedia of Dairy Sciences*. 4: Elsevier; 2022; 206-17.

[3] Bartkiene E., Zavistanaviciute P., Lele V., Ruzauskas M., Bartkevics V., Bernatoniene J., Gallo P., Tenore G.C., Santini A. *Lactobacillus plantarum* LUHS135 and paracasei LUHS244 as functional starter cultures for the food fermentation industry: Characterisation, mycotoxin-reducing properties, optimisation of biomass growth and sustainable encapsulation by using dairy by-products. *Lwt*. 2018; 93:649-58.

[4] Krasaekoopt W., Bhandari B., Deeth H. Evaluation of encapsulation techniques of probiotics for yoghurt. *International dairy journal*. 2003;13 (1):3-13.

[5] Karimi N., Jabbari V., Nazemi A., Ganbarov K., Karimi N., Tanomand A., Karimi S., Abbasi A., Yousefi B., Khodadadi E., Kafil H. S. Thymol, cardamom and Lactobacillus plantarum nanoparticles as a functional candy with high protection against Streptococcus mutans and tooth decay. *Microb Pathog*. 2020;148:104481.

[6] Ren Loi H., Abbasiliasi S., Bothi Raja P., Shamzi Mohamed M., Tan W.-N., Suan Ng H., Chi-Wei Lan J., Shun Tan J. Biosynthesis of silver nanoparticles using nitrate reductase produced by *Lactobacillus plantarum* CAM 4: Characterization and in vitro evaluation of its antimicrobial efficiency. *Journal of Molecular Liquids*. 2023;376:121476.

[7] Wang M., Li Y., Yang J., Shi R., Xiong L., Sun Q. Effects of food-grade inorganic nanoparticles on the probiotic properties of Lactobacillus plantarum and Lactobacillus fermentum. *Lwt*. 2021;139:110540-.

[8] Abouloifa H., Rokni Y., Hasnaoui I., Bellaouchi R., Gaamouche S., Ghabbour N., Karboune S., Ben Salah R., Brasca M., D'Hallewin G., Saalaoui E., Asehraou A. Characterization of antimicrobial compounds obtained from the potential probiotic *Lactiplantibacillus plantarum* S61 and their application as a biopreservative agent. *Braz J Microbiol*. 2022;53(3):1501-13.

[9] Chang H. M., Foo H. L., Loh T. C., Lim E. T. C., Abdul Mutalib N. E. Comparative Studies of Inhibitory and Antioxidant Activities, and Organic Acids Compositions of Postbiotics Produced by Probiotic Lactiplantibacillus plantarum Strains Isolated From Malaysian Foods. *Front Vet Sci*. 2020;7:602280.

[10] Coda R., Cassone A., Rizzello C. G., Nionelli L., Cardinali G., Gobbetti M. Antifungal activity of Wickerhamomyces anomalus and Lactobacillus plantarum during sourdough fermentation: identification of novel compounds and long-term effect during storage of wheat bread. *Appl Environ Microbiol*. 2011;77(10):3484-92.

[11] Li Q., Zeng X., Fu H., Wang X., Guo X., Wang M. *Lactiplantibacillus plantarum*: A comprehensive review of its antifungal and anti-mycotoxic effects. *Trends in Food Science & Technology*. 2023;136:224-38.

[12] Kareem K. Y., Loh T. C., Foo H. L., Akit H., Samsudin A. A. Effects of dietary postbiotic and inulin on growth performance, IGF1 and GHR mRNA expression, faecal microbiota and volatile fatty acids in broilers. *BMC Vet Res*. 2016;12 (1):163.

[13] Panigrahi P., Parida S., Pradhan L., Mohapatra S. S., Misra P. R., Johnson J. A., Chaudhry R., Taylor S., Hansen N.I., Gewolb I.H. Long-term colonization of a

Lactobacillus plantarum synbiotic preparation in the neonatal gut. *J Pediatr Gastroenterol Nutr*. 2008;47 (1):45-53.

[14] Dhewa T., Pant S., Mishra V. Development of freeze dried synbiotic formulation using a probiotic strain of Lactobacillus plantarum. *J Food Sci Technol*. 2014; 51(1):83-9.

[15] Echegaray N., Yilmaz B., Sharma H., Kumar M., Pateiro M., Ozogul F., Lorenzo J. M. A novel approach to *Lactiplantibacillus plantarum*: From probiotic properties to the omics insights. *Microbiol Res*. 2023;268:127289.

[16] Russo P., Arena M. P., Fiocco D., Capozzi V., Drider D., Spano G. *Lactobacillus plantarum* with broad antifungal activity: A promising approach to increase safety and shelf-life of cereal-based products. *Int J Food Microbiol*. 2017;247:48-54.

[17] Cuevas-Gonzalez P. F., Liceaga A. M., Aguilar-Toala J. E. Postbiotics and paraprobiotics: From concepts to applications. *Food Res Int*. 2020;136:109502.

[18] Divyashree S., Shruthi B., Vanitha P. R., Sreenivasa M. Y. Probiotics and their postbiotics for the control of opportunistic fungal pathogens: A review. *Biotechnol Rep (Amst)*. 2023;38:e00800.

[19] Zamani N., Fazeli M. R., Sepahi A. A., Shariatmadari F. A new probiotic Lactobacillus plantarum strain isolated from traditional dairy together with nanochitosan particles shows the synergistic effect on aflatoxin B1 detoxification. *Archives of Microbiology*. 2022; 204 (10):624.

[20] Min Hsiu C., Shu Feng H., Jiau Hua C., Mei Fang L., Chin Shuh C., Shu Chen W. Antibacterial activity Lactobacillus plantarum isolated from fermented vegetables and investigation of the plantaricin genes. *African Journal of Microbiology Research*. 2016;10 (22):796-803.

[21] Khemariya P., Singh S., Jaiswal N., Chaurasia S. Isolation and identification of Lactobacillus plantarum from vegetable samples. *Food biotechnology*. 2016; 30 (1):49-62.

[22] Oguntoyinbo F. A., Narbad A. Multifunctional properties of Lactobacillus plantarum strains isolated from fermented cereal foods. *Journal of Functional Foods*. 2015;17:621-31.

[23] Goel A., Halami P. M., Tamang J. P. Genome analysis of Lactobacillus plantarum isolated from some Indian fermented foods for bacteriocin production and probiotic marker genes. *Frontiers in microbiology*. 2020:40.

[24] Hassan M. U., Nayab H., Shafique F., Williamson M.P., Almansouri T. S., Asim N., Shafi N., Attacha S., Khalid M., Ali N., Akbar N. Probiotic Properties of *Lactobacillus helveticus* and *Lactobacillus plantarum* Isolated from Traditional Pakistani Yoghurt. *Biomed Res Int*. 2020;2020:8889198.

[25] Hu C. H., Ren L. Q., Zhou Y., Ye B. C. Characterization of antimicrobial activity of three Lactobacillus plantarum strains isolated from Chinese traditional dairy food. *Food Sci Nutr*. 2019;7(6):1997-2005.

[26] Centurion F., Basit A. W., Liu J., Gaisford S., Rahim M. A., Kalantar-Zadeh K. Nanoencapsulation for Probiotic Delivery. *ACS Nano*. 2021;15 (12):18653-60.

[27] Dahiya D., Nigam P.S. Clinical Potential of Microbial Strains, Used in Fermentation for Probiotic Food, Beverages and in Synbiotic Supplements, as

Psychobiotics for Cognitive Treatment through Gut–Brain Signaling. *Microorganisms*. 2022;10 (9):1687.

[28] Ducrotte P., Sawant P., Jayanthi V. Clinical trial: *Lactobacillus plantarum* 299v (DSM 9843) improves symptoms of irritable bowel syndrome. *World J Gastroenterol*. 2012;18(30):4012-8.

[29] Hosseinifard E. S., Bavafa-Valenlia K., Saghafi-Asl M., Morshedi M. Antioxidative and metabolic effects of *Lactobacillus plantarum*, inulin, and their synbiotic on the hypothalamus and serum of healthy rats. *Nutrition and Metabolic Insights*. 2020;13:1178638820925092.

[30] Peñalva R., Martínez-López A. L., Gamazo C., Gonzalez-Navarro C. J., González-Ferrero C., Virto-Resano R., Brotons-Canto A., Vitas A. I., Collantes M., Peñuelas I., Irache J. M. Encapsulation of Lactobacillus plantarum in casein-chitosan microparticles facilitates the arrival to the colon and develops an immunomodulatory effect. *Food Hydrocolloids*. 2023;136.

[31] Luz C., Saladino F., Luciano F. B., Mañes J., Meca G. In vitro antifungal activity of bioactive peptides produced by *Lactobacillus plantarum* against *Aspergillus parasiticus* and *Penicillium expansum*. *LWT - Food Science and Technology*. 2017; 81:128-35.

[32] Topić Božič J., Butinar L., Bergant Marušič M., Korte D., Mozetič Vodopivec B. Determination of biogenic amines formation by autochthonous lactic acid bacteria from 'Refošk' grapes using different analytical methods. *Lwt*. 2022;156.

[33] Organization F. A. Guidelines for the evaluation of probiotics in food. FAO Rome; 2002.

[34] Passariello A., Agricole P., Malfertheiner P. A critical appraisal of probiotics (as drugs or food supplements) in gastrointestinal diseases. *Curr Med Res Opin*. 2014; 30 (6):1055-64.

[35] Mayo B., Fiórez A. B. Lactic acid bacteria: *Lactobacillus plantarum*. *Encyclopedia of Dairy Sciences: Third edition*. 2021;4:206-17.

[36] Maidana L., de Souza M., Bracarense A. *Lactobacillus plantarum* and Deoxynivalenol Detoxification: A Concise Review. *J Food Prot*. 2022; 85 (12):1815-23.

[37] Vatascinova T., Pipova M., Fraqueza M. J. R., Mala P., Dudrikova E., Drazovska M., Laukova A. Short communication: Antimicrobial potential of Lactobacillus plantarum strains isolated from Slovak raw sheep milk cheeses. *J Dairy Sci*. 2020;103(8):6900-3.

[38] Nualkaekul S., Cook M. T., Khutoryanskiy V. V., Charalampopoulos D. Influence of encapsulation and coating materials on the survival of Lactobacillus plantarum and Bifidobacterium longum in fruit juices. *Food Research International*. 2013; 53 (1):304-11.

[39] Saniani M., Nateghi L., Hshemiravan M. Investigation of microencapsulated *Lactobacillus plantarum* survival in alginate microsphere incorporated with inulin and dextran in order to produce a novel probiotic whey beverage. *Journal of Food Measurement and Characterization*. 2023:1-12.

[40] Nualkaekul S., Charalampopoulos D. Survival of *Lactobacillus plantarum* in model solutions and fruit juices. *Int J Food Microbiol*. 2011;146 (2):111-7.

[41] Bartkiene E., Lele V., Ruzauskas M., Domig K. J., Starkute V., Zavistanaviciute P., Bartkevics V., Pugajeva I., Klupsaite D., Juodeikiene G., Mickiene R., Rocha J. M. Lactic Acid Bacteria Isolation from Spontaneous Sourdough and Their Characterization Including Antimicrobial and Antifungal Properties Evaluation. *Microorganisms*. 2019; 8 (1).

[42] Petreska Ivanovska T., Jurhar Pavlova M., Mladenovska K., Petrushevska-Tozi L. Probiotics, prebiotics, synbiotics in prevention and treatment of inflammatory bowel diseases. *Macedonian Pharmaceutical Bulletin*. 2014; 60 (02):3-19.

[43] Sudheendra C. V., Patel A. Carrier Materials for Encapsulation. *Encapsulation in Food Processing and Fermentation*: CRC Press; 2022. p. 21-36.

[44] Steele J. A., Halle J. P., Poncelet D., Neufeld R. J. Therapeutic cell encapsulation techniques and applications in diabetes. *Adv Drug Deliv Rev*. 2014;67-68:74-83.

[45] Csatlos N. I., Simon E., Teleky B. E., Szabo K., Diaconeasa Z.M., Vodnar D. C., Ciont Nagy C., Pop O. L. Development of a Fermented Beverage with *Chlorella vulgaris* Powder on Soybean-Based Fermented Beverage. *Biomolecules*. 2023;13 (2):245.

[46] Giraffa G., Chanishvili N., Widyastuti Y. Importance of lactobacilli in food and feed biotechnology. *Res Microbiol*. 2010;161(6):480-7.

[47] Zotta T., Parente E., Ricciardi A. Aerobic metabolism in the genus *Lactobacillus*: impact on stress response and potential applications in the food industry. *J Appl Microbiol*. 2017; 122 (4):857-69.

[48] Ebrahimi Monfared K., Gharachorloo M., Jafarpour A., Varvani J. Effect of storage and packaging conditions on physicochemical and bioactivity of matcha-enriched muesli containing probiotic bacteria. *Journal of Food Processing and Preservation*. 2022; 46 (10):e16878.

[49] Douillard F. P., de Vos W. M. Biotechnology of health-promoting bacteria. *Biotechnol Adv*. 2019; 37 (6):107369.

[50] Bustamante M., Oomah B. D., Rubilar M., Shene C. Effective *Lactobacillus plantarum* and Bifidobacterium infantis encapsulation with chia seed (*Salvia hispanica* L.) and flaxseed (*Linum usitatissimum* L.) mucilage and soluble protein by spray drying. *Food Chem*. 2017;216:97-105.

[51] Quintana G., Gerbino E., Gomez-Zavaglia A. Valorization of okara oil for the encapsulation of *Lactobacillus plantarum*. *Food Res Int*. 2018;106:81-9.

[52] Li H., Turner M.S., Dhital S. Encapsulation of *Lactobacillus plantarum* in porous maize starch. *Lwt*. 2016;74:542-9.

[53] Kaur G., Kaur R., Rani N., Kaur S. Nanoencapsulation of Probiotics in Food Packaging. *Nanotechnology in Intelligent Food Packaging*. 2022:175-202.

[54] Atraki R., Azizkhani M. Survival of probiotic bacteria nanoencapsulated within biopolymers in a simulated gastrointestinal model. *Innovative Food Science & Emerging Technologies*. 2021;72:102750.

[55] Pateiro M., Gómez B., Munekata P. E., Barba F. J., Putnik P., Kovačević D. B., Lorenzo J. M. Nanoencapsulation of promising bioactive compounds to improve their absorption, stability, functionality and the appearance of the final food products. *Molecules*. 2021; 26 (6):1547.

[56] Moghadam F. V., Pourahmad R., Mortazavi A., Davoodi D., Azizinezhad R. Use of Fish Oil Nanoencapsulated with Gum Arabic Carrier in Low Fat Probiotic Fermented Milk. *Food Sci Anim Resour*. 2019; 39 (2):309-23.

[57] Bartkiene E., Lele V., Sakiene V., Zavistanaviciute P., Ruzauskas M., Bernatoniene J., Jakstas V., Viskelis P., Zadeike D., Juodeikiene G. Improvement of the antimicrobial activity of lactic acid bacteria in combination with berries/fruits and dairy industry by-products. *J Sci Food Agric*. 2019;99(8):3992-4002.

[58] Teanpaisan R., Piwat S., Dahlen G. Inhibitory effect of oral *Lactobacillus* against oral pathogens. *Lett Appl Microbiol*. 2011; 53 (4):452-9.

[59] Yang B., Yue Y., Chen Y., Ding M., Li B., Wang L., Wang Q., Stanton C., Ross R.P., Zhao J., Zhang H., Chen W. *Lactobacillus plantarum* CCFM1143 Alleviates Chronic Diarrhea via Inflammation Regulation and Gut Microbiota Modulation: A Double-Blind, Randomized, Placebo-Controlled Study. *Front Immunol*. 2021;12:746585.

[60] Yue Y., He Z., Zhou Y., Ross R. P., Stanton C., Zhao J., Zhang H., Yang B., Chen W. *Lactobacillus plantarum* relieves diarrhea caused by enterotoxin-producing *Escherichia coli* through inflammation modulation and gut microbiota regulation. *Food Funct*. 2020;11(12):10362-74.

[61] González E., Paisano Y., Ramos M.I. P-552 Pilot study to determine efficacy of *L. rhamnosus* BPL205, *L. plantarum* BPL207 and *L.crispatus* BPL209 in normalizing the vaginal environment (study PROSALVAG). *Human Reproduction*. 2023;38 (Supplement_1).

[62] Lele V., Ruzauskas M., Zavistanaviciute P., Laurusiene R., Rimene G., Kiudulaite D., Tomkeviciute J., Nemeikstyte J., Stankevicius R., Bartkiene E. Development and characterization of the gummy–supplements, enriched with probiotics and prebiotics. *CyTA - Journal of Food*. 2018;16 (1):580-7.

[63] Quattrini M., Bernardi C., Stuknyte M., Masotti F., Passera A., Ricci G., Vallone L., De Noni I., Brasca M., Fortina M. G. Functional characterization of *Lactobacillus plantarum* ITEM 17215: A potential biocontrol agent of fungi with plant growth promoting traits, able to enhance the nutritional value of cereal products. *Food Res Int*. 2018;106:936-44.

[64] Riolo M., Luz C., Santilli E., Meca G., Cacciola S. O. Antifungal activity of selected lactic acid bacteria from olive drupes. *Food Bioscience*. 2023;52:102422-
.

[65] Kareem K. Y., Hooi Ling F., Teck Chwen L., May Foong O., Anjas Asmara S. Inhibitory activity of postbiotic produced by strains of Lactobacillus plantarum using reconstituted media supplemented with inulin. *Gut Pathog*. 2014; 6 (1):23.

[66] Wollschlaeger B. The Dietary Supplement and Health Education Act and supplements: dietary and nutritional supplements need no more regulations. *International journal of toxicology*. 2003; 22 (5):387-90.

[67] Cencic A., Chingwaru W. The role of functional foods, nutraceuticals, and food supplements in intestinal health. *Nutrients*. 2010; 2 (6):611-25.

[68] Tucker J., Fischer T., Upjohn L., Mazzera D., Kumar M. Unapproved Pharmaceutical Ingredients Included in Dietary Supplements Associated With US Food and Drug Administration Warnings. *JAMA Netw Open*. 2018;1(6):e183337.

[69] Simon E., Calinoiu L.F., Mitrea L., Vodnar D. C. Probiotics, Prebiotics, and Synbiotics: Implications and Beneficial Effects against Irritable Bowel Syndrome. *Nutrients*. 2021;13 (6):2112.

[70] Gibson G. R., Hutkins R., Sanders M.E., Prescott S. L., Reimer R. A., Salminen S. J., Scott K., Stanton C., Swanson K. S., Cani P. D., Verbeke K., Reid G. Expert consensus document: The International Scientific Association for Probiotics and Prebiotics (ISAPP) consensus statement on the definition and scope of prebiotics. *Nat Rev Gastroenterol Hepatol*. 2017;14 (8):491-502.

[71] de Sire A., de Sire R., Curci C., Castiglione F., Wahli W. Role of Dietary Supplements and Probiotics in Modulating Microbiota and Bone Health: The Gut-Bone Axis. *Cells*. 2022; 11 (4):743.

[72] Manigandan T., Mangaiyarkarasi S. P., Hemalatha R., Hemalatha V. T., Murali N. P. Probiotics, Prebiotics and Synbiotics - A Review. *Biomedical & Pharmacology Journal*. 2012; 5 (2):295-304.

[73] Wang M., Chen X., Zhou L., Li Y., Yang J., Ji N., Xiong L., Sun Q. Prebiotic effects of resistant starch nanoparticles on growth and proliferation of the probiotic *Lactiplantibacillus plantarum* subsp. *plantarum*. *Lwt*. 2022; 154:112572.

[74] Prete R., Alam M. K., Perpetuini G., Perla C., Pittia P., Corsetti A. Lactic Acid Bacteria Exopolysaccharides Producers: A Sustainable Tool for Functional Foods. *Foods*. 2021;10 (7).

[75] Saulnier D. M., Molenaar D., de Vos W. M., Gibson G. R., Kolida S. Identification of prebiotic fructooligosaccharide metabolism in Lactobacillus plantarum WCFS1 through microarrays. *Appl Environ Microbiol*. 2007; 73 (6):1753-65.

[76] Fuhren J., Rosch C., Ten Napel M., Schols H.A., Kleerebezem M. Synbiotic Matchmaking in *Lactobacillus plantarum:* Substrate Screening and Gene-Trait Matching To Characterize Strain-Specific Carbohydrate Utilization. *Appl Environ Microbiol*. 2020; 86 (18).

[77] Swanson K. S., Gibson G. R., Hutkins R., Reimer R. A., Reid G., Verbeke K., Scott K. P., Holscher H. D., Azad M. B., Delzenne N. M., Sanders M. E. The International Scientific Association for Probiotics and Prebiotics (ISAPP) consensus statement on the definition and scope of synbiotics. *Nat Rev Gastroenterol Hepatol*. 2020;17 (11):687-701.

[78] Jia M., Luo J., Gao B., Huangfu Y., Bao Y., Li D., Jiang S. Preparation of synbiotic milk powder and its effect on calcium absorption and the bone microstructure in calcium deficient mice. *Food Funct*. 2023;14(7):3092-106.

[79] Hijova E., Strojny L., Bertkova I., Bomba A., Stofilova J. Dietary *Lactobacillus plantarum* LS/07 and inulin in the management of chronic disease risk factors. *Acta Biochim Pol*. 2020; 67 (4):447-51.

[80] Roth G. A., Forouzanfar M. H., Moran A. E., Barber R., Nguyen G., Feigin V. L., Naghavi M., Mensah G. A., Murray C. J. Demographic and epidemiologic drivers of global cardiovascular mortality. *N Engl J Med*. 2015; 372 (14):1333-41.

[81] Wang Y., Xing X., Ma Y., Fan Y., Zhang Y., Nan B., Li X., Wang Y., Liu J. Prevention of High-Fat-Diet-Induced Dyslipidemia by Lactobacillus plantarum LP104 through Mediating Bile Acid Enterohepatic Axis Circulation and Intestinal Flora. *Journal of Agricultural and Food Chemistry*. 2023.

[82] Wang W., Chen J., Zhou H., Wang L., Ding S., Wang Y., Song D., Li A. Effects of microencapsulated Lactobacillus plantarum and fructooligosaccharide on growth performance, blood immune parameters, and intestinal morphology in weaned piglets. *Food and Agricultural Immunology*. 2017; 29 (1):84-94.

[83] Prabawati E., Hu S. Y., Chiu S. T., Balantyne R., Risjani Y., Liu C. H. A synbiotic containing prebiotic prepared from a by-product of king oyster mushroom, Pleurotus eryngii and probiotic, *Lactobacillus plantarum* incorporated in diet to improve the growth performance and health status of white shrimp, Litopenaeus vannamei. *Fish Shellfish Immunol*. 2022;120:155-65.

[84] Hayisama-ae W., Kantachote D., Bhongsuwan D., Nokkaew U., Chaiyasut C. A potential synbiotic beverage from fermented red seaweed (Gracilaria fisheri) using *Lactobacillus plantarum* DW12. *International Food Research Journal*. 2014;21(5):1789-96.

[85] Li X., Wang N., Yin B., Fang D., Zhao J., Zhang H., Wang G., Chen W. *Lactobacillus plantarum* X1 with α-glucosidase inhibitory activity ameliorates type 2 diabetes in mice. *RSC Advances*. 2016; 6 (68):63536-47.

[86] Dicks L. M. T., Dreyer L., Smith C., van Staden A. D. A Review: The Fate of Bacteriocins in the Human Gastro-Intestinal Tract: Do They Cross the Gut-Blood Barrier? *Front Microbiol*. 2018;9:2297.

[87] Liu Y., Yu X., Yu L., Tian F., Zhao J., Zhang H., Qian L., Wang Q., Xue Z., Zhai Q., Chen W. *Lactobacillus plantarum* CCFM8610 Alleviates Irritable Bowel Syndrome and Prevents Gut Microbiota Dysbiosis: A Randomized, Double-Blind, Placebo-Controlled, Pilot Clinical Trial. *Engineering*. 2021;7 (3):376-85.

[88] Kelly J. R., Kennedy P. J., Cryan J. F., Dinan T. G., Clarke G., Hyland N.P. Breaking down the barriers: the gut microbiome, intestinal permeability and stress-related psychiatric disorders. *Front Cell Neurosci*. 2015; 9:392.

[89] Suez J., Korem T., Zeevi D., Zilberman-Schapira G., Thaiss C. A., Maza O., Israeli D., Zmora N., Gilad S., Weinberger A., Kuperman Y., Harmelin A., Kolodkin-Gal I., Shapiro H., Halpern Z., Segal E., Elinav E. Artificial sweeteners induce glucose intolerance by altering the gut microbiota. *Nature*. 2014; 514 (7521):181-6.

[90] Champagne C. P., Gomes da Cruz A., Daga M. Strategies to improve the functionality of probiotics in supplements and foods. *Current Opinion in Food Science*. 2018; 22:160-6.

[91] Huang W. C., Pan C. H., Wei C. C., Huang H. Y. *Lactobacillus plantarum* PS128 Improves Physiological Adaptation and Performance in Triathletes through Gut Microbiota Modulation. *Nutrients*. 2020;12 (8).

[92] Rahayu E. S., Mariyatun M., Putri Manurung N. E., Hasan P. N., Therdtatha P., Mishima R., Komalasari H., Mahfuzah N. A., Pamungkaningtyas F. H., Yoga W. K., Nurfiana D. A., Liwan S. Y., Juffrie M., Nugroho A. E., Utami T. Effect of probiotic *Lactobacillus plantarum* Dad-13 powder consumption on the gut microbiota and intestinal health of overweight adults. *World J Gastroenterol*. 2021; 27 (1):107-28.

[93] Huang E., Kim S., Park H., Park S., Ji Y., Todorov S. D., Lim S. D., Holzapfel W. H. Modulation of the Gut Microbiome and Obesity Biomarkers by *Lactobacillus*

plantarum KC28 in a Diet-Induced Obesity Murine Model. *Probiotics Antimicrob Proteins*. 2021;13 (3):677-97.

[94] Seddik H. A., Bendali F., Gancel F., Fliss I., Spano G., Drider D. *Lactobacillus plantarum* and Its Probiotic and Food Potentialities. *Probiotics Antimicrob Proteins*. 2017; 9 (2):111-22.

[95] Pradhan D., Singh R., Tyagi A., H. M. R., Batish V. K., Grover S. Assessing safety of *Lactobacillus plantarum* MTCC 5690 and *Lactobacillus fermentum* MTCC 5689 using in vitro approaches and an in vivo murine model. *Regul Toxicol Pharmacol*. 2019;101:1-11.

[96] Additives E. P. O., Products or Substances used in Animal F., Bampidis V., Azimonti G., Bastos M.L., Christensen H., Dusemund B., Fasmon Durjava M., Kouba M., Lopez-Alonso M., Lopez Puente S., Marcon F., Mayo B., Pechova A., Petkova M., Ramos F., Sanz Y., Villa R. E., Woutersen R., Brozzi R., Galobart J., Innocenti M., Lopez-Galvez G., Pettenati E., Revez J., Vettori M. V., Gregoretti L. Safety and efficacy of a feed additive consisting on *Lactiplantibacillus plantarum* (formerly *Lactobacillus plantarum*) CECT 8350 and *Limosilactobacillus reuteri* (formerly *Lactobacillus reuteri*) CECT 8700 (AQ02) for suckling piglets (AQUILON CYL S.L.). *EFSA J*. 2021;19 (6):e06631.

[97] Todorov S. D., Perin L. M., Carneiro B. M., Rahal P., Holzapfel W., Nero L.A. Safety of *Lactobacillus plantarum* ST8Sh and Its Bacteriocin. *Probiotics Antimicrob Proteins*. 2017; 9 (3):334-44.

[98] Jin Y. H., Lee J. H., Park Y. K., Lee J. H., Mah J. H. The Occurrence of Biogenic Amines and Determination of Biogenic Amine-Producing Lactic Acid Bacteria in Kkakdugi and Chonggak Kimchi. *Foods*. 2019;8(2).

[99] Ye H., Lang X., Ji Y., Li S., Xin N., Meng X., Zhang T., Shen X., Zhao C. The interaction between Lactobacillus plantarum SC-5 and its biogenic amine formation with different salt concentrations in Chinese Dongbei Suancai. *Food Res Int*. 2021;150(Pt B):110813.

[100] Wang S. Y., Zhu H. Z., Lan Y. B., Liu R. J., Liu Y. R., Zhang B. L., Zhu B.-Q. Modifications of Phenolic Compounds, Biogenic Amines, and Volatile Compounds in Cabernet Gernishct Wine through Malolactic Fermentation by *Lactobacillus plantarum* and Oenococcus oeni. *Fermentation*. 2020;6 (1).

[101] Ruiz-Capillas C., Herrero A. M. Impact of Biogenic Amines on Food Quality and Safety. *Foods*. 2019;8(2).

[102] Snydman D. R. The safety of probiotics. *Clin Infect Dis*. 2008;46 Suppl 2:S104-11; discussion S44-51.

[103] Michail S., Abernathy F. *Lactobacillus plantarum* inhibits the intestinal epithelial migration of neutrophils induced by enteropathogenic Escherichia coli. *J Pediatr Gastroenterol Nutr*. 2003;36(3):385-91.

[104] Jang S. E., Han M. J., Kim S. Y., Kim D. H. *Lactobacillus plantarum* CLP-0611 ameliorates colitis in mice by polarizing M1 to M2-like macrophages. *Int Immunopharmacol*. 2014; 21(1):186-92.

[105] Probi A., Lund S. Generally Recognized as Safe (GRAS) determination for the use of Lactobacillus plantarum strain 299v in conventional foods. Submission by Probi AB to the United States Food and Drug Administration; 2016.

[106] Van Zyl W., Deane S., Dicks L. *Enterococcus mundtii* ST4SA and *Lactobacillus plantarum* 423 excludes Listeria monocytogenes from the GIT, as shown by bioluminescent studies in mice. *Beneficial Microbes*. 2016; 7 (2):227-35.

[107] van Zyl W. F., Deane S. M., Dicks L. M. Use of the mCherry Fluorescent Protein To Study Intestinal Colonization by Enterococcus mundtii ST4SA and Lactobacillus plantarum 423 in Mice. *Appl Environ Microbiol*. 2015; 81 (17):5993-6002.

[108] Dreyer L., Smith C., Deane S.M., Dicks L. M. T., van Staden A. D. Migration of Bacteriocins Across Gastrointestinal Epithelial and Vascular Endothelial Cells, as Determined Using In Vitro Simulations. *Sci Rep*. 2019; 9 (1):11481.

[109] Biesiada G., Krycinska R., Czepiel J., Stazyk K., Kedzierska J., Garlicki A. Meningoencephalitis caused by Lactobacillus plantarum - case report. *Int J Neurosci*. 2019;129(7):715-8.

[110] Tavernese A., Stelitano M., Mauceri A., Mollace R., Uccello G., Romeo F., Cammalleri V. Progression of Lactobacillus plantarum prosthetic valve endocarditis followed by transesophageal echocardiogram. *Int J Infect Dis*. 2020; 97:160-1.

[111] Smith D. A., Nehring S. M. Bacteremia. *StatPearls*. Treasure Island (FL): StatPearls Publishing Copyright © 2023, StatPearls Publishing LLC.; 2023.

[112] de Vos P., Mujagic Z., de Haan B. J., Siezen R. J., Bron P. A., Meijerink M., Wells J. M., Masclee A. A. M., Boekschoten M. V., Faas M. M., Troost F. J. *Lactobacillus plantarum* Strains Can Enhance Human Mucosal and Systemic Immunity and Prevent Non-steroidal Anti-inflammatory Drug Induced Reduction in T Regulatory Cells. *Front Immunol*. 2017; 8:1000.

[113] Wang Q., Guo H., Mao W., Qian X., Liu Y. The Oral Delivery System of Modified GLP-1 by Probiotics for T2DM. *Pharmaceutics*. 2023;15 (4).

[114] Oh M. R., Jang H. Y., Lee S. Y., Jung S. J., Chae S. W., Lee S. O., Park B. H. *Lactobacillus plantarum* HAC01 Supplementation Improves Glycemic Control in Prediabetic Subjects: A Randomized, Double-Blind, Placebo-Controlled Trial. *Nutrients*. 2021; 13 (7).

[115] Pellaton C., Nutten S., Thierry A. C., Boudousquie C., Barbier N., Blanchard C., Corthesy B., Mercenier A., Spertini F. Intragastric and Intranasal Administration of *Lactobacillus paracasei* NCC2461 Modulates Allergic Airway Inflammation in Mice. *Int J Inflam*. 2012; 2012:686739.

[116] Rather I. A., Choi K. H., Bajpai V. K., Park Y. H. Antiviral mode of action of <i>*Lactobacillus plantarum*</i> YML009 on Influenza virus H1N1. *Bangladesh Journal of Pharmacology*. 2015; 10 (2).

[117] Vladareanu R., Mihu D., Mitran M., Mehedintu C., Boiangiu A., Manolache M., Vladareanu S. New evidence on oral *L. plantarum* P17630 product in women with history of recurrent vulvovaginal candidiasis (RVVC): a randomized double-blind placebo-controlled study. *Eur Rev Med Pharmacol Sci*. 2018; 22 (1):262-7.

[118] Ahren I. L., Bjurberg M., Steineck G., Bergmark K., Jeppsson B. Decreasing the Adverse Effects in Pelvic Radiation Therapy: A Randomized Controlled Trial Evaluating the Use of Probiotics. *Adv Radiat Oncol*. 2023; 8 (1):101089.

[119] Cianci A., Cicinelli E., De Leo V., Fruzzetti F., Massaro M.G., Bulfoni A., Parazzini F., Perino A. Observational prospective study on *Lactobacillus plantarum* P 17630 in the prevention of vaginal infections, during and after systemic antibiotic therapy or in women with recurrent vaginal or genitourinary infections. *J Obstet Gynaecol*. 2018; 38 (5):693-6.

[120] D'Orazio G., Di Gennaro P., Boccarusso M., Presti I., Bizzaro G., Giardina S., Michelotti A., Labra M., La Ferla B. Microencapsulation of new probiotic formulations for gastrointestinal delivery: *in vitro* study to assess viability and biological properties. *Appl Microbiol Biotechnol*. 2015; 99 (22):9779-89.

[121] Stevenson C., Blaauw R., Fredericks E., Visser J., Roux S. Randomized clinical trial: effect of Lactobacillus plantarum 299 v on symptoms of irritable bowel syndrome. *Nutrition*. 2014; 30 (10):1151-7.

[122] Fuentes M. C., Lajo T., Carrion J. M., Cune J. Cholesterol-lowering efficacy of Lactobacillus plantarum CECT 7527, 7528 and 7529 in hypercholesterolaemic adults. *Br J Nutr*. 2013;109 (10):1866-72.

[123] Hazards E. P. B. Scientific opinion on risk based control of biogenic amine formation in fermented foods. *Efsa Journal*. 2011; 9 (10):2393.

Chapter 5

Lactobacillus plantarum in Bakery and Pastry Products

Simona Maria Man*
Adriana Păucean
Anamaria Pop
and Maria Simona Chiș
Department of Food Engineering, Faculty of Food Science and Technology,
University of Agricultural Sciences and Veterinary Medicine of Cluj-Napoca, Romania

Abstract

Sourdough is widely used as a natural leavening agent in the modern biotechnology of bakery and pastry products due to the advantages over baker's yeast, such as improving texture and flavour of bread and leading to a final product with high sensory quality. The unique properties of sourdough derive from the metabolic activity of the naturally present or inoculated LAB. Among the outstanding processes during sourdough fermentation by LAB are lactic fermentation, proteolysis, synthesis of volatile compounds and anti-mold activity. The most important group of bacteria involved in sourdough fermentation belong to the *Lactobacillus* genus being responsible for improving nutritional quality and stability in continuous sourdough refreshment. From the *Lactobacillus* species, *Lactobacillus plantarum* (*L. Plantarum*), is one of the most widely studied species which is used in the bakery and pastry industry as a probiotic microorganism and/or microbial starter in order to improve texture and flavour of products and prolong the shelf-life. Additionally, *L. plantarum* species are extremely versatile because they are able to

* Corresponding Author's Email: simona.man@usamvcluj.ro.

In: Lactobacillus plantarum and Its Role in Human Health
Editors: Maria Simona Chiș, Adriana Paucean
ISBN: 979-8-89113-696-0

ferment gluten-free flours to produce functional bread enriched with bioactive compounds and adequate textural characteristics. Thus, L. plantarum was find to ferment a variety of substrates, including wheat flour (*Triticum aestivum*), flour of ancient wheat species (einkorn, spelt, emmer), flour of sorghum, rye, maize, oats, buckwheat, rice, amaranth, millet, chickpeas, quinoa, chia, lentils and soybeans, in order to improve the final quality of bakery products in term of texture and sensory features. Also, various studies have emphasized the capacity of *L. plantarum* strains to improve the nutritional profile, antioxidant activity and to give a better digestibility to the final baked goods. In this regard, it was shown that sourdough fermentation with *L. plantarum* (single strain or co-culture) lead to enhanced content of soluble dietary fibre amino-acids, minerals, ABTS scavenging capacity, total antioxidant capacity in different bread dough formulations, but in the case of some pastry products, too.

Other studies have shown the potential of this starter culture to control spoilage microorganisms in bread production, prolonging the product shelf-life without adding any chemical preservatives. Organic acids, mainly lactic and acetic one, phenolic compounds, carbon dioxide, ethanol, hydrogen peroxide, fatty acids, acetoin, diacetyl, and cyclic dipeptides were found to have antifungal activity.

Maltogenic amylase originated from *L. plantarum* was find to have antistaling effect by inducing a slower starch retrogradation rate together with lower hardness in white wheat bread.

The increased consumers attention for fermented foods have produced the renascence of the sourdough technology which nowadays it is considered as an economic, feasible and biotechnological approach that led to nutritional enriched products. In this context, *L. plantarum* strain is a powerful toll mainly because of its adaptability, flexibility and versatility, having a larger genome with probiotic future.

The purpose of this chapter is to stress out the applicability of L. plantarum species in the production of bakery and pastry products, as well as the beneficial role that microbial fermentation plays in the development of foods with high nutritional value, improved texture and taste, and longer shelf life.

Keywords: *L. plantarum*, bakery, pastry, functional products, antimicrobial activity

1. Introduction

Sourdough fermentation is a centuries-old technique for fermenting cereal flour, which improves bread quality while also providing nutritional and health benefits (Akamine et al., 2023). Consuming bread, particularly sourdough bread, represent a decision of civilization, this being an essential component of peasant diets. Maintaining consumption habits shows us that sensory and nutritional alterations, which are also implemented by sourdough fermentation, were empirically observed by the rural people (Cappelle et al., 2023). Sourdough is a flour-water mixture that has been fermented with lactic acid bacteria (LAB) and yeasts (Dallagnol et al., 2013; De Vuyst et al., 2009) producing chemical reactions and metabolites which provide the product distinct properties (better nutritional quality, increased shelf life) and a high sensory quality (Akamine et al., 2023). As well, the qualities of sourdough are determined by the synthesis of organic acids (lactic and acetic acids) and the proteolytic activity of LAB throughout the fermentation process.

Lactiplantibacillus plantarum, formerly known as *Lactobacillus plantarum* (*L. plantarum*), is one of the most flexible and adaptable lactic acid bacteria, with a long history of use in foods and claims of probiotic benefits. This species has demonstrated encouraging results in post-harvest fruit protection and mold prevention in the products such as drinks and bread (Seddik et al., 2017; De Simone et al., 2022; Akamine et al., 2023) also, maintaining its probiotic effect even after the baking and storage processes (Zhang et al., 2015). Many in vitro and in vivo investigations have shown that *L. plantarum* possesses health-promoting characteristics in addition to its functional properties in the food business (Arasu et al., 2016; Prete et al., 2017; Tang et al., 2017). Therefore, probiotic *L. plantarum* strains may improve gut microbiota, control the immune system, lower blood cholesterol levels, and reduce the risk of some malignancies (Abdelazez et al., 2018; Yilmaz et al., 2022).

Sourdough fermentation, in general, has a good effect on wheat flour-based products due to the effect of low pH on the structural creation of dough constituents such as arabinoxylans, starch and gluten (Teleky et al., 2020). Moreover, may reduce the glycemic response of baked goods, improve the characteristics and bioavailability of dietary fiber complex and phytochemicals, and may increase mineral uptake. As well during sourdough fermentation, microbial metabolism may also produce new nutritionally active substances like as peptides and amino acid derivatives, as well as potentially prebiotic exo-polysaccharides (Gobbetti et al., 2014; Chiş et al., 2020).

LAB have a favorable impact on bread quality; due to their metabolic features, carbohydrates' consumption lead to the growth of LAB microbial load and increase the organic acids production causing a pH reduction (Chiş et al., 2020). These bacteria adapts easily, has a faster sourdough acidification rate, and are adaptable in cocultures with other bacteria or yeasts (Paucean et al., 2013). A variety of products, including short-chain fatty acids, amines, bacteriocins, vitamins, and exopolysaccharides, can be produced by *L. plantarum* ATCC 8014 during metabolic activity, according to studies (Wang et al., 2021; Păucean et al., 2021; Serban et al., 2023). This includes decomposing macromolecular substances in food, including the degradation of indigestible polysaccharides and transformation of undesirable flavor components. *L. plantarum* can therefore produce amylase, which hydrolyzes starch into dextrin and then glucose (De Vuyst et al., 2009; Oguntoyinbo & Narbad, 2012; Wang et al., 2021).

The degradation of macromolecular proteins during food processing is an important process that influences food quality, food safety, and food nutrition. Protein allergies in food can be eliminated via the breakdown of proteins by lactic acid bacteria. Thus, some strains of LAB isolated from sourdough can hydrolyze wheat proteins such as albumins, globulins, and gliadins (Stefańska et al., 2016) and could produce a variety of small molecule peptides or free amino acids. Thus, LAB can improve the food protein digestibility and might enhance the food nutritional protein value through proteolysis. For example, fermentation of faba bean flour with a strain of *L. plantarum* VTT E-133328 can improve *in vitro* protein digestibility, particularly the level of essential amino acids and free amino acids (Coda et al., 2015). Another study highlighted that after LAB fermentation combined with xylanase treatment, the *in vitro* protein digestibility of pigmented wheat varieties, hull-less barley, and emmer was 87%, and the product had high free radical scavenging activity and a high concentration of peptides and free amino acids (Pontonio et al., 2020). Furthermore, LAB can produce a wide range of vitamins, including folic acid, riboflavin, vitamin C, pyridoxal (Capozzi et al., 2012), and others. For instance, Capozzi et al., 2012, showed that *L. plantarum* WCFS1 strain is able to produce during sourdough fermentation of wheat flour (for bread production) and semolina flour (prefermentation step for pasta manufacturing) a water soluble vitamin such as riboflavin, also known as B_2 vitamin. Therefore, authors highlighted a new biotechnological approach able to fortified bread and pasta in vitamin content, using an economic and efficient process such as LAB fermentation. Vitamins generated during the fermentation of LAB might lead to nutritional fortification of food in the food industry, being able to obtain food for special nutrition (Wang et al., 2021).

A variety of LAB, among which is *L. plantarum*, can synthesize different kinds of exopolysaccharides. Sasikumar et al., 2017, showed that the high molecular weight exopolysaccharides synthesized by *L. plantarum* BR2 has strong antioxidant activity, radical scavenging activity, and no cytotoxicity. Also, Chen et al., 2016 claimed that adding sucrose to the dough can stimulate glucan formation, and the particular effect of the glucan structure may extend the pores of the crumbs and increase bread texture. Valerio et al., 2020, showed that fermentation with *Weiss Ella cibaria* and *L. plantarum* produced exopolysaccharides mainly in the presence of pseudocereals amaranth or quinoa and hydrolyzed proteins during fermentation. Moreover, using *L. plantarum* sourdough strain ITM21B in wheat/quinoa formulations, more efficient proteolysis, including the glutenin and gliadin portion of wheat, was produced. Nowadays, many exopolysaccharides produced during LAB fermentation such as pullulan, dextran, alginate and xanthan are claimed to have commercial applications in industries such as food, cosmetic, biomedicine or even pharmaceutical sector (Erdem et al., 2023).

LAB contributed to the synthesis of flavour compounds in fermented sourdough. During the fermentation of bread sourdough, the combination of lactic acid bacteria (*Lactiplantiacillus plantarum*, *Furfurilactobacillus rossiae*, and *Lacticaseibacillus casei*) and yeast produced compounds related to sour aromas of bread and contributed to bread aroma characteristics (Winters et al., 2019). Moreover, Liu et al., 2019, claimed that *L. plantarum* may promote the production of more C4-C6 alcohols in sourdough.

Additionally, LAB in fermented foods could be able to increase the antioxidant activity of some bioactive compounds emphasizing some therapeutic benefits on the human body. Although, some LAB (such as *Levilactobacillus brevis*, *Limosilactobacillus fermentum* and *Lactiplantibacillus plantarum*) can metabolize phenolic acid through decarboxylase and reductase (Filannino et al., 2015), meantime, the decarboxylation and reduction reaction of phenolic acid can decompose hydroxycinnamic acids (p-coumaric acid, caffeic acid, ferulic acid, and m-coumaric acid) and certain hydroxybenzoic acids (gallic acid and protocatechuic acid) (Rodríguez et al., 2009).

The majority of LAB identified in sourdough microflora are considered to have probiotic effect, and therefore sourdough bread might be considered as a product with probiotic effects (Bircan et al. 2017; Seddik et al., 2017; Abdelazez et al., 2018; Kezer G., 2022). The presence of LAB varies depending on the type of flour, the dough ingredients and technological conditions during bread making process. LAB have been found to create antifungal substances such as lactic and acetic acid, carbon dioxide, di-acetyl, hydrogen peroxide, caproic acid, 3-hydroxy fatty acids, phenyl lactic acid, cyclin dipeptides, roterin, and fungicines in sourdough breads. These organic antibacterial compounds, which are generated during sourdough fermentation, protect bread from ageing, stalling, spoilage and thus increase its shelf life (Kezer G., 2022).

Also, it has been shown that the fermentation with *L. plantarum* could lead to the reduction of anti-nutritional compounds level in physically processed legume and pulse flours and positively influences the nutrient availability. Thus, Byanju et al., 2021, studied the effect of combined physical process (sonication or precooking) and fermentation with *L. plantarum* and *Pediococcus acidilactici* on the anti-nutritional factors (phytic acid, tannins, and enzyme inhibitors) of some legumes (soybean flour, green pea flour, and lentil flour). *L. plantarum* and *P. acidilactici* grew well in both modified and unmodified soybean flour, green pea flour, and lentil flour. The fermentation of these physically processed legumes and pulse flours influenced the reduction of numerous antinutritional compounds while also improved nutritional quality.

Cereal-based fermented products are globally important food resources for human nutrition because they are high in protein, dietary fiber, carbs, and minerals (Guyot, 2012). In recent years, functional fermented foods of ancient cereals have gained global interest due to their versatility to face to the major consumer trends-focused in consuming food with improved nutritional content (Todorov et al. 2010; Russo, Arena, et al., 2017).

L. plantarum was mentioned to ferment a variety of substrates, including wheat flour, flour of ancient wheat species (einkorn, spelt, emmer), flour of sorghum, rye, maize, oats, buckwheat, rice, quinoa, amaranth, millet, chickpeas, lentils, and soybeans, in order to improve bakery product quality.

1.1. Ancient and Durum Wheat Species in Relation with *L. plantarum*

Worldwide, *Triticum aestivum L. subsp. aestivum*, the “common” wheat, is the major wheat species grown and used for human consumption. On the second place is *Triticum turgidum var. durum* (the durum wheat), a tetraploid species which is adapted for the Mediterranean climate and which is mainly used for pasta making. However, other wheat species known as "ancient wheat species" are gaining more and more attention especially due to their rich content in biologically active compounds and consequently, their health beneficial properties (Shewry and Hey, 2015). The three types of ancient wheat species that were used as whole grains by people for millennia before being substituted by contemporary bread wheat include einkorn, emmer, and spelt (Kulathunga et al., 2021).

Einkorn (*Triticum monococcum var. monococcum*) is a diploid wheat, while emmer (*T. turgidum var. dicoccum*) and spelt (*T. aestivum var. spelta*) are tetraploid and hexaploid, respectively. Another difference of emmer, spelt and most types of einkorn comparing to common and durum wheat is the necessity to be dehulled in special equipment during milling. Einkorn is a separate species, but emmer and spelt are cultivars of *T. turgidum* and *T. aestivum*, respectively (Shewry et al., 2022). Khorasan wheat (Kamut®) is also promoted as "ancient wheat" type. It is known to be a Khorasan wheat genotype, a kind of *T. turgidum* linked to emmer and current durum wheats. Kamut® is a recognized brand of Kamut International Ltd, and it is farmed exclusively on certified organic farms. Similarly, the tetraploid Italian wheat Graziella Ra® is said to have originated in an Egyptian tomb (Shewry et al., 2017).

Because of their complex nutritional content, ancient grains have grown in popularity as a primary source of proteins, lipids (mostly unsaturated fatty acids), soluble fibers, minerals, vitamins, and bioactive substances with antioxidant activity. Even so, based on their bioactive compounds composition, some studies report only minor differences when compared to modern wheat varieties. The health benefits of ancient wheat are reported, primarily due to the antioxidant activity of some compounds naturally present or formed during baking, such as polyphenols and melanoidins (Şerban et al., 2021).

Many researchers are now focused on the study of sourdough fermentation and its implications on bioactive component content. Ancient wheat sourdough is gaining popularity due to its ability to synthesize new functionally active molecules with increased bioaccessibility, resulting in bread with improved nutritional content.

A large number of LAB strains were used to produce spelt, emmer, einkorn and Kamut sourdoughs. Between them, *L. plantarum, L. brevis, L. sanfranciscensis, L. paracasei, L. alimentarius* were mostly successfully used. According to these research studies, the selected LAB strains contribute to baked goods with increased sensory quality, but they can also serve other functions, such as the production of peptides with antioxidant activity (Şerban et al., 2021).

Thus, when the LAB microbiota of emmer and spelt were characterized, the most biodiversity was found in spelt flour, while *L. plantarum* predominated in emmer flour (Coda et al., 2010). Also, Van Der Meulen et al., 2007, reported that *L. plantarum* was present in spelt sourdough ecosystems along with other identified microorganisms, while Korcari et al., 2020 found in their study six strains of *L. plantarum* during the spontaneous fermentation of wholemeal spelt sourdough.

L. plantarum is commonly found in sourdough ecosystems, and its dominance in cereal fermentations is mostly owing to its versatile carbohydrate metabolism (Luc De Vuyst and Neysens, 2005). It was also stated that endogenous strains of *L. plantarum* are preferred over those isolated from other matrices to produce a quick and vigorous acidification process with a good impact on nutritional and technical qualities of sourdough bread (Di Cagno et al., 2008). However, to utilize, combined starters were regarded functional in order to fully use the potential of spelt and emmer flours. A mixture of strains with varying carbohydrate metabolism could be utilized due to the capacity to provide appropriate acidity and sensory qualities (Gobbetti, 1998). Between the *L. plantarum* strains isolated from emmer and spelt flours, three of them (31S, 6E and 10E) were found with the best performance and were selected to be used to ferment spelt and emmer sourdoughs. The kinetics of growth and acidification, the quotient of fermentation and the release of free amino acids during sourdough fermentation were the main indicators used for their selection (Coda et al., 2010).

L. plantarum ATCC 8014 was used to ferment einkorn, spelt and emmer sourdoughs with good results (Serban et al., 2023). The highest bacterial cell growth was found for einkorn flour, followed by spelt and emmer flours, while the cells concentrations ranged between 9.6 log cfu/g and 9.0 log cfu/g. The same study revealed for common wheat sourdough a final bacterial cell count of 9.4 log cfu/g after 24h. The good microbial adaptability of *L. plantarum* in the ancient wheat species is a result of the nutrients availability in these matrices. High proteins and amino-acids content along with vitamin E, vitamin B-group, calcium, magnesium, iron, zinc support the bacterial growth during sourdough fermentation. For this purpose, free amino-acids, vitamins and simple carbohydrates are firstly consumed and then the proteolytic enzymes assure the nitrogen requirements by breaking down the protein chains. The higher protein content of einkorn and spelt could be the reason of a better microbial growth of *L. plantarum* compared to emmer and common wheat

(Şerban et al., 2021). Nevertheless, the changes in the final cell count, might be attributed to variances in flour quality based on origin, environment, production processes, and storage conditions (Korcari et al., 2020). The metabolic profiles of ancient wheat and common wheat sourdoughs revealed significant variations. As a result of the interaction between ancient wheat flours and *L. plantarum* ATCC 8014, unique metabolites may be identified. Emmer demonstrated different fermentation behavior in terms of cell dynamics, sugar metabolization, and lactic acid production. This might be explained by its higher proportion of resistant starch, but also by the lower quantities of Zn and Mn, both of which are required for microbial cell proliferation (Serban et al., 2023). Maltose, glucose and fructose were consumed differently in emmer sourdough compared to einkorn, spelt and common wheat. As a result, lactic acid content was also smaller than in the other ancient wheat sourdoughs. Emmer's higher starch content together with higher resistant starch amount might be the reason of this difference. However, since some important minerals were found in a smaller concentration in emmer compared to einkorn and spelt, this also could be an explanation for smaller cell growth *of L. plantarum.* One of the important influences of *L. plantarum* metabolism in interaction with the raw matrix is the volatile derivatives synthetization. Because of this interaction, the volatile profile of emmer sourdough differed. The largest concentrations of volatiles generated in emmer sourdough fermented with *L. plantarum* were for 1 butanol-3 methyl, 1-heptanol, 1 hexanol, 2 butanone-3 hydroxy, hexanoic acid, acetic acid, hexyl ester, and acetic acid, pentyl ester. The volatile derivatives found in highest amounts in einkorn sourdough were: -2-nonanone, 3-buten-1-ol, 3-methyl, 1-butanol, 3-methyl, 2-heptanone and 1-butanol, 2-methyl. In the case of common wheat, the major aroma compounds found in sourdough were: butanoic acid, butanoic acid, ethyl ester, butanoic acid, propyl ester, disulfide, dimethyl, dimethyl trisulfide, 1-butanol, 3-methyl and 1-Penten-3-ol, 4-methyl. With respect to spelt flour sourdough the clustering showed high levels of 1-butanol-2 methyl, furan-2 pentyl, citric acid, benzene-acetaldehyde, benzoic acid, 2 octen-1-ol, 2-hexanol-5 methyl.

The interactions between durum wheat and KAMUT® Khorasan wheat flours and *L. plantarum* strains isolated from bread and wine (collection of the Department of Agri-Food Science and Technologies from University of Bologna, Bologna, Italy) were studied by (Ferri et al., 2016). Volatile, polyphenols, flavonoids, phenolic compounds and antioxidant activity were analysed in the fermented sourdoughs with the specific aim to improve sensorial and functional properties of cereal-fermented products. Ten strains of *L. plantarum* were chosen due to the increased content of polyphenols identified in the foods from which it was isolated. The methodology used by the authors associated the metabolic profiles with heat maps and the hierarchical clustering. By this approach it was possible to obtain important information and conclusions in order to choose the optimal combination between the raw flour and the relevant bacterial strain of *L. plantarum*. For KAMUT® Khorasan sourdough 5 alcohols, 6 carbonyls, dodecanoic acid and 1,3-hexadiene were found correlated with the polyphenolic compounds (gallic acid, epigallocatechin-gallate, epigallocatechin, flavonoids, protocatechuic acid) and total polyphenols. For the case of durum sourdough, the results were different in term of correlations. Thus, from the group of volatiles, 10 alcohols, 5 carbonyls, 3 acids and 3 hydrocarbons showed high correlation with epigallocatechin, epigallocatechin-gallate, flavonoids and total polyphenols. Moreover, the results indicated that volatiles, especially alcohols and carbonyls compounds, were more correlated with polyphenols, while antioxidant activity was highly correlated with hydrocarbons and ester. Also, this approach highlighted specific interactions between the raw flour and the bacterial strain based on the correlated compounds belonging to different chemical classes. The selected strains of *L. plantarum* showed increased capacity to produce phenolics and flavonoids with antioxidant activity as a result of depolymerization reactions. It is also worth to be mentioned that the metabolic profile in durum sourdough was richer than in the case of KAMUT® Khorasan sourdough.

The modern durum wheat and ancient KAMUT® Khorasan whole grains (immature and fully ripped) were also tested by Saa et al., 2017 by fermenting these flours with a co-culture of *L. plantarum* 98a, *L. sanfranciscensis* BB12, *L. brevis* 3BHI and *Saccharomyces cerevisiae* LBS (Department of Agricultural and Food Science and Technology of the University of Bologna, Italy).The combined influence of sourdough fermentation and baking intensity on the content of the dietary fiber and phenolics of bread was studied. The results showed that the highest amount of insoluble fibers was found in fully ripe KAMUT® Khorasan sourdough bread, while high content of soluble fiber was determined in durum sourdough. For the insoluble fiber content of KAMUT® Khorasan a lower release of fermentable sugars by endogenous enzymes could be an explanation since it is known that insoluble fibers are poorly fermented by LAB. On the contrary, a higher hydrolytic solubilisation activity of endogenous enzymes at lower pH value determined the higher amount of dietary soluble fiber. Moreover, LAB sourdough bread provided higher concentrations of insoluble dietary fiber comparing to the yeast fermented bread showing a low degradation activity of the bakery yeast (*S. cerevisiae*).

With respect to the total polyphenols, sourdough fermentation positively influenced their content in all bread samples without being affected by the ripe degree of the grains. When unripe flour was fermented to sourdough, the KAMUT® Khorasan bread kept a larger proportion of free flavonoids. Gianotti et al., 2011 described the preservation of total phenolic components in KAMUT® Khorasan wheat bread throughout sourdough fermentation. The level of total phenolic compounds determined after baking was comparable to that found in the KAMUT® Khorasan flour used as raw material. These findings showed that sourdough fermentation might mitigate the heat loss of phenolic chemicals during the baking process.

The same mix culture of *L. plantarum* 98a, *L. sanfranciscensis* BB12, *L. brevis* 3BHI and *Saccharomyces cerevisiae* LBS and the same flours (durum and KAMUT® Khorasan) were used by Saa et al., 2019 to determine the volatile profile of breads. For this aim a metabolomic approach was used and the analytical methods were E-nose and SPME-GC-MS. The relationship between the LAB strain and the wheat composition clearly established that various flours yield varied volatile profiles of sourdough. As a result of the greater protein content of KAMUT® Khorasan flour, a broader spectrum of sulphur compounds was found in the associated sourdough. KAMUT® Khorasan sourdough and fermented breads have greater levels of volatile chemicals such as acetic acid, pentanoic acid, hexanol, ethanol, heptanal, hexanal, and decanal. The interactions between the substrate composition in nutrients and the LAB strains resulted in a larger level of acetic acid in this sourdough. The oxidative breakdown of unsaturated fatty acids yielded heptanal, hexanal, and decanal (Păucean et al., 2021).

Di Renzo et al., 2018 studied the volatile profile of quinoa and Kamut® sourdoughs fermented with *L. paracasei*, *L. plantarum* and *L. brevis*. The results were compared to wheat sourdough obtained by using the same strains. Significant changes in the volatile profiles of the sourdough samples were found in the groups of aldehydes, sulphur compounds, ketones, esters and acetates, alcohols, furans, pyrazines, and acids. The generation of volatile chemicals was higher in Kamut and quinoa sourdoughs than in wheat doughs, which had a mild scent. High levels of pentanal, hexanal, trans (E)-2-heptanal, nonanal, 2-octenal, 2,4-nonadienal, and 2,4-decadienal were identified when Kamut flour was fermented with *L. plantarum M4* and *L. paracasei I1*.

1.2. Application of *L. plantarum* in Sourdough and Baked Goods

Arora et al., 2021, states that during the last 30 years sourdough baked goods underwent characterization in almost 50 countries and all continents, mainly dealing with salty (breads and substitutes) and in a smaller proportion sweet products. These studies discussed the microbiological, biochemical and technological features of typical/traditional sourdough baked goods. Sourdough has been claimed as an indispensable starter for increasing the sensory, rheology, and shelf life qualities of baked goods due to its unique microbial composition and functionality. Sourdough fermentation also raised mineral bioavailability, allowed the fiber fortification, improved protein digestibility, and decreased anti-nutritional amount (Arora et al., 2021; Apostol et al., 2020; Di Biase et al., 2019; Hu et al., 2023). Various studies who analysed the addition of selected *L. plantarum* strains to dough, in order to improve the final quality of bakery products are presented in table 1:

Beldean et al., 2022, studied the adaptability of *L. plantarum* strain on a mix of wheat flour and insect flour fermentation. The results showed that fermentation of insect flour with *L. plantarum* ATCC 8014 strain increases the value of organic acids such as lactic, acetic, and oxalic acid, whereas citric acid diminishes its value. The pH value decrease during sourdough fermentation, meantime TTA (total titrable acidity) increased it value at least twice. Saturated and monounsaturated fatty acid groups were positively impacted by *L. plantarum* fermentation, however polyunsaturated fatty acid groups decreased. During insect sourdough fermentation, a positive trend for amino acid, aroma volatile content, and mineral enhancement was observed, primarily at 24 h of fermentation. For instance, magnesium increased its value after 24 h of fermentation from 10.31 mg/100g to 15.33 mg/100g, meantime Zinc reached a final value of 6.52 mg/100g.

Teleky et al., 2020b aimed to compare the efficiency of two *Lactobacillus* strains, *L. plantarum* ATCC 8014 and *L. casei* ATCC 393, in metabolizing different white wheat flour (WF) and soybean flour (SF) combinations for sourdough fermentation with and without *Saccharomyces cerevisiae* (100% WF, 95% WF + 5% SF and 90% WF + 10%). The viability, pH, organic acids, and secondary metabolite synthesis, as well as the dynamic rheological properties of the sourdough throughout 24 h fermentation after frozen storage, were studied in this study. The results showed that LAB grew faster during sourdough fermentation, and the pH dropped dramatically from over pH 6 at 0 h to under 4 at 24 h for each experiment. Co-cultures of LAB and yeast produced more lactic acid than single cultures, notably in soy-enriched sourdough. Also, acetic acid developed in sourdoughs was found only in co-cultures enhanced by the soy-flour addition. Sourdoughs in general exhibited a stable, elastic-like behavior, the addition of soy flour conferring greater elasticity than sourdoughs without soy flour. This effect may be linked to the fact that soy proteins have a higher water holding capacity during frozen storage.

Table 1. Effect of *L. plantarum* in sourdough and baked goods

Products	Fermentable substrate	*L. plantarum* strain	Influences of product properties	References
Sourdough	Wheat and insect flour	*L. plantarum* ATCC 8014	↑ the value of organic acids such as lactic, acetic, and oxalic acid; ↓ citric acid; ↓ polyunsaturated fatty; ↑ amino-acids, and minerals; ↑ aroma volatile compounds.	Beldean et al., 2022
Bread	Wheat flour	*L. plantarum* AR524	- *Fusarium graminearum* growth was strongly inhibited; - deoxynivalenol (DON) was eliminated; ↑ the bread's textural attributes; ↑ shelf life from three to six days.	Cao et al., 2021
Sourdough and bread	Wheat and amaranth flour	*L. plantarum* and *Saccharomyces cerevisiae*	- improved sourdough fermentation; ↑ specific volume and total titratable acidity; ↓ water activity and hardness bread; ↑ sensory properties and shelf life of bread; - softer texture of bread.	Karimi et al., 2021
Bread	Wheat flour and 30,%, 35% and 40% sorghum seed flour	*L. plantarum* (*Aurum Plantarum*), 0.3 g/100 g flour	↑ minerals content (K, Mg, Fe); ↑ sensorial characteristics in bread samples in which lactic acid bacteria was used; ↑ acidity for the bread samples with the addition of *Lb. plantarum;* ↓ porosity and elasticity with increasing degree of sorghum replacement and *L. plantarum.*	Apostol et al., 2020
Breads	Wheat flour	*L. plantarum*	- slower retrogradation rate with 25%, during storage for 7 days at 4°C; - lower hardness relative with 63%, during storage for 7 days at 4°C.	Woo et al., 2020

Table 1. (Continued)

Products	Fermentable substrate	*L. plantarum* strain	Influences of product properties	References
Sourdough	Wheat and soy flour	*L. plantarum* ATCC 8014 and *Lactobacillus casei* ATCC 393	- pH decreased significantly; ↑ lactic, acetic, and citric acid production; - improved rheological qualities.	Teleky et al., 2020ab
Sourdough	Wheat flour	*L. plantarum* L14	↑ growth rate and biomass production; ↑ acidity during fermentation; - more cohesive and sticky dough formation was detected.	Üçok and Sert, 2020
Bread	Chickpea and wheat flour	*L. plantarum* ITM21	↑ nutritional profile (amino acid and protein content); ↑ digestibility; ↑ sensory properties.	Di Biase et al., 2019
White pan bread	Wheat flour	*L. plantarum* SPC-SNU 72-2 (KCTC13315BP) isolated from kimchi	- good baking capabilities; - rich aroma during dough fermentation; ↑ probiotic properties; - immunostimulating effect.	Park et al., 2019
Breads and doughs	whole-grain wheat and rye	*Candida milleri*, *Lactobacillus brevis*, and *L. plantarum*	- changes in metabolite profiles in the whole-grain wheat and rye; ↑ quantities for microbial metabolites of phenolic acids, phenolic acid derivatives, sugars or sugar derivatives, phosphatidylcholines and fatty acids.	Koistinen et al., 2018
Bread	Wheat flour	*L. plantarum* P8	- the bacteria in the bread crust, more thermo-stable than those in the crumb; ↑ bacterial viability, during storage.	Zhang et al., 2018
Bread	Wheat flour and 20% chia flour	*L. plantarum* C8	↓ consistency of the chia sourdough; ↑ viscous character of the chia sourdough; ↑ phenolic compound concentration and antioxidant activity of the sourdough and bread fermented by *L. plantarum* the specific; ↓ volume of the loaves; ↓ firmness and chewiness of the crumb; ↑ cohesiveness.	Bustos et al., 2017

Products	Fermentable substrate	*L. plantarum* strain	Influences of product properties	References
Bread	Wheat flour	*L. plantarum* UFG 121	- totally prevented the growth of *Fusarium culmorum*; - inhibited mold development in bread samples contaminated with *Aspergillus flavus, Penicillium chrysogenum*, and *Penicillium expansum*; - not inhibited mold development in bread samples contaminated with *Aspergillus niger* or *Penicillium roqueforti*.	Russo et al., 2017
Sourdough	Quinoa and wheat flour	*L. plantarum* CRL 778	↑ proteolytic activity (the release of organic acids, peptides, and amino acids from the breakdown of quinoa proteins by LAB); ↑ the level antifungal substances (phenyllactic and hydroxyphenyl lactic acids) in quinoa	Dallagnol et al., 2013
Bread	Wheat and oat flour	*L. plantarum*	- significant effects on the texture and crumb characteristics; ↑ flavour of the bread; -b-glucan decreased slightly.	Flander et al., 2011
Dough	Wheat and amaranth flour	*L. plantarum* AL30 and *L. paralimentarius* AL28	↑ rheological behavior	Houben et al., 2010
Bread	Wheat flour	*L. plantarum* FST 1.7	- *Fusarium culmorum* and *Fusarium graminearum* growth was strongly inhibited; ↑ shelf life; - good fermentation capacity of the sourdough; - produces bread of good quality.	Dal Bello et al., 2007
Crackers	Wheat flour and whole wheat flour	*L. plantarum* HLJ29L2 and yeast	↓ decreased the pH; ↓ protein digestibility; ↑ amino acid content.	Hu et al., 2023
Noodles	Oat flour	*L. bulgaria, L. plantarum, L. brevis, L. sanfrancisco*	↓ decreased the pH; ↓↑ gel strength and amylose content; ↓ viscosity; ↑ hardness and springiness; ↑ cooking quality.	Wan et al., 2011

The authors concluded that sourdough fermentation with single and co-cultures of LAB and yeast has various favorable effects, and the addition of soy flour increased sourdough quality. Sourdough containing 10% soy flour demonstrated improved rheological qualities as well as increased lactic, acetic, and citric acid production.

Recently, IIIlueca et al., 2023 showed that *L. plantarum* 5L1 strain could be successfully used for wheat sourdough fermentation influencing the drop of the pH value and the increase of the TTA value, mainly because of the acid metabolism production by *L. plantarum* 5L1 strain. On the other side, the antioxidant activity and the total phenolic content of the fermented sourdough improved through fermentation, meantime organic acids such as lactic increased its value. It is also important to mentioned that during wheat sourdough fermentation with *L. plantarum* 5L1 strain the protein hydrolysis plays a key role. Using SDS page *(Sodium Dodecyl Sulphate-Polyacrylamide Gel Electrophoresis)* authors demonstrated that *L. plantarum* 5L1 strain was able to realize a complete hydrolysis of the proteins with a molecular weight of 50 kDa entitled α-gliadins, which are mainly involved in causing celiac disease. Therefore, through wheat sourdough fermentation with *L. plantarum* 5L1 strain α-gliadins could be reduced, allowing the manufacturing of bread with low gluten free content.

Dallagnol et al., 2013, studied fermentative and proteolytic activities of *L. plantarum* CRL 778 in slurries prepared from wheat and quinoa flours. The release of organic acids, peptides, and amino acids from the breakdown of quinoa proteins by LAB may promote the growth and metabolic activity of these microorganisms. Thus, proteolytic activity of both slurries was indirectly activated by lactic fermentation. The results of this study showed that, while wheat protein hydrolysis was only 0–20%, quinoa protein hydrolysis was faster, reaching 40–100% after 8 hours of incubation. Furthermore, quinoa was shown to have higher concentrations of peptides and free amino acids than wheat. As a result, the antifungal strain *L. plantarum* CRL 778 produced higher levels of antifungal substances (phenyllactic and hydroxyphenyl lactic acids), about 2.6-fold higher in quinoa than in wheat slurry. These promising results showed that *L. plantarum* CRL 778 strain may be utilized in the quinoa sourdough manufacturing aiming to produce baked goods with enhanced nutritional quality and extended shelf life, able to be consumed by people diagnosed with celiac disease.

In another study, the addition of soy flour (SF) to wheat flour (WF) via fermentation using *L. plantarum* and *L. casei* cocultures was studied by Teleky et al., 2020a. Three different tests were performed: with 0% SF, 5% SF and 10% SF. The fermentation with these two LAB produced various favourable effects, which, when combined with increased SF content, improved the rheological and physicochemical properties of the dough. So, the dynamic rheological investigation revealed that doughs with soy flour had more stable elastic-like behaviour, while the dough fermentation with *L. plantarum* and *L. casei* cocultures produced excellent results in organic acid development, particularly increased lactic, citric, and tartaric acid generation.

Metabolic profiling of sourdough fermented wheat and rye bread, were studied by Koistinen et al., 2018. The authors used LC-QToF-MS (*Liquid Chromatography Quadrupole Time-of-Flight Mass Spectrometry*) to evaluate whole-grain wheat and rye breads and doughs produced with baker's yeast or with sourdough starter containing *Candida milleri, L. brevis*, and *L. plantarum*.

High concentrations of six sugars or sugar derivatives, two phosphatidylcholines [PC (18:2/18:2) and PC (18:2/18:3)], two fatty acids, and three microbial metabolites of phenolic acids (dihydroferulic acid, dihydrocaffeic acid, and dihydrosinapic acid) were found in the whole-grain rye sourdough and the corresponding bread. Additionally discovered as possibly bioactive substances in much larger amounts were 2-benzoxazolinone (benzoxazinoid), 2-hydroxyvaleric acid, isorhamnetin (flavonoid), N-acetylspermidine, and phenylethanolamine. Branched chain amino acids such as leucine and isoleucine, methionine and phenylalanine as well as small peptides increased their amounts mainly in rye sourdough and rye bread respectively, due to its intensive proteolysis process. The aforementioned amino-acids are involved in the insulin response process whilst the small peptides are claimed to have antioxidant potential and positive effect on antihypertensive activity. The impact of fermentation on the metabolic profile of whole rye grain was more significant compared with the wheat grain likely attributable to their different available range of chemical compounds and endogenous enzymes (Koistinen et al., 2018).

In the study conducted by Bustos et al., 2017 the rheological behavior, organic acid production, phenolic compound content and antioxidant activity of wheat/chia sourdough fermented by a selected *L. plantarum* strain were assessed. The wheat flour and chia flour ratio were 4:1 in both formulations (unfermented and fermented samples). Moreover, chia sourdough was used in the wheat bread manufacturing process and a functional and technological profile was carried out aiming to highlight the benefits of using fermented chia sourdough instead of unfermented one. Chia sourdough lost firmness and had a more viscous texture after 24 hours of lactic acid fermentation. The increase in proteolytic activity was observed in the chia dough fermented by the C8 strain which may be partially responsible for these rheological changes, as previously emphasised for wheat and rye sourdough (Clarke et al., 2004;

Thiele et al., 2012). Moreover, the authors argued that comparing to unfermented chia flour dough, lactic acid fermentation increased the organic acid mass fraction (lactic, acetic, and phenyl lactic acids to 12.3, 1.0, and 23.8 µg per kg of dough, respectively) and antioxidant activity by about 33 - 40%. Additionally, after 24 hours of fermentation by *L. plantarum* C8, the total phenolic content increased by 25% and its composition underwent significant modification. Also, the use of chia sourdough enhanced the physical and antioxidant qualities of conventional wheat bread, which were even better than those seen in the bread manufactured with unfermented chia flour.

In comparison to wheat bread, the inclusion of sourdough or chia flour decreased the specific volume of the loaves. Since pH steadily decreased during fermentation, enabling the activation of amylolytic and proteolytic enzymes, among others, to modify the dough components, it has been hypothesized that the influence of sourdough on bread volume is mostly caused by enzymatic processes that arise during fermentation. While the cohesiveness (textural parameter that is linked to the integration of components of a sample when it is subjected to deformation) of the wheat bread with chia sourdough and the wheat bread with chia flour both significantly increased, the addition of chia sourdough significantly decreased the stiffness and chewiness of the crumb compared to that of wheat bread. So, these researchers suggest that chia sourdough can be a promising substitute for wheat bread in terms of enhancing its technological and antioxidant properties (Bustos et al., 2017).

In the study performed by Üçok & Sert, 2020 the authors aimed to determine the growth kinetics and biomass properties of *L. plantarum* isolated from sourdough and to investigated the effects of the fermentation time on the technological performance of the sourdough dominated by *L. plantarum* strain. The kinetics growth of *L. plantarum* L14 were studied at 37°C for 28 hours in MRS medium, and wheat doughs fermented with *L. plantarum* L14 biomass were fermented for 1, 15, 20, and 25 hours, respectively. The doughs' acidity, cell number, and machinability were studied. The results of the study emphasized a positive trend between the increased acidity amount and dough cohesiveness and stickiness characteristics. This is also due to the higher acid tolerance of *L. plantarum* strain compared with other LAB. In addition, as compared to the literature, *L. plantarum* L14 had a high growth rate and biomass production.

Amaranth selective hydrolyzed protein (ASPH) could potentially enhance the characteristics of sourdough and bread quality. In this regard, Karimi et al., 2021, investigated the effect of ASPH on sourdough fermentation with *L.*

plantarum and *Saccharomyces cerevisiae* and on wheat bread qualities. The authors concluded that, ASHP further improved sourdough fermentation, in addition, the prepared sourdough using ASHP increased the specific volume and total titratable acidity, whereas it decreased the water activity and hardness bread. Also, bread with sourdough (S-ASPH) showed a softer texture, and the sensory properties and shelf life of bread increased with the ASHP addition.

In line with this, Houben et al., 2010 studied the influence of chemical acidification by lactic acid and the fermentation by two different lactobacilli strains (*L. plantarum* AL30 and *L. paralimentarius* AL28) on the amaranth dough rheological characteristics. The addition of lactic acid to the wheat-amaranth dough only had a positive effect in the dough firmness but there was no really satisfying changes on its rheological behaviour. In the case of wheat-amaranth dough fermentation with different lactobacillus strains the rheological behaviour has been improved. The use of *L. plantarum* AL30 had the greatest influence. The authors concluded that the rheological parameters of sourdough addition in the case of amaranth dough were not only based on the amount of acid but as well as on their metabolic activity.

The effect of the sorghum seed flour and fermentation with *L. plantarum* was studied by Apostol et al., 2020 for six bread samples. In this study six bread formulation based on sorghum seed flour and wheat flour (30:70; 33:55 and 40:40), salt, dried yeast and water was proposed, from which three samples were fortified with *L. plantarum* compared to the other three bread samples without the addition of any LAB. A control bread sample made with wheat flour was compared to each of the six bread samples. By this approach, authors reported that the porosity decreased with increasing degree of sorghum seeds flour replacement from 75,7% to 68,6%, respectively. On the other hand, there was a negative trend regarding the porosity parameter which decreased, as the addition of *L. plantarum* increased reaching values from 75.7% to 71.3%, from 71.8% to 66.7%, or from 68.6% to 64%, respectively. Every time sorghum seed flour or *L. plantarum* was added, the porosity value was less than the control sample's (77.8%). The same effects of adding sorghum seeds flour were observed on the elasticity since the value obtained in the case of the control sample (97%) was considerably higher than experimental variants (92%, 76% and 74%). Similarly, *L. plantarum* led to a decrease in the elasticity of the product from 92% to 90%, respectively from 76% to 75%, or from 74% to 72%. The acidity was significantly influenced by the presence of *L. plantarum*, the values being higher that of samples without *L. plantarum*, however within normal limits according to the standards in force. Magnesium, potassium, and iron concentrations were also higher than in wheat flour.

Besides, in bread samples containing LAB, there was a noticeable improvement in the sensory properties.

Woo et al., 2020 investigated the application of maltogenic amylase derived from *L. plantarum* (LpMA) as an antistaling enzyme. Furthermore, in order to boost the expression level of LpMA in *L. plantarum*, it was grown on a modified medium (De Man, Rogosa, and Sharpe (MRS) medium supplemented with an additional 6% glucose), and the cell extract - CELP (crude enzyme) was then used to bake the bread and delay staling. By changing the growth conditions, the expression of the LpMA in *L. plantarum* increased 54 times, causing an antistaling action of the cell extract. During the 7 day storage at 4°C, the CELP- treated bread displayed a 25% slower retrogradation rate and a 63% lower hardness than the control bread.

Flander et al., 2011 studied how sourdough fermentation of wheat flour with *L. plantarum* affected the quality features of mixed oat-wheat bread (51 g whole grain oat flour and 49 g/100 g white wheat flour). The emphasis was placed on both ß-glucan stability bread structure and sensory quality. The amount of sourdough used and the temperature at which was fermented had a considerable impact on the texture and crumb qualities of the oat-wheat bread. Also, a slight degradation of ß-glucan occurred during proofing and baking, but it was not affected by the bread acidity variation. The authors of this study demonstrated that the use of an optimized sourdough process in the production of oat bread provides a feasible technology for producing new tasty variants of oat bread with a high ß-glucan content.

The effects of LAB fermentation on gel strength, pasting properties, and the amylose content of oat flour using different LAB (*L. bulgaria, L. plantarum, L. brevis, L. sanfrancisco*) and different fermentation times were studied by Wan et al., 2011. Likewise, authors also studied the suitability of oat flour for noodle making process by investigating the texture and cooking quality of the fermented oat noodles produced. The results of the study showed that fermented samples had a significantly lower pH, gel strength and amylose content which initially increased and then decreased, whilst viscosity decreased with fermentation time. Furthermore, fermented noodles demonstrated improved hardness and springiness values, samples fermented with *L. plantarum* highlighting the greatest springiness, cohesiveness, gumminess, chewiness, and resilience values after 12 hours of fermentation. Regarding to cooking quality, fermentation was found to improve the quality of oat starch noodles. When compared to noodles prepared from fresh flour, noodles manufactured from fermented oats had lower cooking loss and higher cooking weight.

Another study Di Biase et al., 2019, had as purpose to improve the nutritional profile of yeast leavened salt reduced sliced bread and puccia type bread fortified with a wheat-based *L. plantarum* ITM21B fermentation product (Bio21B). Thus, the protein content of bread prepared in the lab was increased by using 15% chickpea flour (CF) addition and wheat-based fermentation product (Bio21B) or Bio21B including a fungal protease to promote gluten hydrolysis. According to the study's results, breads with peculiar sensory properties were produced at both laboratory and industrial scales, along with improved amino acid, protein content and high digestibility degree. In comparison to the control bread, the laboratory bread made with Bio21B and CF had more total free amino acids content and acidic metabolites, primarily phenyllactic (PLA) and hydroxy-phenyllactic (OH-PLA) ones. The addition of CF to the bread formula significantly increased the protein content, mainly acidic GG (glutenins + gliadins) and AG (albumin + globulins) fractions. Remarkably, the acidity caused by the fermentation product *L. plantarum* ITM21 allowed for the complete digestion of AG fractions, which include the legume's storage proteins, which are normally poorly hydrolyzed by digestive enzymes. As a result, the authors argue that this research represents a strategy for overcoming the disadvantages of using legume flour in bread products due to the low digestion of proteins, to their structure and the presence of antinutritional compounds (Di Biase et al., 2019).

Sourdough fermentation has been widely used in bakery products. However, there has been limited study of the effect of fermentation on the dough and cracker products. The influence of co-fermentation with *L. plantarum* HLJ29L2 and yeast on wheat protein digestibility of cracker was studied by Hu et al., 2023. During co-fermentation with *L. plantarum* HLJ29L2 and yeast, *L. plantarum* HLJ29L2 developed quickly and produced a considerable amount of organic acids in the sourdough. This drastically organic acid production decreased the pH value and stimulated the sourdough's protease activity, promoting protein breakdown. So, the protein digestibility of cracker was greatly increased by co fermentation with *L. plantarum* HLJ29L2 and yeast. At the same time, the free amino acid content of crackers increased by 20%.

Recently, Demirkesen-Bicak et al., 2021 showed that glycemic index, textural and sensory properties of the bread could be influenced by the type of fermentation and temperature used for sourdough manufacturing. The authors manufactured bread with sourdough made from wheat and whole wheat flour using a fermentation temperature of 25°C and 30°C, respectively, and two type of fermentations (type 1 and type 2). The type 1 fermentation was made through spontaneous fermentation, whilst, type 2 fermentation was made with the help of the following LAB: *L. plantarum* ELB75, *L. brevis ELB99* and *Saccharomyces cerevisiae* TGM55 strain. The results highlighted that type 2 fermentation together with controlled temperature, emphasised better results regarding the resistant starch content, glycemic index value, textural and sensory properties compared with spontaneous fermentation. Higher specific volume of the bread and improved hardness values was obtained with sourdough fermented at 30°C and type-2 fermentation. The improved textural parameters were justified by the presence of lactic acid generated by LAB which can lead to hydrolysis, enlargement, and improved solubility gluten protein whilst, LAB strains could produce exopolysaccharides, another crucial element that influence in a positive way the texture of the bread. The reduction of the bread glycemic index value may be due to the presence of organic acids which are a result of the controlled LAB and yeast strain fermentation. For instance, lactic acid is involved in lowering the starch digestion rate, meantime the propionic and acetic acids dropped the pH value of the small intestine which may reduce the α-amylase and α-glucosides starch digestion enzymes (Demirkesen-Bicak et al., 2021).

In line with this, Akamine et al., 2023 defined the glycemic index as the speed that sugar is able to enter in our bloodstream and mentioned that probiotic can positively affect glycemic index value. Moreover, Akamine et al., 2023 claimed that acetic acid is able to bring out a delayed gastric emptying rate whilst, lactic acid diminished insulinemic responses.

Costantini et al., 2022 concluded that in the digestibility degree of the final baked products several factors are involved, such as the antinutritional factors amount, hydrolysis of protein during food manufacturing and digestion process, satiety level and gastrointestinal symptoms after the food intake. The authors identified that long time fermentation sourdough improved in a positive way the bread digestibility and that breads manufactured with whole cereals such as wheat, spelt or rye fermented with selected LAB with high peptidase activity, at an optimal temperature of 37°C with the addition of fungal proteases increased their *in vitro* digestibility level. Furthermore, the consumption of the aforementioned sourdough breads is correlated with a high quality protein level and with a low glycemic post-prandial response.

In the study made by Park et al., 2019, the feasibility of using of *L. plantarum* SPC-SNU 72-2 (KCTC13315BP) as a sourdough starter to produce functional breads was evaluated. The *L. plantarum* 72-2 strain demonstrated probiotic properties like as food safety, high tolerance to gastrointestinal stress, and high adherence to human epithelial cells. Furthermore, the baking characteristics of the 72-2 strain were identical to the commercial sourdough starter, *Lallemand* L73, and the usage of this strain produced better physicochemical results than the use of yeast alone. Authors concluded that *L. plantarum* 72-2 strain had good baking capabilities, generating a rich aroma during dough fermentation and helping to improve bread quality thus, highlighting a great potential in manufacturing functional breads with immunostimulating effect.

Probiotics are considered live microorganisms that have several positive effects on human health such as improving gut microbiota, preventing bone health diseases, respiratory tract infection, several allergies, obesity and even mental health. Even if sourdough probiotics are not naturally present in the intestine environment, they are able to provide gastrointestinal benefits, such as pre-digestion of the anti-nutritional factors like phytic acid (Akamine et al., 2023).

Zhang et al., 2018 investigated the effect of different baking settings and subsequent storage on the survival of a model strain *L. plantarum* P8. Bread samples varied in dough weights (5, 30, and 60 g) were baked for 8 minutes at different temperatures (175, 205, and 235°C), with the residual viability of bacteria evaluated every 2 minutes. Bacterial viability was assessed for both bread crust and crumb since they have different temperature-moisture parameters during baking with related microstructural features. The results showed that despite the increased temperature in the crust during baking under specific conditions, bacteria in the crust were found to be more thermo-stable than those in the crumb. The decreased moisture level of the crust, as well as its dense and glassy microstructure, may benefit the thermo-stability of bacteria in the crust during baking. The population of probiotic bacteria recovered to greater than 10^6 cfu/g in the crumb and 10^8 cfu/g in the crust after 4 day storage, correlating to the changing pH and titratable acidity (TTA) of bread during storage.

L. plantarum UFG 121, a strain with documented wide antifungal activity (Crowley et al., 2013; Russo et al., 2017), was investigated as a potential protective culture for bread production by Russo et al., 2017. The study was carried out on artificially contaminated bread after one week of storage, evaluating the ability of *L. plantarum* UFG 121 to control the growth of six different species of filamentous fungi belonging to three different genera: *Aspergillus* spp., *Penicillium* spp., and *Fusarium culmorum*. Wheat bread was manufactured in two ways: (a) with a commercial *Saccharomyces cerevisiae* strain inoculated into the dough (control) and (b) with a commercial

Saccharomyces cerevisiae strain and *L. plantarum* UFG 121 inoculated into the dough.

After one week of storage, *L. plantarum* strain totally prevented the growth of *Fusarium culmorum*. The LAB inhibited mold development in samples contaminated with *Aspergillus flavus*, *Penicillium chrysogenum*, and *Penicillium expansum*, but not in the bread with *Aspergillus niger* or *Penicillium roqueforti*. These research supports the potential of *L. plantarum* UFG 121 as a biocontrol agent in bread production and reveal that mold sensitivity varies by species or strain. Furthermore, it is suggested that a new generation of mixed starting protection cultures, active against several fungus species, may be better able to significantly extend the shelf life of baked goods (Russo, Arena, et al., 2017).

In the study carried out by Dal Bello et al., 2007, the ability of *L. plantarum* FST 1.7 to produce antifungal chemicals during sourdough fermentation and to create bread with good quality and longer shelf life was investigated. *In vitro* testing for antimicrobial activity revealed that *L. plantarum* FST 1.7 is effective against deteriorating bacteria and fungi, the studies being carried out on *Fusarium culmorum* and *Fusarium graminearum* two fungi found on breads. The three principal components identified as being responsible for antimicrobial activity were lactic acid, phenyllactic acid, and the two dipeptides cycle (L-Leu-L-Pro) and cycle (L-Phe-L-Pro).

In this study a biologically acidified (using *Lactobacillus sanfranciscensis* ferment sourdough), a chemically acidified, and a non-acidified loaf were compared to bread made with *L. plantarum* fermented sourdough. The total titratable acidity (TTA) value of bread made with *L. plantarum* was equivalent to that of both sourdough using *L. sanfranciscensis* and artificially acidified breads, although having a substantially higher pH than the other breads. Compared to either the nonacidified or the chemically acidified treatments, the addition of *L. plantarum* fermented sourdough produced breads with higher specific loaf volumes and displayed a softer crumb. Thus, in this study it was demonstrated that *L. plantarum* FST 1.7 was able to controlled sourdough fermentation, yields bread of high quality, and had inhibitory action against *Fusarium* in both sourdough and bread produced with the strain. Moreover, has the potential to lengthen the shelf-life of bread under normal conditions without the use of mold spores.

Russo et al., 2017 studied growth inhibition of *Fusarium graminearum* and deoxynivalenol detoxification (DON) by lactic acid bacteria and their application in sourdough bread. For this research, eight LAB were taken into study: *Lactobacillus casei* LC2W, *Bifidobacterium animalis* AR668, *L.*

plantarum AR113, *L. plantarum* AR523, *L. plantarum* AR524, *L. plantarum* AR526, *L. plantarum* AR527, and *L. plantarum* AR528, respectively. Additionally, the selected LAB strains were applied as starter cultures to their performance during the bread-making process, using a standard recipe, made up of 200 g of wheat flour, 100 g of sourdough, 2 g of salt, 18 g of sucrose, 12 g of oil, and 100 mL of water. The growth of *Fusarium graminearum* was strongly inhibited by *L. plantarum* AR524 in a pH-dependent manner, and up to 40.9% of the DON was eliminated. Its antifungal action was mostly due to the antifungal chemical compounds produced by LAB and the resulting pH lowering (such as acetic acid, propionic acid, and phenyllactic acid). The addition of *L. plantarum* AR524 to sourdough considerably reduced DON levels (50.53%) and development of *Fusarium graminearum* (60.19%). *L. plantarum* AR524 also significantly improved the bread's textural attributes, extending its shelf life from three to six days without the use of any chemical preservatives. Thus, it can be stated that *L. plantarum* AR524 exhibits high potential for use as a bioprotective starter culture in bread products, according to this study's argument (Cao et al., 2021).

1.3. Application of *L. plantarum* in Gluten-Free Bakery Products

When it comes to discuss about gluten-free products, *L. plantarum* was found to have been used since ancient times, LAB being considered as cell factories capable of delivering bioactive substances and food ingredients, resulting in higher quality of gluten free (GF) goods (Arent et al., 2011; Zannin et al., 2012). It is important to note that *L. plantarum* itself does not have any direct impact on gluten content. Gluten is a protein found in grains like wheat, barley, and rye, and it is responsible for the elasticity and structure of dough in baked goods. Gluten-free products are specifically formulated to be free of gluten-containing ingredients or cross-contamination with gluten. These products often use alternative flours and binders to achieve similar textures and structures with conventional products but without the need for gluten (Moghaddam et al., 2020).

Studies have shown that the application of sourdough biotechnology to naturally gluten-free ingredients, such as GF cereals, pseudocereals, and legumes, improved the sensory, technological, nutritional, and functional properties of final products, similar to the positive effects described for the samples containing gluten flours (Moroni et al., 2009; Nionelli and Rizzello, 2016).

Raw matrix carbohydrates play an important function in LAB's adaptability into a new environment. These make up the majority of flour, with starch, simple sugars, and fiber being the most important components. Starch granules are broken during milling, and the amylose and amylopectin glucose polymers can be hydrolyzed to simple molecules like maltose and glucose (Chiş et al., 2020).

L. plantarum may be added to gluten-free products for various reasons.

Regarding the fermentation, *L. plantarum* can aid in fermentation processes, contributing to the flavour and texture of gluten-free products. It can enhance the development of desirable flavors and textures during fermentation, such as in gluten-free bread or sourdough.

Regarding, the shelf life and food safety, *L. plantarum* has antimicrobial properties and can help extend the shelf life of gluten-free products by inhibiting the growth of harmful bacteria or molds. This is explained by the fact that during the fermentation process, LAB convert carbohydrates into organic acids, primarily lactic acid. The accumulation of lactic acid leads to a decrease in the pH of the food, creating an acidic environment. This lowered pH inhibits the growth and activity of spoilage microorganisms, such as certain bacteria, yeasts, and molds (de Sousa Moraes et al., 2014; Moghaddam et al., 2020; Wang et al., 2021).

Regarding the probiotic benefits, *L. plantarum* is considered a beneficial bacteria and is known to support gut health. Adding it to gluten-free products can provide the potential health benefits associated with probiotics (Ghasemi et al., 2022).

The use of millet in the production of gluten-free sourdough can offer significant benefits, particularly for individuals with gluten sensitivity. Many studies highlighted that LAB and yeasts were screened for their functional properties in sourdough preparation using both unmalted and malted millet (Banwo et al., 2020). The selection of the LAB and yeast starters in the study was based on two specific properties: acidification and exopolysaccharide production (EPS). Starters with strong acidification properties were likely chosen to ensure the desired characteristics in the resulting sourdough bread. These EPS played a significant role in dough rheology, texture, and overall sensory properties of bread. Starters capable of producing exopolysaccharides were likely selected to enhance the texture and sensory profile of the gluten-free millet sourdough bread, as shown in the study. Overall, the sourdough bread samples were acceptable in terms of sensory evaluation. The bread made from malted flour and spontaneously fermented showed the highest overall acceptability rating, indicating that this particular combination was favoured by the sensory panel. This suggested that the fermentation process and the specific combination of microorganisms used can influence the taste, aroma, and texture of the final product. Moreover, the nutritional composition of the gluten-free bread samples varied in terms of protein, ash, and fiber content. These values ranged from 10.1 to 11.4 g/100 g for protein, 2.2 to 4.5 g/100 g for ash, and 1.45 to 1.74 g/100 g for fiber. Millet itself is known to be a good source of protein and dietary fiber, which contributes to the nutritional value of the sourdough gluten free-bread (Banwo et al., 2020).

The study conducted by Chiş et al., 2020, supports the use of controlled fermentation with lactic acid bacteria, specifically *L. plantarum ATCC 8014*, for the production of gluten-free baked products using quinoa flour. It highlighted the beneficial effects of fermentation on the nutritional profile and antioxidant activity of muffins final product. The study utilized two types of sourdough: quinoa sourdough fermented with *L. plantarum* ATCC 8014 and quinoa sourdough spontaneously fermented. The results indicated that the use of *L. plantarum ATCC 8014* influenced the chemical composition of the muffins. Specifically, it led to a decrease in carbohydrate content, higher levels of organic acids, and increased folic acid content. Furthermore, the fermentation with *L. plantarum ATCC 8014* resulted in higher levels of flavonoids, total phenols, and increased radical scavenging activity in the muffins. These findings suggest that the use of this strain in the fermentation process positively affects the nutritional composition and antioxidant properties of quinoa-based baked gluten free goods.

Buckwheat flour fermented by *L. plantarum* has been shown to improve the functional qualities of gluten-free muffins, according to Zielinski et al.'s, 2017 study. When compared to control muffins prepared from commercially available gluten-free maize flour, the functional characteristics of four samples of gluten-free muffins made from unfermented and fermented (by *L. plantarum*) buckwheat flour were evaluated. In comparison to muffins made with unfermented buckwheat flour, those made with fermented buckwheat flour displayed a significantly higher antioxidant capacity, increased activity against the formation of advanced glycation end products (AGEs), increased available lysine content, and a higher browning index. The study discovered that gluten-free muffins' functional characteristics might be enhanced by using buckwheat flour that has been fermented by *L. plantarum*.

Considering the excellent fermentation performance and favourable nutritional composition, buckwheat and quinoa flours could be utilized as sourdough substrates to enhance gluten-free bread. The results of the study conducted by Wolter et al., 2014, indicated that the mentioned flours, can be effectively fermented by *L. plantarum FST 1.7.* Among the flours tested, quinoa and buckwheat showed the strongest acidification performance during sourdough fermentation. These flours are nutritionally beneficial, as they contain high levels of lysine and methionine. However, the study did not observe any improvement in the microbial shelf life of the bread. It was concluded that the sensory quality of gluten-free bread with mentioned flours still needs to be improved considering that 20% sourdough addition was insufficient to degrade odorants with negative aromas in the flour or generate positive odorants during fermentation. Alternatively, the study suggests that sprouting and toasting gluten-free grains could be used to create favourable toasted and nutty flavours in the bread. This process may also increase the release of amino acids through proteolysis, which can serve as flavour precursors.

Other study results demonstrate the possibility of developing gluten-free breads using 100% fermented quinoa. Fermentation with *L. plantarum* (JC5 and JCM1149) strains improved the characteristics of the quinoa dough, leading to breads with desirable texture, sensory attributes, and nutritional composition (Ceballos-González et al., 2018). The results indicated that after 2 days of fermentation with either strain, the dough exhibited higher levels of soluble protein content and improved textural properties compared to unfermented quinoa dough. This suggests that the fermentation process helped enhance the protein content and overall texture of the dough. Furthermore, the breads produced from the fermented quinoa dough showed desirable characteristics. They had a homogeneous porous crumb, good sensory quality, and high nutritional value. These findings suggest that fermented quinoa can be a valuable option for individuals with gluten sensitivities or celiac disease.

Svensson et al., 2010, demonstrates that microbial fermentation of red sorghum variety PAN 3860, fermented with *Lactobacilli*, affected the content of polyphenols and influenced the nutritional value and antimicrobial activity of sorghum. The authors investigated sorghum sourdoughs fermented with two binary strain combinations, *L. plantarum* and *L. casei* or *L. fermentum* and *L. reuteri*, compared to chemically acidified sample controls. Thus, caffeoylglycerol, dicaffeoylglycerol, coumaroyl-caffeoylglycerol, and coumaroyl-feruloylglycerol, four previously undetected glycerol esters in sorghum, were tentatively found. Phenolic acids, phenolic acid esters, and flavonoid glucosides were all broken down during lactic fermentation. Both phenolic acid decarboxylases and phenolic acid reductases are responsible for the breakdown of phenolic acids in lactic fermented sorghum doughs. Both binary strain combinations metabolized caffeine, coumaric acid, and ferulic acid, however, *Lb. plantarum* and *Lb. casei* did not metabolize protocatechuic acid. Ferulic acid decreased but not decarboxylated by *L. plantarum* and *L. fermentum* during single strain fermentations in MRS. Although flavonoid hexoxides were only partially hydrolyzed in chemically acidified doughs, they were quantitatively metabolized during lactic fermentations. Eriodictyol and naringenin concentrations were significantly greater in lactic fermented doughs than they were in flour for the flavonoid hexoxides, indicating that flavonoids bound to insoluble cell wall components had been released.

The potential of *L. plantarum* FST 1.7, a strain known for producing antifungal compounds, to improve the quality and shelf life of gluten-free bread has also been reported by the researchers Moore et al., 2008. The strain's antifungal properties were shown to inhibit mold growth, which is beneficial for enhancing the bread's overall preservation. The effects of incorporating sourdough fermented by *L. plantarum FST 1.7* into a gluten-free bread mixture (brown rice flour, corn starch, buckwheat, soya flour) were compared to sourdough fermented by a non-antifungal strain, *L. sanfranciscensis* TMW 1.52, as well as chemically or non-acidified batters. The researchers conducted fundamental rheological tests to assess the dough's characteristics and observed an increase in firmness and elasticity over time ($p < 0.05$) when sourdough was added to the gluten-free mix. The results showed that the gluten-free breads acidified using sourdough fermentation were softer compared to those chemically acidified ($p < 0.001$). Furthermore, the researchers conducted antifungal challenge tests using a fungal species called *Fusarium culmorum*. The results demonstrated that *L. plantarum* FST 1.7, in comparison to the control groups, inhibited the growth rate of the fungal species, suggesting its potential as an antifungal agent in gluten-free bread (Moore et al., 2008).

The lactic acid bacteria *L. brevis* E139 and *L. plantarum* E138 were also experimentally selected by Parakhina et al., 2021 for new gluten-free sourdoughs which are based on corn starch, rice flour, extruded corn starch, soy protein isolate. Bread made with sourdoughs had more pronounced taste and flavour, brighter crust colour and better texture compared with bread without sourdough. The authors concluded that both of sourdough composition may be recommended for applications in the gluten-free bread-making process.

The corn sourdough lactic acid bacteria were assessed by Moghaddam, 2019 to manufacture gluten-free bread, and the combination of rice and corn flour was investigated to see if it could improve the quality and organoleptic qualities of bread. *L. plantarum* ATCC 20179 and *L. fermentum* ATCC 9338 were employed as starter cultures to make corn sourdough. The study concluded that fermented sourdough affects all positive aspects including stiffness and staling, flavour, shelf-life against microbial spoilage, and other useful properties of bread. Therefore, fermented sourdough can have a favourable impact on sensory and rheological characteristics of bread.

LAB-inoculated sourdough and olive leaf extract can be considered as viable alternatives to gluten, contributing to the improvement of the structure and acceptability of gluten-free bread (Moghaddam et al., 2020). The study highlights the potential of these ingredients in enhancing the quality, nutritional value, and shelf-life of gluten-free bread, based on using corn-based and rice-based sourdough inoculated with *L. plantarum* (ATCC 14917) and *L. fermentum* (ATCC 9338) providing alternatives for individuals with celiac disease or gluten intolerance. Overall, the utilization of LAB-inoculated sourdough and olive leaf extract positively influenced various quality aspects of the bread, including taste, staleness, odor, chewability, softness, moisture content, pH, acidity, and texture. Moreover, these ingredients were found to enhance the antifungal properties of the bread, leading to an extended shelf-life.

Several notable findings revealed how microencapsulation affects the physicochemical properties, staling, and viability of probiotic bacteria in gluten-free sorghum bread (Ghasemi et al., 2022). Specifically, *L. acidophilus* and *L. plantarum* were chosen as the probiotic bacteria, and tragacanth gum and sago starch were employed for encapsulation purposes. The encapsulation of probiotic bacteria improved moisture retention in the bread during both the baking and storage processes. This, in turn, resulted in a reduction in the intensity of staling, which refers to the deterioration of bread quality over time. The encapsulation process also had a positive impact on the survival of probiotic bacteria during baking and storage, increasing their viability by more than 2 log cycles. These findings suggest that microencapsulation can be a valuable technique for improving the quality and functionality of probiotic-enriched gluten-free bread products.

Conclusion

Sourdough fermentation is an old technique for fermenting cereal flour, which improves bakery products quality, providing also nutritional and health benefits. The fermented dough has a diverse microbiome primarily formed by lactic acid bacteria and yeasts. The metabolic activity of the naturally occurring or inoculated LAB is responsible for the distinctive features of sourdough. Among the outstanding processes during sourdough fermentation by LAB are lactic fermentation, proteolysis, synthesis of volatile compounds and anti-mold activity. In this chapter was summarized the applicability of *L. plantarum* species in the production of bakery and pastry products, as well as the beneficial role that microbial fermentation plays in the development of bakery products with high nutritional value, improved texture and taste, and a longer shelf life. Therefore, *L. plantarum*, is one of the most widely studied species which is used in the bakery and pastry industry as a probiotic microorganism and/or microbial starter in order to improve texture and flavour of products and prolong the shelf-life. Furthermore, *L. plantarum* species are extremely adaptable, as they can ferment gluten-free flours to generate functional bread rich in bioactive components and with adequate texture features. *L. plantarum* was frequently used in bakery products to ferment a variety of substrates, including wheat flour (*Triticum aestivum*), flour of ancient wheat species (einkorn, spelt, emmer), flour of sorghum, rye, maize, oats, buckwheat, rice, amaranth, millet, chickpeas, quinoa, chia, lentils and soybeans. These products support growth of heterofermentative LAB to improve the final quality of bakery products in terms of texture and sensory features (impart a distinctive flavour and aroma to the final products), the nutritional profile, antioxidant activity but also for to give a better digestibility degree.

Other studies have shown the potential of this starter culture to control spoilage microorganisms in bread production, prolonging the product shelf-life without adding any chemical preservatives. Lactic acid and other organic acids, phenolic compounds, carbon dioxide, ethanol, hydrogen peroxide, fatty acids, acetoin, diacetyl, and cyclic dipeptides were found to have antifungal activity. Additionally, synergistic interactions between various bioactive molecules may significantly boost the total antimicrobial activity of LAB. According to research, *L. plantarum* AR524 exhibits high potential for use as a bioprotective starter culture in bread products, considerably reduced DON levels (50.53%) and development of *Fusarium* graminearum (60.19%), also significantly improved the bread's textural attributes, extending its shelf life from three to six days without the use of any chemical preservatives.

Also, *L. plantarum* UFG 121, a strain with wide antifungal activity was investigated as a potential protective culture for bread production. After one week of storage, the *L. plantarum* strain totally prevented the growth of *Fusarium culmorum*. The lactic acid bacterium inhibited mold development in samples contaminated with *Aspergillus flavus*, *Penicillium chrysogenum*, and *Penicillium expansum*, but not in the bread with *Aspergillus niger* or *Penicillium roqueforti*. This research supported the potential of *L. plantarum* UFG 121 as a biocontrol agent in bread production and revealed that mold sensitivity varies by species or strain. Furthermore, studies suggest that a new generation of mixed starting protection cultures, active against several fungus species, may be better able to significantly extend the shelf life of baked goods. Another study claimed that *L. plantarum* FST 1.7 dominated sourdough fermentation, yields bread of high quality, and had inhibitory action against *Fusarium* in both sourdough and bread. Moreover, had the potential to prolonged the shelf-life of bread under normal conditions without the use of mold spores.

Maltogenic amylase originated from *L. plantarum* was found to have antistaling effect by inducing a slower starch retrogradation rate together with lower hardness in white wheat bread. *L. plantarum*, it was grown on a modified medium (De Man, Rogosa, and Sharpe (MRS) medium supplemented with an additional 6% glucose), and the cell extract - CELP (crude enzyme) was then used to bake the bread and delay staling. During the 7 day storage at 4°C, the CELP- treated bread displayed a 25% slower retrogradation rate and a 63% lower hardness than the control bread.

Moreover, fermentation with *L. plantarum* strains revealed increasing firmness and elasticity even in the case of gluten-free bread. Sourdough fermentation, in particular, has been found to be highly effective in enhancing the flavour, shelf life, and structure of gluten-free bread but also in improving the quality of some pastry products. Thus, *L. plantarum* ATCC 8014 influenced the chemical composition of the muffins based on quinoa flour. Specifically, it led to a decrease in carbohydrate content, higher levels of organic acids, and increased folic acid content. Furthermore, the fermentation with *L. plantarum* ATCC 8014 resulted in higher levels of flavonoids, total phenols, and increased radical scavenging activity in the muffins. These findings suggest that the use of this strain in the fermentation process positively affects the nutritional composition and antioxidant properties of baked gluten free goods.

Sourdough offers undeniable advantages over conventional leavening agents in terms of sensory, rheology, shelf life, and many nutritional properties due to its unique and diverse microbial composition.

References

[1] Abdelazez, A., Heba, A., Zhu, Z., and Sami, R. (2018). Potential benefits of *Lactobacillus plantarum* as probiotic and its advantages in human health and industrial applications: A review. *Advances in Environmental Biology*, 12 (1). https://doi.org/10.22587/aeb.2018.12.1.4.

[2] Akamine, I. T., Mansoldo, F. R. P., and Vermelho, A. B. (2023). Probiotics in the sourdough bread fermentation: Current Status. *Fermentation*, *9*(2). https://doi.org/10.3390/fermentation9020090.

[3] Apostol, L., Belc, N., Gaceu, L., Oprea, O. B., and Popa, M. E. (2020). Sorghum flour: A valuable ingredient for bakery industry? *Applied Sciences (Switzerland)*, *10*(23), 1–16. https://doi.org/10.3390/app10238597.

[4] Arasu, M. V., Al-Dhabi, N., Ilavenil, S., Choi, K. C., and Srigopalram, S. (2016). In vitro importance of probiotic Lactobacillus plantarum related to medical field. *Saudi Journal of Biological Sciences*, *23*(1), S6–S10. https://doi.org/10.1016/j.sjbs.2015.09.022.

[5] Arena, M. P., Russo, P., Spano, G., and Capozzi, V. (2020). From microbial ecology to innovative applications in food quality improvements: The case of sourdough as a model matrix. *J. Multidiscip. Sci. J.* 3, 3. doi:10.3390/j3010003.

[6] Arendt, E. K., Moroni, A., and Zannini, E. (2011). Medical nutrition therapy: Use of sourdough lactic acid bacteria as a cell factory for delivering functional biomolecules and food ingredients in gluten free bread. *Microb. Cell Fact.* 10 (Suppl. 1), 1–9. doi:10.1186/1475-2859-10-S1-S15.

[7] Arora, K., Ameur, H., Polo, A., Di Cagno, R., Rizzello, C. G., and Gobbetti, M. (2021). Thirty years of knowledge on sourdough fermentation: A systematic review. *Trends in Food Science and Technology*, *108*, 71–83. https://doi.org/10.1016/j.tifs.2020.12.008.

[8] Axel, C., Brosnan, B., Zannini, E., Peyer, L. C., Furey, A., Coey, A., and Arendt, E. K. (2016). Antifungal activities of three dierent Lactobacillus species and their production of antifungal carboxylic acids in wheat sourdough. *Appl. Microbiol. Biotechnol.* 2016, 100, 1701–1711.

[9] doi: 10.1007/s00253-015-7051-x.

[10] Banwo, K., Fasuyi, T. O., and Olojede, A. O. (2020). Potentials of *Lactobacillus plantarum* and *Pichia kudriavzevii* in co-fermentation of sourdough from millet. *International Journal of Food Science and Technology*, 0–3. https://doi.org/10.1111/ijfs.14729.

[11] Bircan, D, Güray, C. T., and Bostan, K. (2017). Studies on Sour Dough Bread Making by Different Methods. *Aydın Gastronomy,* 1: 1-8.

[12] Beldean, B. V., Chiș, M. S., Alexa, E., Pop, C., Păucean, A., Man, S., Igual, M., Haydee, K. M., Dalma, K. E., Stănilă, S., Socaci, S., Fărcaș, A., Berbecea, A., Popescu, I., and Muste, S. (2022). The impact of insect flour on sourdough fermentation-fatty acids, amino-acids, minerals and volatile profile. *Insects*, *13*(7). https://doi.org/10.3390/insects13070576.

[13] Bustos, A. Y., Gerez, C. L., Mohtar Mohtar, L. G., Paz Zanini, V. I., Nazareno, M. A., Taranto, M. P., and Iturriaga, L. B. (2017). Lactic acid fermentation improved

textural behaviour, phenolic compounds and antioxidant activity of Chia (*Salvia hispanica* L.) dough. *Food Technology and Biotechnology*, *55*(3), 381–389. https://doi.org/10.17113/ft b.55.03.17.5133.

[14] Byanju, B., Hojilla-Evangelista, M. P., and Lamsal, B. P. (2021). Fermentation performance and nutritional assessment of physically processed lentil and green pea flour. *Journal of the Science of Food and Agriculture*, *101*(14), 5792–5806. https://doi.org/10.1002/jsfa.11229.

[15] Cao, H., Meng, D., Zhang, W., Ye, T., Yuan, M., Yu, J., Wu, X., Li, Y., Yin, F., Fu, C., and Xu, F. (2021). Growth inhibition of Fusarium graminearum and deoxynivalenol detoxification by lactic acid bacteria and their application in sourdough bread. *International Journal of Food Science and Technology*, *56*(5), 2304–2314. https://doi.org/10.1111/ijfs.14852.

[16] Cappelle, S., Guylaine, L., Gänzle, M., and Gobbetti, M. (2023). *History and Social Aspects of Sourdough. Handbook on Sourdough Biotechnology* (pp.1-13). DOI:10.1007/978-3-031-23084-4_1.

[17] Capozzi, V., Russo, P., Dueñas, M. T., López, P., and Spano, G. (2012). Lactic acid bacteria producing B-group vitamins: A great potential for functional cereals products. *Applied Microbiology and Biotechnology*, *96*(6), 1383–1394. https://doi.org/10.1007/s00253-012-4440-2.

[18] Ceballos-González, C., Bolívar-Monsalve, J., Ramírez-Toro, C., and Bolívar, G. A. (2018). Effect of lactic acid fermentation on quinoa dough to prepare gluten-free breads with high nutritional and sensory quality. *Journal of Food Processing and Preservation*, *42*(3). https://doi.org/10.1111/jfpp.13551.

[19] Chen, L., Zhang, Y., Sha, O., Xu, W., and Wang, S. (2016). Hypolipidaemic and hypoglycaemic activities of polysaccharide from *Pleurotus eryngii* in Kunming mice. *International Journal of Biological Macromolecules*, *93*, 1206–1209. https://doi.org/10.1016/j.ijbiomac.2016.09.094.

[20] Chiş, M. S., Păucean, A., Man, S. M., Vodnar, D. C., Teleky, B. E., Pop, C. R., Stan, L., Borsai, O., Kadar, C. B., Urcan, A. C., and Muste, S. (2020). Quinoa sourdough fermented with *Lactobacillus plantarum* ATCC 8014 designed for gluten-free muffins—a powerful tool to enhance bioactive compounds. *Applied Sciences (Switzerland)*, *10*(20), 1–23. https://doi.org/10.3390/app10207140.

[21] Clarke, C. I., Schober, T. J., Dockery, P., O'Sullivan, K., and Arendt, E. K. (2004). Wheat sourdough fermentation: eff ects of time and acidifi cation on fundamental rheological properties. *Cereal Chem,* 81:409–17.https://doi.org/10.1094/ CCHEM.2004.81.

[22] Coda, R., Nionelli, L., Rizzello, C. G., De Angelis, M., Tossut, P., and Gobbetti, M. (2010). Spelt and emmer flours: Characterization of the lactic acid bacteria microbiota and selection of mixed starters for bread making. *Journal of Applied Microbiology*, *108*(3), 925–935. https://doi.org/10.1111/j.1365-2672.2009.04497.x.

[23] Coda, R., Melama, L., Rizzello, C. G., Curiel, J. A., Sibakov, J., Holopainen, U., Pulkkinen, M., and Sozer, N. (2015). Effect of air classification and fermentation by Lactobacillus plantarum VTT E-133328 on faba bean (*Vicia faba* L.) flour nutritional properties. *International Journal of Food Microbiology*, *193*, 34–42. https://doi.org/10.1016/j.ijfoodmicro.2014.10.012.

[24] Constantini, A., Da Ros, A., Nikoloudaki O., Montemurro, M., Di Cahno, R., Genot, B., Gobbetti, M., and Rizzello, C. G. (2022). How cereal flours, starters, enzymes, and process parameters affect the in vitro digestibility of sourdough bread. *Food Research International,* 159, 1-12. https://doi.org/10.1016/j.foodres.2022.111614.

[25] Crowley, S., Mahony, J., and Van Sinderen, D. (2013). Current perspectives on antifungal lactic acid bacteria as natural bio-preservatives. *Trends in Food Science and Technology*, *33*(2), 93–109. https://doi.org/10.1016/j.tifs.2013.07.004.

[26] Dal Bello, F., Clarke, C. I., Ryan, L. A. M., Ulmer, H., Schober, T. J., Ström, K., Sjögren, J., van Sinderen, D., Schnürer, J., and Arendt, E. K. (2007). Improvement of the quality and shelf life of wheat bread by fermentation with the antifungal strain *Lactobacillus plantarum* FST 1.7. *Journal of Cereal Science*, *45*(3), 309–318. https://doi.org/10.1016/j.jcs.2006.09.004.

[27] Dallagnol, A. M., Pescuma, M., De Valdez, G. F., and Rollán, G. (2013). Fermentation of quinoa and wheat slurries by *Lactobacillus plantarum* CRL 778: Proteolytic activity. *Applied Microbiology and Biotechnology*, *97*(7), 3129–3140. https://doi.org/10.1007/s00253-012-4520-3.

[28] De Simone, N., Rocchetti, M. T., la Gatta, B., Spano, G., Drider, D., Capozzi, V., Russo, P., and Fiocco, D. (2022). Antimicrobial Properties, Functional Characterisation and Application of *Fructobacillus fructosus* and *Lactiplantibacillus plantarum* Isolated from Artisanal Honey. *Probiotics and Antimicrobial Proteins*, *0123456789*. https://doi.org/10.1007/s12602-022-09988-4.

[29] Demirkesen-Bicak., H., Arici, M., Yaman., M., Karasu., S., and Sagdic., O. (2021). Effect of Different Fermentation Condition on Estimated Glycemic Index, In Vitro Starch Digestibility, and Textural and Sensory Properties of Sourdough Bread. *Foods,* 10 (514), 1-13. https://doi.org/10.3390/foods10030514.

[30] De Sousa Moraes, L. F., Grzeskowiak, L. M., De Sales Teixeira, T. F., and Do Carmo Gouveia Peluzio, M. (2014). Intestinal microbiota and probiotics in celiac disease. *Clinical Microbiology Reviews*, *27*(3), 482–489. https://doi.org/10.1128/CMR.00106-13.

[31] De Vuyst, L., Vrancken, G., Ravyts, F., Rimaux, T., and Weckx, S. (2009). Biodiversity, ecological determinants, and metabolic exploitation of sourdough microbiota. *Food Microbiology*, *26*(7), 666–675. https://doi.org/10.1016/j.fm.2009.07.012.

[32] De Vuyst, L., and Neysens, P. (2005). The sourdough microflora: Biodiversity and metabolic interactions. *Trends in Food Science and Technology*, *16*(1–3), 43–56. https://doi.org/10.1016/j.tifs.2004.02.012.

[33] Di Biase, M., Bavaro, A. R., Lonigro, S. L., Pontonio, E., Conte, A., Padalino, L., Minisci, A., Lavermicocca, P., and Valerio, F. (2019). *Lactobacillus plantarum* ITM21B fermentation product and chickpea flour enhance the nutritional profile of salt reduced bakery products. *International Journal of Food Sciences and Nutrition*, *70*(6), 701–713. https://doi.org/10.1080/09637486.2019.1567699.

[34] Di Cagno, R., Rizzello, C. G., De Angelis, M., Cassone, A., Giuliani, G., Benedusi, A., Limitone, A., Surico, R. F., and Gobbetti, M. (2008). Use of selected sourdough strains of *Lactobacillus* for removing gluten and enhancing the nutritional properties

of gluten-free bread. *Journal of Food Protection*, *71*(7), 1491–1495. https://doi.org/10.4315/0362-028X-71.7.1491.

[35] Di Renzo, T., Reale, A., Boscaino, F., and Messia, M. C. (2018). Flavoring production in Kamut®, Quinoa and wheat doughs fermented by *Lactobacillus paracasei*, *Lactobacillus plantarum,* and *Lactobacillus brevis*: A SPME-GC/MS study. *Frontiers in Microbiology*, *9*(MAR). https://doi.org/10.3389/fmicb.2018.00429.

[36] Ferri, M., Serrazanetti, D. I., Tassoni, A., Baldissarri, M., and Gianotti, A. (2016). Improving the functional and sensorial profile of cereal-based fermented foods by selecting *Lactobacillus plantarum* strains via a metabolomics approach. *Food Research International*, *89*, 1095–1105. https://doi.org/10.1016/j.foodres.2016.08.044.

[37] Filannino, P., Bai, Y., Di Cagno, R., Gobbetti, M., and Gänzle, M. G. (2015). Metabolism of phenolic compounds by *Lactobacillus spp*. during fermentation of cherry juice and broccoli puree. *Food Microbiology*, *46*, 272–279. https://doi.org/10.1016/j.fm.2014.08.018.

[38] Flander, L., Suortti, T., Katina, K., and Poutanen, K. (2011). Effects of wheat sourdough process on the quality of mixed oat-wheat bread. *Lwt*, *44*(3), 656–664. https://doi.org/10.1016/j.lwt.2010.11.007.

[39] Ghasemi, L., Leila Nouri, L., and Nafchi, A. M. (2022). The impact Encapsulation exerted by Tragacanth Gum on Viability and Staling of *Lactobacillus Plantarum* and *Lactobacillus acidophilus* During Baking and Storing Gluten-free Sorghum Bread. *Journal of Chemical Health Risks* 12, https://doi.org/10.22034/jchr.2022.1913164.1210.

[40] Gianotti, A., Danesi, F., Verardo, V., Serrazanetti, D. I., Valli, V., Russo, A., Riciputi, Y., Tossani, N., Caboni, M. F., Guerzoni, M. E., and Bordoni, A. (2011). Role of cereal type and processing in whole grain in vivo protection from oxidative stress. *Frontiers in Bioscience*, *16*(5), 1609–1618. https://doi.org/10.2741/3808.

[41] Gobbetti, M., Rizzello, C. G., Di Cagno, R., and De Angelis, M. (2014). Zhang. *Food Microbiology*, *37*, 30–40. https://doi.org/10.1016/j.fm.2013.04.012.

[42] Gobbetti, M. (1998). The sourdough microfora:Interactions of lactic acid bacteria and yeasts. *Trends in Food Science & Technology* 9(7), 267-274. https://doi.org/10.1016/S0924-2244(98)00053-3.

[43] Guyot, J. P. (2012). Cereal-based fermented foods in developing countries: Ancient foods for modern research. *International Journal of Food Science and Technology*, *47*(6), 1109–1114. https://doi.org/10.1111/j.1365-2621.2012.02969.x.

[44] Houben, A., Götz, H., Mitzscherling, M., and Becker, T. (2010). Modification of the rheological behavior of amaranth (*Amaranthus hypochondriacus*) dough. *Journal of Cereal Science*, *51*(3), 350–356. https://doi.org/10.1016/j.jcs.2010.02.003.

[45] Hu, L., Li, Y., Huang, X., Du, C., Huang, D., and Tao, X. (2023). The effect of co-rermentation with *Lactobacillus plantarum* HLJ29L2 and yeast on wheat protein characteristics in sourdough and crackers. *Foods*, *12*(3). https://doi.org/10.3390/foods12030555.

[46] Illueca, F., Moreno, A., Calpe, J., de Melo Nazareth, T., Dopzazo, V., Meca, G., Quiles, J. M., and Luz., C. (2023). Bread Biopreservation through the Addition of Lactic Acid Bacteria in Sourdough. *Foods,* 12 /864), 1-26.

[47] Karimi, N., Zeynali, F., Rezazad Bari, M., Nikoo, M., Mohtarami, F., and Kadivar, M. (2021). Amaranth selective hydrolyzed protein influence on sourdough fermentation and wheat bread quality. *Food Science and Nutrition*, *9*(12), 6683–6691. https://doi.org/10.1002/fsn3.2618.

[48] Kezer, G. (2022). Functional Perspective on Sourdough Bread. *Turk. J. Agric. Food Sci. Technol.* 10, 1410–1414.doi: https://doi.org/10.24925/turjaf.v10i8.1410-1414.4860.

[49] Koistinen, V. M., Mattila, O., Katina, K., Poutanen, K., Aura, A. M., and Hanhineva, K. (2018). Metabolic profiling of sourdough fermented wheat and rye bread. *Scientific Reports*, *8*(1), 1–12. https://doi.org/10.1038/s41598-018-24149-w.

[50] Korcari, D., Ricci, G., Quattrini, M., and Fortina, M. G. (2020). Microbial consortia involved in fermented spelt sourdoughs: dynamics and characterization of yeasts and lactic acid bacteria. *Letters in Applied Microbiology*, *70*(1), 48–54. https://doi.org/10.1111/lam.13241.

[51] Kulathunga, J., Reuhs, B. L., Zwinger, S., and Simsek, S. (2021). Comparative study on kernel quality and chemical composition of ancient and modern wheat species: Einkorn, emmer, spelt and hard red spring wheat. *Foods*, *10*(4). https://doi.org/10.3390/foods10040761.

[52] Liu, Y., Van Bennekom, E. O., Zhang, Y., Abee, T., and Smid, E. J. (2019). Long-chain vitamin K2 production in *Lactococcus lactis* is influenced by temperature, carbon source, aeration and mode of energy metabolism. *Microbial Cell Factories*, *18*(1), 1–14. https://doi.org/10.1186/s12934-019-1179-9.

[53] Moghaddam, M. F. T., Jalali, H., Nafchi, A. M., and Nouri, L. (2020). Evaluating the effects of lactic acid bacteria and olive leaf extract on the quality of gluten-free bread. *Gene Reports*, *21*(August), 100771. https://doi.org/10.1016/j.genrep.2020.100771.

[54] Moghaddam, M. F. T. (2019). Evaluating the properties of gluten-free bread produced using corn sourdough lactic acid bacteria. *Infection Epidemiology and Microbiology*. 5(2):41-51.

[55] Moore, M. M., Dal Bello, F., and Arendt, E. K. (2008). Sourdough fermented by *Lactobacillus plantarum* FST 1.7 improves the quality and shelf life of gluten-free bread. *European Food Research and Technology*, *226*(6), 1309–1316. https://doi.org/10.1007/s00217-007-0659-z.

[56] Moroni, A. V., Dal Bello, F., and Arendt, E. K. (2009). Sourdough in gluten-free bread-making: An ancient technology to solve a novel issue? *Food Microbiology* 26, 676–684. doi:10.1016/j.fm.2009.07.001.

[57] Nionelli, L., and Rizzello, C. G. (2016). Sourdough-based biotechnologies for the production of gluten-free foods. *Foods*, 5, 65; doi:10.3390/foods5030065.

[58] Oguntoyinbo, F. A., and Narbad, A. (2012). Molecular characterization of lactic acid bacteria and in situ amylase expression during traditional fermentation of cereal foods. *Food Microbiology*, *31*(2), 254–262. https://doi.org/10.1016/j.fm.2012.03.004.

[59] Parakhina, O., Lokachuk, M., Kuznetsova, L., Savkina, O., Pavlovskaya, E., and Gavrilova, E. (2021). Evaluation of selected lactic acid bacteria as starter cultures for gluten-free sourdough bread production. *Agronomy Research* 19(S3), 1260–1272. https://doi.org/10.15159/AR.21.087.

[60] Park, D. M., Bae, J. H., Kim, M. S., Kim, H., Kang, S. D., Shim, S., Lee, D., Seo, J. H., Kang, H., and Han, N. S. (2019). Suitability of *Lactobacillus plantarum* SPC-SNU 72-2 as a probiotic starter for sourdough fermentation. *Journal of Microbiology and Biotechnology*, *29*(11), 1729–1738. https://doi.org/10.4014/jmb.1907.07004.

[61] Păucean, A., Mureșan, V., Man, S. M., Chiș, M. S., Mureșan, A. E., Șerban, L. R., Pop, A., and Muste, S. (2021). Metabolomics as a tool to elucidate the sensory, nutritional and safety quality of wheat bread—a review. *International Journal of Molecular Sciences*, *22*(16). https://doi.org/10.3390/ijms22168945.

[62] Păucean, A., Vodnar, D. C., Socaci, S. A., and Socaciu, C. (2013). Carbohydrate metabolic conversions to lactic acid and volatile derivatives, as influenced by *Lactobacillus plantarum* ATCC 8014 and *Lactobacillus casei* ATCC 393 efficiency during in vitro and sourdough fermentation. *European Food Research and Technology*, *237*(5), 679–689. https://doi.org/10.1007/s00217-013-2042-6.

[63] Pontonio, E., Dingeo, C., Di Cagno, R., Blandino, M., Gobbetti, M., and Rizzello, C. G. (2020). Brans from hull-less barley, emmer and pigmented wheat varieties: From by-products to bread nutritional improvers using selected lactic acid bacteria and xylanase. *International Journal of Food Microbiology*, *313* (February 2019). https://doi.org/10.1016/j.ijfoodmicro.2019.108384.

[64] Prete, R., Tofalo, R., Federici, E., Ciarrocchi, A., Cenci, G., and Corsetti, A. (2017). Food-associated *Lactobacillus plantarum* and yeasts inhibit the genotoxic effect of 4-nitroquinoline-1-oxide. *Frontiers in Microbiology*, *8*(NOV), 1–9. https://doi.org/10.3389/fmicb.2017.02349.

[65] Rodríguez, H., Curiel, J. A., Landete, J. M., De las Rivas, B., De Felipe, F. L., Gómez-Cordovés, C., Mancheño, J. M., and Muñoz, R. (2009). Food phenolics and lactic acid bacteria. *International Journal of Food Microbiology*, *132*(2–3), 79–90. https://doi.org/10.1016/j.ijfoodmicro.2009.03.025.

[66] Russo, P., Arena, M. P., Fiocco, D., Capozzi, V., Drider, D., and Spano, G. (2017). *Lactobacillus plantarum* with broad antifungal activity: A promising approach to increase safety and shelf-life of cereal-based products. *International Journal of Food Microbiology*, *247*, 48–54. https://doi.org/10.1016/j.ijfoodmicro.2016.04.027.

[67] Russo, P., Fares, C., Longo, A., Spano, G., and Capozzi, V. (2017). *Lactobacillus plantarum* with broad antifungal activity as a protective starter culture for bread production. *Foods*, *6*(12). https://doi.org/10.3390/foods6120110.

[68] Saa, D. L. T., Nissen, L., and Gianotti, A. (2019). Metabolomic approach to study the impact of flour type and fermentation process on volatile profile of bakery products. *Food Research International*, *119*, 510–516. https://doi.org/10.1016/j.foodres.2019.01.024.

[69] Saa, D. T., Di Silvestro, R., Dinelli, G., and Gianotti, A. (2017). Effect of sourdough fermentation and baking process severity on dietary fibre and phenolic compounds

of immature wheat flour bread. *Lwt*, *83*, 26–32. https://doi.org/10.1016/j.lwt.2017.04.071.

[70] Sasikumar, K., Kozhummal Vaikkath, D., Devendra, L., and Nampoothiri, K. M. (2017). An exopolysaccharide (EPS) from a *Lactobacillus plantarum* BR2 with potential benefits for making functional foods. *Bioresource Technology*, *241*, 1152–1156. https://doi.org/10.1016/j.biortech.2017.05.075.

[71] Seddik, H. A., Bendali, F., Gancel, F., Fliss, I., Spano, G., and Drider, D. (2017). *Lactobacillus plantarum* and its probiotic and food potentialities. *Probiotics and Antimicrobial Proteins*, *9*(2), 111–122. https://doi.org/10.1007/s12602-017-9264-z.

[72] Șerban, L. R., Păucean, A., Chis, M. S., Pop, C. R., Man, S. M., Pușcaș, A., Ranga, F., Socaci, S. A, Alexa, E., Semeniuc, C. A., and Mureșan, V. (2023). Metabolic Profile of Einkorn , Spelt , Emmer Ancient Wheat Species Sourdough Fermented with Strain of *Lactiplantibacillus plantarum* ATCC 8014. *Foods*. 4;12(5):1096. doi: 10.3390/foods12051096.

[73] Șerban, L. R., Păucean, A., Man, S. M., Chiş, M. S., and Mureșan, V. (2021). Ancient wheat species: Biochemical profile and impact on sourdough bread characteristics—a review. *Processes*, *9*(11). https://doi.org/10.3390/pr9112008.

[74] Shewry, P. R., America, A. H. P., Lovegrove, A., Wood, A. J., Plummer, A., Evans, J., Van den Broeck, H. C., Gilissen, L., Mumm, R., Ward, J. L., Proos, Z., Kuiper, P., Longin, C. F. H., Andersson, A. A. M., Philip van Straaten, J., Jonkers, D., and Brouns, F. (2022). Comparative compositions of metabolites and dietary fibre components in doughs and breads produced from bread wheat, emmer and spelt and using yeast and sourdough processes. *Food Chemistry*, *374*(November 2021), 131710. https://doi.org/10.1016/j.foodchem.2021.131710.

[75] Shewry, P. R., Corol, D. I., Jones, H. D., Beale, M. H., and Ward, J. L. (2017). Defining genetic and chemical diversity in wheat grain by 1H-NMR spectroscopy of polar metabolites. *Molecular Nutrition and Food Research*, *61*(7), 1–9. https://doi.org/10.1002/mnfr.201600807.

[76] Shewry, P. R., and Hey, S. (2015). Do "ancient" wheat species differ from modern bread wheat in their contents of bioactive components? *Journal of Cereal Science*, *65*, 236–243. https://doi.org/10.1016/j.jcs.2015.07.014.

[77] Stefańska, I., Piasecka-Jóźwiak, K., Kotyrba, D., Kolenda, M., and Stecka, K. M. (2016). Selection of lactic acid bacteria strains for the hydrolysis of allergenic proteins of wheat flour. *Journal of the Science of Food and Agriculture*, *96*(11), 3897–3905. https://doi.org/10.1002/jsfa.7588.

[78] Svensson, L., Sekwati-Monang, B., Lutz, D. L., Schieber, R., and Gänzle, M. G. (2010). Phenolic acids and flavonoids in nonfermented and fermented red sorghum (*Sorghum bicolor* (L.) Moench). *Journal of Agricultural and Food Chemistry*, *58*(16), 9214–9220. https://doi.org/10.1021/jf101504v.

[79] Tang, W., Xing, Z., Li, C., Wang, J., and Wang, Y. (2017). Molecular mechanisms and in vitro antioxidant effects of *Lactobacillus plantarum* MA2. *Food Chemistry*, *221*, 1642–1649. https://doi.org/10.1016/j.foodchem.2016.10.124.

[80] Teleky, B. E., Martău, G. A., and Vodnar, D. C. (2020a). Physicochemical effects of *Lactobacillus plantarum* and *Lactobacillus casei* cocultures on soy–wheat flour dough fermentation. *Foods*, *9*(12). https://doi.org/10.3390/foods9121894.

[81] Teleky, B. E., Martău, A. G., Ranga, F., Chețan, F., and Vodnar, D. C. (2020b). Exploitation of lactic acid bacteria and Baker's yeast as single or multiple starter cultures of wheat flour dough enriched with soy flour. *Biomolecules,* 10(5). https://doi.org/10.3390/biom10050778.

[82] Thiele, C., Gänzle M. G, and Vogel, R. F. (2002). Contribution of sourdough lactobacilli, yeast, and cereal enzymes to the generation of amino acids in dough relevant for bread fl avor. *Cereal Chem.* 79:45–51. https://doi.org/10.1094/CCHEM.2002.79.1.45.

[83] Todorov, S. D., and Gombossy De Melo Franco, B. D. (2010). *Lactobacillus Plantarum*: characterization of the species and application in food production. *Food Reviews International*, 26:205–229. doi: 10.1080/87559129.2010.484113.

[84] Üçok, G., and Sert, D. (2020). Growth kinetics and biomass characteristics of *Lactobacillus plantarum* L14 isolated from sourdough: Effect of fermentation time on dough machinability. *Lwt, 129*, 109516. https://doi.org/10.1016/j.lwt.2020.109516.

[85] Valerio, F., Bavaro, A. R., Di Biase, M., Lonigro, S. L., Logrieco, A. F., and Lavermicocca, P. (2020). Effect of Amaranth and quinoa flours on exopolysaccharide production and protein profile of liquid sSourdough fermented by *Weissella cibaria* and *Lactobacillus plantarum. Frontiers in Microbiology, 11*(May), 1–16. https://doi.org/10.3389/fmicb.2020.00967.

[86] Van Der Meulen, R., Scheirlinck, I., Van Schoor, A., Huys, G., Vancanneyt, M., Vandamme, P., and De Vuyst, L. (2007). Population dynamics and metabolite target analysis of lactic acid bacteria during laboratory fermentations of wheat and spelt sourdoughs. *Applied and Environmental Microbiology*, *73*(15), 4741–4750. https://doi.org/10.1128/AEM.00315-07.

[87] Wan, J., Huang, W., Zhong, J., Huang, L., Rayas-Duarte, P., and Liu, B. (2011). Effects of LAB fermentation on physical properties of oat flourand its suitability for noodle making. *Cereal Chemistry*, *88*(2), 153–158. https://doi.org/10.1094/CCHEM-12-09-0160.

[88] Wang, Y., Wu, J., Lv, M., Shao, Z., Hungwe, M., Wang, J., Bai, X., Xie, J., Wang, Y., and Geng, W. (2021). Metabolism cCharacteristics of lactic acid bacteria and the expanding applications in food industry. *Frontiers in Bioengineering and Biotechnology*, *9*(May), 1–19. https://doi.org/10.3389/fbioe.2021.612285.

[89] Winters, M., Panayotides, D., Bayrak, M., Rémont, G., Viejo, C. G., Liu, D., Le, B., Liu, Y., Luo, J., Zhang, P., and Howell, K. (2019). Defined co-cultures of yeast and bacteria modify the aroma, crumb and sensory properties of bread. *Journal of Applied Microbiology*, *127*(3), 778–793. https://doi.org/10.1111/jam.14349.

[90] Wolter, A., Hager, A. S., Zannini, E., Czerny, M., and Arendt, E. K. (2014). Impact of sourdough fermented with *Lactobacillus plantarum* FST 1.7 on baking and sensory properties of gluten-free breads. *European Food Research and Technology*, *239*(1), 1–12. https://doi.org/10.1007/s00217-014-2184-1.

[91] Woo, S. H., Shin, Y. J., Jeong, H. M., Kim, J. S., Ko, D. S., Hong, J. S., Choi, H. D., and Shim, J. H. (2020). Effects of maltogenic amylase from *Lactobacillus plantarum* on retrogradation of bread. *Journal of Cereal Science*, *93*(April), 102976. https://doi.org/10.1016/j.jcs.2020.102976.

[92] Yilmaz, B., Bangar, S. P., Echegaray, N., Suri, S., Tomasevic, I., Lorenzo, J. M., Melekoglu, E., Rocha, J. M., and Ozogul, F. (2022). The Impacts of *Lactiplantibacillus plantarum* on the functional properties of fermented Foods: A Review of Current Knowledge. *Microorganisms*, *10*(4), 1–18. https://doi.org/10.3390/microorganisms10040826.

[93] Zannini, E., Pontonio, E., Waters, D. M., and Arendt, E. K. (2012). Applications of microbial fermentations for production of gluten-free products and perspectives. *Appl. Microbiol. Biotechnol.* 93, 473–485. doi:10.1007/s00253-011-3707-3.

[94] Zhang, L., Taal, M. A., Boom, R. M., Chen, X. D., and Schutyser, M. A. I. (2018). Effect of baking conditions and storage on the viability of *Lactobacillus plantarum* supplemented to bread. *Lwt*, *87*, 318–325. https://doi.org/10.1016/j.lwt.2017.09.005.

[95] Zhang, L., Taal, M., Boom, R. M., Chen, X. D., Schutyser, M. A. I., (2015). Viability of *Lactobacillus plantarum P8* in Bread during Baking and Storage. The 20th International Drying Symposium, Gifu, JAPAN.

[96] Zielinski, H., Ciesarova, Z., Kukurova, K., Zielinska, D., Szawara-Nowak, D., Starowicz, M., and Wronkowska, M. (2017). Effect of fermented and unfermented buckwheat flour on functional properties of gluten-free muffins. *J Food Sci Technol.* doi:10.1007/s13197-017-2561-4.

Chapter 6

Lactobacillus plantarum and Its Role in Milk and Dairy Products Manufacturing

Delia Michiu[1]
Mirela Anamaria Jimborean[1,*]
Cristina Anamaria Semeniuc[1]
Elena Suzana Biriş-Dorhoi[2]
and Liana Claudia Salanţă[2]
[1]Department of Food Engineering, Faculty of Food Science and Technology, University of Agricultural Sciences and Veterinary Medicine of Cluj-Napoca, Romania
[2]Department of Food Science, Faculty of Food Science and Technology, University of Agricultural Sciences and Veterinary Medicine of Cluj-Napoca, Romania

Abstract

This chapter provides an overview of the current trends in using *Lactobacillus plantarum* as a source of functional compounds in developing dairy products. Probiotics play an essential role in improving health and well-being, including their antimicrobial activity and modulation of the immune system. There is a considerable amount of literature on *L. plantarum*, a strain of probiotic bacteria in the intestines revealing that it stimulates the digestive system, fights disease-causing bacteria and helps the body produce vitamins. Moreover, *L. plantarum* has gained much attention due to its significant probiotic and antioxidant activities. As dairy products are a good source of different live lactic acid bacteria species, more recent evidence highlights that *L. plantarum* represents an essential part of the natural microflora of many dairy

[*] Corresponding Author's Email: mirela.jimborean@usamvcluj.ro.

In: Lactobacillus plantarum and Its Role in Human Health
Editors: Maria Simona Chiş, Adriana Paucean
ISBN: 979-8-89113-696-0

products and plays a relevant role in developing the final products' sensory and organoleptic properties. *L. plantarum* is spread worldwide and is the dominant species in the last step of natural raw-material fermentation, including meat, fish, dairy products, and plant-based fermented foods. In literature, the genus *Lactobacillus* usually refers to safe use in the food industry, especially in dairy products with a prolonged shelf life, due to their bio-preservative capabilities and positive health impact.
As a contribution to this approach, this chapter will provide a comprehensive overview of the dairy production environment as a source of *L. plantarum* strains with probiotic potential, emphasising the characterisation and application in controlled fermentations. There is perfect agreement between the desirable properties enhancing the quality of dairy products and the associated health benefits; most *L. plantarum* strains can produce pleasant flavour due to their proteolytic activity.

Keywords: *Lactobacillus plantarum*, literature review, dairy products, probiotics

1. Introduction

One of the top research priorities for the food industry is the development of foods that promote health and well-being because there is a significant trend for consumers to purchase foods that offer excellent nutrition and health benefits, especially those that can prevent illness and/or maintain health (Daneshi et al., 2013). A rising body of research has shown the importance of gut microbiota to human health and the advantages of probiotic microbes, which, when taken consistently and in sufficient doses, have a favourable impact on host health (Dos Santos et al., 2015). Probiotics are live organisms that offer health advantages when ingested in the body in a sufficient quantity. Probiotic bacteria have shown a positive impact on human health after being ingested by having the capacity to withstand acid and bile, exhibit antimicrobial activity, adapt to the gastrointestinal environment, and retain high viability of at least 10^6–10^8 cfu/g (Nuraida, 2015; Li et al., 2017; Meidistria et al., 2020). They might help manage and lessen the body's metabolic abnormalities (Ngamsomchat et al., 2022). When taken, probiotic bacteria may temporally colonize the gut, aiding in the direct competitive exclusion of pathogens or impacting the immune system. In addition, they may modify microbiota composition and functional activity in advantageous ways, such as lactose digestion for lactose intolerant persons, constipation relief, increased mineral absorption, and vitamin production (Pereira de Souza et al., 2013). According to research on both people and experimental animals, functional food can alter microbiota metabolic profile in addition to enhancing the host's metabolism. (Hütt et al., 2015). Probiotics are also a significant source of antioxidants, which help to lower the risk of many chronic illnesses brought on by oxidative reactions. Instead of using antibiotics when the immune system is compromised by different pathogenic microbes, boosting probiotic consumption is a suitable alternative (Ngamsomchat et al., 2022). Moreover, according to Dallagnol et al. (2013), using *Lactobacillus plantarum* in food is safe. It has been a popular choice in creating innovative functional products due to its dual purpose as a native human gut resident and a safe fermenting culture in food (De Vries et al., 2006; Li et al., 2017). Many authors that employed various agro-residue substrates for biomass synthesis explored this probiotic for its interesting metabolites, mainly lactic acid (Kacho, 2019).

The *Lactobacillus* genus has a long history of safe usage (especially in the dairy industry) and is crucial in creating fermented milk products (Isa and Razavi, 2017). *L. plantarum* is a member of the facultative hetero-fermentative group of lactobacilli under the genus *Lactobacillus. L. plantarum*, a non-pathogenic mesophilic lactic acid bacterium, is routinely isolated from food items and is employed extensively in manufacturing fermented foods (Isa and Razavi, 2017). Probiotic strains must be cultured in a product at the proper concentrations. In addition, they must sustain cell viability during shelf life, which is the critical difficulty posed by the rising demand for probiotics on the global market (Tripathi and Giri, 2014; Fonseca et al., 2020). The cornerstones of dietary living worldwide are fermented milk and dairy products. The health advantages of fermented dairy products are well-established and extend beyond their nutritional and organoleptic qualities (Agagündüz et al., 2021). Milk products are the finest probiotic species matrix carriers for lactic acid bacteria (Fonseca et al., 2020). The main lactic acid bacteria in food fermentation are the starter, additive, and probiotic cultures. Thus, the dairy sector is developing innovative functional products by adding probiotic bacteria to fermented milk (Georgieva et al., 2009). As it is defined, fermented milk is a dairy product that undergoes nutritional, physical, and chemical sensory changes during fermentation. Many microorganisms that utilize milk as a substrate and various dairy products, such as whole milk, skim milk, partially skim milk, fortified milk, or modified milk, all contribute to this process (Pereira de Souza et al., 2013).

The inclusion of these microbes in fermented milk has yielded products with high cell viability and functioning, and therefore, probiotic-containing foods have been studied as probiotic delivery systems (Chaucheyras-Durand and Durand, 2010; Champagne et al., 2014). In addition, the production of numerous naturally occurring antimicrobial compounds by *L. plantarum*, including bacteriocins, organic acids (primarily lactic and acetic acid), and hydrogen peroxide, helps to create recognizable tastes and improves final product quality (Tremonte et al., 2017).

1.1. Influence of *Lactobacillus plantarum* on Yoghurt Fermentation

Lactic acid bacteria (LAB) generate fermented milk by acting as an acidifier during metabolism, which causes significant physicochemical, sensory, and microbiological changes in the milk. Starter, additive, and probiotic cultures comprise the main LAB in food fermentation (Casarotti et al., 2014). One of the most popular fermented milk products due to its high nutritional content, distinct flavour, and beneficial health properties is yoghurt. *S. thermophilus* and *L. delbrueckii ssp. bulgaricus* have historically been grown for the production of yoghurt. Therefore, a significant priority in the dairy business is the creation of innovative functional products by adding probiotic bacteria to fermented milk (Zhang et al., 2020).

Jang et al., in their study from 2018, analysed the starter cultures of ginseng extract powder (GEP), *L. plantarum NK181*, and *S. thermophilus* in yoghurt to determine its composition, pH, titratable activity, microbial characteristics, and antioxidant impact. The yoghurt exhibited various GEP concentrations (0%, 0.5%, 1%, 1.5%, and 2% (w/v)). The pH of yoghurt declined while titratable acidity and viable cell counts grew during the fermentation process. Moreover, yoghurt moisture content dropped when GEP was added, but its fat, ash, and total solid contents rose instead. With the addition of GEP, the antioxidant effect and β-carotene bleaching assays gradually increased. Overall, the cell viability of yoghurt fermented with 1% GEP was adequate and it was thus established that the probiotic *L. plantarum NK181* and GEP enhance dairy product qualities and antioxidant activity.

In was also in Hokkaido, Japan, that well-pickled vegetables were used to isolate *L. plantarum HOKKAIDO* (HOKKAIDO strain). Nishimura et al., in 2016, examined the impact of *L. plantarum HOKKAIDO* on stress indicators and immunological function in 171 adult participants, and they concluded that Neutrophils were lower in those who consumed the yoghurt-like dessert against those who consumed the HOKKAIDO strain yoghurt. In addition, NLR (neutrophil-to-lymphocyte ratio), a stress-related marker, trended lower in the yoghurt made with the HOKKAIDO strain than in the yoghurt-like dessert group. Finally, yoghurt made with the HOKKAIDO strain could boost immune system activity and lower stress-related indicators.

The possibility of producing low-sugar yoghurt by co-cultivating *L. plantarum* with yoghurt starter cultures was therefore highlighted by Zhang et al. in their study from 2020, where initially, *L. plantarum WCFS1* was co-cultured with *S. thermophilus* or *L. bulgaricus* in lactose-based medium to verify this theory. According to the findings, galactose was well digested, and lactose was entirely absorbed. Compared to conventional fermentation methods, co-cultivation of *L. plantarum WCFS1* with yoghurt starter cultures resulted in a more significant reduction of the total sugar content. Furthermore, the sensory evaluation revealed that yoghurt appearance, texture, and flavour were acceptable to customers after being fermented using yoghurt starter cultures and *L. plantarum WCFS1*.

The effects of nine *L. plantarum* strains were assessed by Li et al. (2017) with broad-spectrum antibacterial activity on fermented milk, taking into account changes in fermentation characteristics (such as pH, titration acidity, and viable counts), texture profile, relative volatile compound content, and sensory evaluation during 28 days of storage at 4°C. The most remarkable result from the data is that *L. plantarum* IMAU80106, IMAU10216, and IMAU70095 showed the highest levels of proteolytic activity and coagulation capacity among the studied strains. In addition, the texture and volatile flavour profiles of IMAU70095 were the closest to those of the control without the addition of the adjunct bacteria, when compared to *L. plantarum* IMAU80106 and IMAU10216, indicating that this strain may be the most appropriate for further use in the development of functional dairy products.

Humans have consumed fermented foods for thousands of years, and the employment of microbial starters may impart food with special tastes and textures. Active free amino acids, peptides, and vitamins created during the fermentation process are drawing interest around the globe in recent decades due to their potential health advantages (Lang et al., 2022). Traditional fermented milk was used to isolate *L. plantarum P-8, a* probiotic bacterium awith high fermentation capabilities. *L. plantarum P-8* can considerably improve gut flora, lower fat levels, and immunological performance. Furthermore, it can be employed as a starter in conjunction with *S. thermophilus* to enhance the flavour and texture of fermented dairy products (Bao et al., 2012b; Zhang et al., 2015). In their investigation of probiotic bacteria *L. plantarum* P-8, Dan et al. 2019) used six ratios of *L. plantarum P-8* to yoghurt starter (1:1, 1:5, 1:10, 1:50, 1:100, and 1:1000). Aldehydes, ketones, acids, alcohols, alcohol esters, and aromatic compounds were among the 66 volatile substances in milk fermented with the six distinct *L. plantarum P-8* to yoghurt starter ratios at 0 days of storage. The 1:100 ratio treatment allowed to identify important taste chemicals, including acetoin, 2-heptanone, 2-nonanone, nonanal, 3-methylbutanal, hexanal and (E)-2-octenal. Additionally, the milk samples viable cell count, pH, titratable acidity, viscosity, and syneresis during fermentation, during 14 days of storage at 4°C were all examined. According to the findings, milk may be fermented using *L. plantarum P-8* together with *L. delbrueckii subsp. bulgaricus* and *S. thermophilus* and the probiotic bacteria did not affect milk physicochemical properties (Dan et al., 2019).

Drinking yoghurt, or Doogh, is a fermented beverage that combines yoghurt with water, salt, and, in certain areas, herbal flavourings. With a yearly output of 120.000 tons of Doogh made from yoghurt, Iran is one of the top manufacturers and consumers in the world. According to Lucey (2002), edible gums can be utilized as thickeners, stabilizers, gelling agents, emulsifiers, suspension stabilizers, and occasionally as prebiotics. Cress seed gum (CSG), an edible gum, has demonstrated a significant potential for use as a stabilizing component in drinkable food systems. In a recent study, Jouki et al. (2013) showed that CSG may be utilized to make edible films as a gelling agent. Cress (*Lepidium sativum*) seeds make cress seed gum when they soak in water, and a clear gel surrounds the whole seed. The viability of *L. plantarum LS5* and the physicochemical characteristics of drinking yoghurt (Doogh), coriander extract (CE) and cress seed gum (CSG) were tested by Shariati et al. in 2019. The levels of additional CSG were 0%, 0.1%, 0.25%, and 0.5%, whereas the levels of added CE were 0%, 0.05%, 0.1%, and 0.25%. After being kept at 4°C for 1, 2, and 3 weeks, Doogh samples were examined. Compared to the other samples, the Doogh sample with 0.05% CE and 0.5% CSG had the highest probiotic count, overall acceptability score, and least amount of lipid oxidation and phase separation.

1.2. Influence of *Lactobacillus plantarum* on Cheese

One of the most well-known white soft skimmed milk cheeses, Karish, is still made the traditional way in Egyptian villages using unpasteurised milk. This method involves storing raw milk in earthenware pots for 24-72 hours (variable depending on the season) until the cream layer is separated. Once it is separated, it is removed, and the remaining fermented skim milk is pressed and transferred into a mat that is hung for 2-3 days to drain the whey. It is then dry salted, cut into cubes, and allowed to drain for 2 hours before consumption (Hammam et al., 2020). To obtain safe pasteurised Karish cheese with improved sensory characteristics, Hegab et a (2021) used probiotics and prebiotics for a synbiotic Karish cheese. Laboratory-made Karish cheese allowed researchers to compare the impact of *L. plantarum* with and without inulin on cheese quality. Treatments like microbiological, chemical, and sensory qualities, as well as their shelf life and *L. plantarum* survival, were all evaluated by the authors. Against *E. aerogenes* in cheese, *L. plantarum* and inulin antibacterial effects were assessed. Karish cheese with *L. plantarum*, received the highest taste rating, while the treatment, which also contained *L. plantarum* and inulin, received the highest body and texture ratings. In addition, *L. plantarum* and inulin dramatically decreased the *E. aerogenes* count during the cold storage of Karish cheese; Inulin also considerably improved *L. plantarum* survivability throughout the storage period.

There have yet to be studies done using strains from non-dairy sources; however, lactobacilli have been utilized as adjunct cultures in the production of several kinds of cheese to expedite ripening and/or increase cheese quality. The effectiveness of 10 dairy and non-dairy *L. plantarum, L. paraplantarum*, and *L. pentosus* strains as additives in cheese production was tested using a tiny cheddar-style cheese model by Ciocia et al., 2013. The outcomes showed that adding *L. plantarum* adjuncts reduces the secondary proteolysis significantly, as indicated by the production of free amino acids, with only a minor impact on the gross composition and primary starter performance. Their findings imply that even adjunct strains isolated from different environments—wine, sourdough or starchy foods, olives—can survive and multiply in cheese, probably due to their capacity to utilize the excess sugars and amino acids as well as their high salt tolerance, which enables them to adapt to the environmental conditions of the cheese during ripening (Ciocia et al., 2013).

Glycolysis, lipolysis, and, most significantly, proteolysis are a few of the numerous chemical and metabolic changes that occurr while cheese ripens (Rasovic et al., 2017). As demonstrated before for Cheddar cheese (Ivens et al., 2017), proteolysis plays a crucial part in defining the usual sensory qualities of each distinct variety of cheese, and it acts as a substantial predictor of quality.

Additionally, adjunct cultures are sources of essential microflora that hasten to ripen and produce a variety of proteases (Marchiani et al., 2016). The effects of adjunct cultures of the *L. plantarum MU12* and *S6-4* strains on the ripening of Cheddar cheese were investigated for survival and proteolytic activity by Duan et al. (2019). Samples were examined after 1, 30, 60, and 90 days of cheese ripening at 48̊C. The authors concluded that postripening hydrolyzed protein, free amino acids, and volatile levels were consistently higher in adjunct-treated cheeses than in the control, which impacted on the flavour. At the same time, no significant variations were identified in composition (fat, protein, and moisture) and texture across cheeses.

Burns et al. (2012) call into question some effects of two cheese-isolated *Lactobacillus* strains on cheese composition, acceptability, and probiotic potential. Prepared soft cheeses included or excluded the inclusion of *L. plantarum I91* or *L. paracasei I90*. The most well-liked cheeses have the highest proteolysis levels and compositional alterations due to *L. plantarum I91*. On the other hand, the composition of cheeses containing *L. paracasei I90*, was comparable to that of the controls. However, these samples were more poorly received than cheeses devoid of lactobacilli.

In the food sector, the new name for FF (functional foods) was "food with naturally occurring or naturally enriched substances with a specific health-promoting effect beyond." thus with a real nutritional benefit (Vukasovic et al., 2017). According to Aadinath et al. (2017), the dairy industry is well-positioned to grow and take advantage of the FF market. There is no question that dairy products serve as the primary vehicle for probiotic supplementation; hence, Granato et al. (2010) and Tripathi and Giri (2014) provided detailed information on probiotics as a source for functional foods. Nahed et al. (2020) aimed at employing *L. helveticus CH5* and *L. plantarum ATCC 14917* in the production of probiotic Gouda cheese. Gouda cheese treated with *L. helveticus*, followed by cheese treated with *L. plantarum*, had the highest values in total bacterial count and count of proteolytic and lipolytic bacteria when fresh and during the ripening period. For body, texture, and flavour, the control cheese and cheese from T3 (with *L. plantarum)* received the highest rankings, and there were statistically significant differences between them. Authors have confirmed that using *L. helveticus CH5* or *L. plantarum ATCC14917* in combination with the traditional Gouda cheese starter culture can produce a high-quality probiotic Gouda cheese effectively.

1.3. Influence of *Lactobacillus plantarum* on Ice Cream

There is indeed a high need for functional foods that might benefit and improve human health (Gadhiya et al., 2015). Because they are GRAS

(Generally Recognized As Safe) species and may demonstrate the efficiency of improving the health of animals as well as the human gut, the *Lactobacillus* and *Bifidobacterium* genera are frequently employed as probiotics (Georgieva et al., 2009). One category of functional food is synbiotic ice cream, which combines prebiotics and probiotics. Prebiotics are sometimes referred to as oligosaccharides, which are resistant, indigestible fiber substances that support the development of probiotic bacteria or yeast in digestive tracts. Prebiotics serve as the probiotic food source and protective carrier in the human digestive tract (Chen et al., 2005). Consuming probiotics has been shown to provide a number of health advantages. For instance, probiotic *L. plantarum* has proven to be effective in treating various symptoms, including diarrhoea and constipation, according to research by Zago et al. (2011). In addition, according to Parvez et al. (2006), it may lower the chance of developing cancer, ease allergy symptoms, and boost immunity. Desai et al. (2005) show that the "microencapsulation technique" refers to consolidating bacterial cells, food, nutritional supplements, or nutraceuticals into little pills that only provide the data at a specific target. This technique protects materials from deterioration and damage caused by environmental factors. In this respect, Nag et al. (2011) reveals that the goal of the probiotic bacteria microencapsulation method is to preserve steadiness and endurance when storing and safeguard the digestive tract from environmental stress, as well as regulate the gastrointestinal release. Since high-temperature encapsulation might destroy the beneficial bacteria (Tripathi and Giri, 2014), freeze-drying has been shown to be one of the most successful microencapsulation strategies for probiotics (Tee et al., 2014).

Omar et al. (2018) presented a new approach to obtaining ice creams (symbiotic) made with three distinct probiotic strains (*L. plantarum that has been capsuled* along with a combination of commercial *Bifidobacteria Sp.*and *L. plantarum*). Their study concluded that incorporating encapsulated probiotics *L. plantarum* within the ice cream may significantly impact the rheological qualities regarding elastic properties and melting speed of ice cream. As a result, the viscoelasticity and melting rate of ice cream made using the freeze-dried encapsulation process may be increased. Furthermore, their sensory data showed that the ice cream prepared with probiotics in capsules had better mean scores for general acceptance among panels, making it appropriate for commercialisation (Omar et al., 2018).

The project of Sabet-Sarvestani et al. (2021) involved the creation of synbiotic ice creams made with fructooligosaccharides. Combining *L. casei* and *L. plantarum*, the ice cream mix was fermented. Compared to unfermented samples, the fermented ones showed a lower pH and higher acidity. Synbiotic ice creams had the highest probiotic viability during storage, proving the value of fructooligosaccharides in the development of lactic acid bacteria (LAB). Fructooligosaccharides and LAB were used to create synbiotic ice creams, with better thermo-functional characteristics and more antioxidant activity than the control ice cream. Due to the elevated acidity caused by LAB development, the sensory study revealed that the fermented ice creams were less generally acceptable than the unfermented ice creams (Sabet-Sarvestani et al., 2021).

In general, the health effects of probiotics depend on their capacity to maintain their viability (concentration of 10^6–10^7 CFU/ml) until they reach their site of action and are resistant to the gastrointestinal environment. It is impossible to prevent the loss of probiotic bacteria in ice cream during product manufacturing, processing, storing, and melting (El-Sayed et al., 2015). Additionally, the nutritional benefits and sensory evaluation of probiotic ice cream made using coconut waste have seldom been studied. The study by Hanafi et al. (2022) set out to produce ice cream with additional coconut waste that contains the probiotic ATCC *L. plantarum* after analysing the impact of coconut waste on the properties of probiotic ice cream during 60 days and to gauge consumer acceptance of the probiotic and coconut residue-enriched ice cream. For their analysis, maltodextrin, nonfatpowdered milk, egg yolk, heavy cream, sugar and milk fat were used to make ice cream. Also, *L. plantarum* 1% and various quantities of coconut leftover fiber (~0.03 g/mL) were used. The leftovers of coconut meat after it has been mechanically squeezed to create a final extract of coconut milk are known as coconut residue, also referred to as coconut milk residue. It contains carbs and much cellulose in it. As a result, it has been recognized as a source of carboxymethyl cellulose (CMC). It also includes crude fiber and carbohydrates that, when combined, can produce additional cellulose through a CMC reaction (Huang et al., 2017). According to Hanafi et al. (2022) data, the optimum formulation for producing probiotic ice cream had 0.02 g/mL coconut leftover. It sustained microbial stability under storage, a creamy consistency, a minimal melting point, a substantial amount of protein with a minimal fat content, a pH that is favorable for probiotics, and good sensory evaluations for overall customer acceptance. A possible unique method for both producing a dessert that is nutrient-rich and also beneficial to human health while reducing any potential agricultural pollution is the beneficial interaction between microorganisms and coconut waste in ice cream.

Another study used microencapsulation with calcium alginate and whey protein concentrate to assess the longevity of three probiotic strains in ice cream: *L. plantarum, L. casei, and B. bifidum.* Additionally, the impact of some prebiotics, including inulin, lactulose, and fructooligosaccharides, was investigated. Six different kinds of synbiotic ice cream, including free and microencapsulated *L. plantarum*, *L. casei*, and *B. bifidum*, were created by EL-Sayed et al. in 2015 by using 2% fructooligosaccharides. Even in the presence of FOS, the survival of all tested strains improved with various sugars. Additionally, compared to free cells, the vitality of microencapsulated strains improved by more than 1 log cycle. In the Free State in ice cream, the viable cell counts of *L. plantarum*, *L. casei*, and *B. bifidum* were 8.344, 8.413 log cfu/ g on day one, and the numbers reduced to 7.841, 6.110, and 6.436 log cfu/ g after 90 days of storage, respectively (EL-Sayed et al., 2015).

1.4. *Lactobacillus plantarum* as Functional Starter Cultures for the Dairy Industry

Due to their technological and practical advantages, lactic acid bacteria (LAB) are highly sought-after on an industrial scale. They could improve biological (by thwarting harmful microbes) and chemical (by lowering acrylamide, polycyclic aromatic hydrocarbons, mycotoxins, etc.) safety, or they might provide one or more benefits, for example, increasing a product's nutritional value or enhancing its sensory and functional qualities (Cizeikiene et al., 2013; Bartkiene et al., 2017). *L. plantarum*, the most adaptable species/strain from the widespread *Lactobacillus*, is commonly present in fermented food items. In industrial fermentation and food processing, *L. plantarum* is often used and is both "generally recognized as safe" (GRAS). It has also a qualified presumption of safety (QPS) status (Ricci et al., 2017). The most significant need for *L. plantarum* strains is that they must be safe for humans and animals (FAO and WHO) and have a high capacity for survival in the GI tract and adhesion to its epithelial cells (Jia et al., 2017). Utilizing *L. plantarum* strains, which have a long history of use in food fermentation, creates a new field and helps develop foods with added value. *L. plantarum* strains have also been employed to create innovative or conventional functional meals and drinks with better nutritional and technical attributes. *L. plantarum* strains were found in a variety of traditional foods, and they were examined for their systematics, molecular taxonomy, enzyme systems and bioactive substances (bacteriocin, dipeptides, and other preservatives) (Behera et al., 2018). Regarding the dairy industry, Quigley et al. (2013) highlighted the infrequent discovery of *L. plantarum* in unprocessed milk and its negligible technological significance in conventional milk processing.

However, strains via probiotic abilities have been isolated from various dairy-related niches, including whey (Ołdak et al., 2017; Pisano et al., 2014; Hulak et al., 2016) cheese made from cow or sheep raw milk and camel milk (Abushelaibi et al., 2017) (Figure 1).

In order to create unique products with improved health advantages, the research of Turchi et al. (2017) has concentrated more on adding probiotic strains of *L. plantarum* to fermented milk drinks or cheeses.

L. plantarum is a multifunctional organism with a diverse lifestyle with a long tradition of safe usage in producing fermented foods, and it plays a significant role in the microflora of the GI tract (De Vries et al., 2006). The ability to survive and positively impact health varies significantly amongst the different strains of *L. plantarum*. Genetic analyses of diverse strains of *L. plantarum* revealed the presence and lack of numerous DNA sections, such as those encoding the synthesis of bacteriocin, exopolysaccharides, and genes involved in sugar metabolism. The organism's adaptability and survival in various environmental niches may be impacted by these genetic variants, which may also affect its capability to function as a probiotic organism (Kaushik et al., 2009).

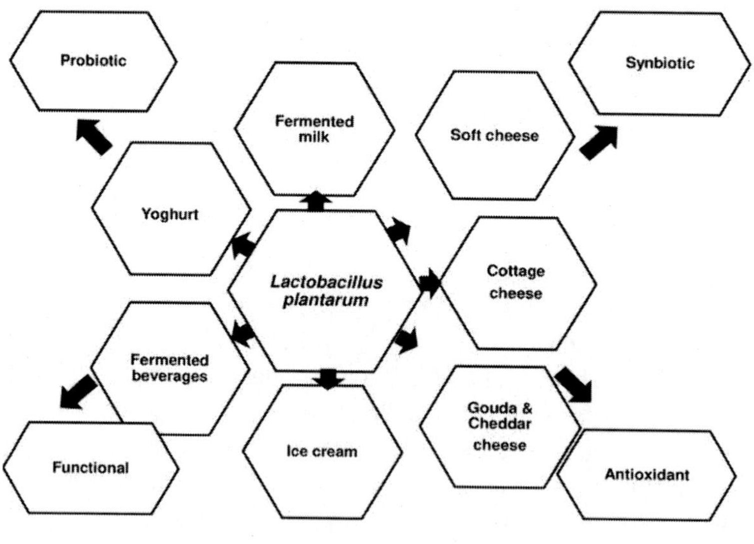

Figure 1. Potential applications and effects of *L. plantarum* for the dairy industry.

In addition, food products of a plant-based origin often include phenolic chemicals. These substances are connected to food taste, astringency, and colour. Additionally, phenolic compounds are good for health because they have anti-inflammatory, anti-proliferative, and antioxidant properties (Cory et al., 2018). Since they can produce differentiated products with a high added value, phenolic compounds with functional properties added to products are of great interest to the food industry. The biological activity of many of these molecules is also likely greatly influenced by the biosynthesis of these phenolic compounds. The fermentative microbiota transforms some dietary phenolics when the food is fermenting (Selma et al., 2009).

The lactic acid bacteria *L. plantarum* is most usually discovered in fermenting food items made from plants where phenolic chemicals are prevalent. This type of bacteria serves as the model for the research of phenolic chemical metabolism (Rodriguez et al., 2009).

By boosting their antioxidant activity, the usage of phenolic components in various dairy products has shown positive results. Additionally, because some phenolic compounds have an antibacterial effect, the ability to convert phenolic esters into their derivatives will increase bacterial survival. It may be necessary for the biological activity of these substances. Since *L. plantarum* esterase genes are involved in the metabolism of phenolic acid derivatives, Landete et al. (2021) investigated the introduction into lactic acid bacteria in their study. Their work demonstrated that the heterologous expression of phenolic acid metabolism-related genes from the lactic acid bacteria *L. plantarum* led to the generation of beneficial chemicals that improved the bioavailability of these dietary components. Furthermore, the capacity to change certain phenolic compounds has been conferred onto several lactic acid bacterial strains by transforming *L. plantarum* esterase genes involved in the metabolism of phenolic compounds. Thus, it increases their metabolic capability (Landete et al., 2021).

Moreover, probiotics are utilized more often as functional dietary components. In their work, Ngamsomchat et al. (2022) isolated and characterized the probiotic bacteria of dairy and fermented products and a chosen strain was used to make probiotic chèvre cheese. First, the ability to tolerate an acidic environment (pH 2.0) and the presence of bile salt (0.4% (w/v)) were examined. Therefore, the isolate of *L. plantarum* and *L. fermentum* was chosen to produce probiotic chèvre cheese from goat's milk, and it was prepared in a lyophilized form with a probiotic culture concentration of 8.6 log CFU/g. The cheese was stored for eight days. The probiotic, starter, and yeast contents were 7.56 ± 0.05,7.81 ± 0.03 and 5.64 log

CFU/g, respectively, on the expiration date. This chèvre cheese contained a high enough concentration of bacteria to qualify as a probiotic cheese.

Prebiotics include a wide range of compounds, including lactose derivatives like lactobionic acid (LBA), which have garnered considerable interest. This ingredient is very useful in the food industry since it is used as an antioxidant, moisturizer, chelating agent, and prebiotic (Cardoso et al., 2019). Furthermore, LBA can be metabolized by gastrointestinal microflora since it is resistant to digestive enzymes and poorly absorbed in the small intestine (Saez-Orviz et al., 2020). Additionally, a synbiotic product is created when probiotic strains and prebiotic substances are combined in a single product in order to produce a synbiotic product directly; probiotic and prebiotic ingredients are frequently included with milk before making cheese in a variety of dairy products (Langa et al., 2019). However, due to LBA's high solubility in water, this procedure is unsuitable for cheese curdling since this molecule tends to be lost to the whey rather than becoming held in the curd (Cardoso et al., 2019). As a result, another method to produce a synbiotic functional food product is to use bioactive coatings containing this prebiotic rather than adding LBA to cheese (Pavli et al., 2017). Experiments on creating a synbiotic coating that contains both a probiotic strain (*L. plantarum CECT 9567*) and a prebiotic substance (LBA) were performed on cottage cheese in 2020 by a group of researchers from Spain. As a result, the creation of bioactive coatings enables the production of synbiotic, helpful, and novel cottage cheeses that may, from a nutritional standpoint, have a high degree of consumer approval (Saez-Orviz et al., 2020).

On the one hand, there are exopolysaccharides (EPS), which can be produced and excreted by some lactic bacterial species, extracellular polysaccharides. Due to the functional characteristics of these bio-polymers and their generally recognized safe (GRAS) status, the generation of exopolysaccharides (EPS) by lactic acid bacteria (LAB) has attracted particular attention over the past ten years. These exopolysaccharides, produced by lactic acid bacteria, can change rheological characteristics by influencing a variety of processes, including viscosity, emulsification, and flocculation. They could also be used in biological, probiotic, and prebiotic processes in the food sector (Silva et al., 2019).

On the other hand, heteropolysaccharides (HePS), which make up the majority of EPS from LAB, are primarily used in the dairy industry when fermentation is taking place in-house to improve emulsifying and thickening properties for syneresis reduction and firmness increase (Ale et al., 2016). It was Wang et al. (2015b) who reported that using EPS produced by *L.*

plantarum YW11 was technically feasible because the substance demonstrated higher viscosity in skim milk and a pH of around 4, both ufavorable for addition in dairy products. According to Ayyash et al. (2018), EPS *L. plantarum* isolated from camel milk produced a good amount of EPS, and the strain also served as a starting culture for cheese manufacturing and displayed EPS production skills equivalent to those of a commercial crop.

More precisely, EPS generated by *L. plantarum* has several advantageous characteristics. The key characteristics of the EPS generated by this bacterium are its rheological and prebiotic qualities. According to a current study, EPS has numerous uses, including health, in terms of anticancer and antioxidant properties, including prebiotic benefits (Silva et al., 2019).

1.5. The Synergistic Impact of Probiotic Bacteria with *Lactobacillus Plantarum*

The fungus species *Aspergillus nomius, Aspergillus favus, and Aspergillus parasiticus* create aflatoxins, a category of significant mycotoxins which are secondary metabolites. Four different aflatoxins (types B1, G1, B2, and G2) are considered to influence the development of cancer for both humans and animals. The strongest hepatotoxic and hepatocarcinogenic of these is B1 (Zamani et al., 2022). Using chemicals, which run the danger of causing environmental pollution is the foundation of strategies to lower aflatoxin contamination. As a result, different alternatives have recently been examined, such as using microorganisms and plant essential oils to inhibit the growth of fungi that produce aflatoxin (Gómez et al., 2018). Experiments on assessing how novel *L. plantarum* strains isolated from dairy products and chitosan nanoparticles affected the toxicity of aflatoxin B1 (AFB1) in vitro were performed in 2022 by a group of researchers from Iran. Lactic acid bacterial strains (LABs) have been identified and isolated, employing biochemical and molecular techniques after collecting and processing yoghurt, cheese, milk, and whey products. In addition, salt, bile, and pH tolerance tests were employed to assess probiotic activity. By evaluating AFB1 using the enzyme-linked immunosorbent assay (ELISA) and high-performance liquid chromatography (HPLC), the effect of cheese-specific strain isolate and chitosan nanoparticles on lowering aflatoxin B1 (AFB1) in the medium was examined. They concluded that combining the novel cheese-specific strain *L. plantarum* strains with chitosan nanoparticles reduced the amount of the AFB1 toxin in food items (Zamani et al., 2022). Yılmaz and Gökmen (2017) focused on the interactions between *S. thermophilus RSKK 04082, L. delbrueckii subsp. bulgaricus DSM 20081,* and *L. plantarum RSKK 02030* to examine the generation of tyramine during yoghurt fermentation. Single strains of these microorganisms or mixed cultures with double- or triple strains were utilized in yoghurt fermentation. Tyramine might be produced by the bacteria *S. thermophilus RSKK 04082 and L. plantarum RSKK 02030*, depending on the fermentation circumstances, but not by *L. delbrueckii subsp. bulgaricus DSM 20081*. Tyramine production was discovered to be influenced by synergistic interactions between the *S. thermophilus and L. delbrueckii subsp. bulgaricus* strains as well as *L. delbrueckii subsp. bulgaricus* and *L. plantarum.*

Since prebiotics are non-digestible dietary components used to improve probiotic functional performance in the gastrointestinal system, they positively impact the host by deliberately promoting healthy colon bacterial development and/or activity (Stoyanova et al., 2010). Inulin and other non-digestible carbohydrates appear to be real prebiotics. Gum acacia is one of several additional non-digestible oligosaccharides that have recently been produced. Gum acacia is highly fermentable in vitro using human intestinal flora and in vivo in humans and rats. For instance, synbiotics are created by combining probiotics and prebiotics to improve microbial control in the gastrointestinal system. Evidence suggests that the survival and activity of the organism are enhanced when proper prebiotics and probiotics are combined. When administered together, synbiotics have been shown to reduce colon carcinogenesis more than when used alone (Nagpal et al., 2007).

In order to create a synbiotic product made with the selected culture and subsequently freeze-dried, the study of Dhewa et al. (2014) assesses the prebiotics impact (acacia gum and inulin) on *L. plantarum.* A freeze-dried synbiotic formulation containing *L. plantarum* and prebiotics was created using nonfat dry milk as a starting point. The product, which can be of significant assistance in producing probiotic food, had substantial quantities of active probiotics even after 90 days of storage at 4°C. Furthermore, viable counts of the probiotic microorganisms in the product remained high for the whole 90 days of refrigeration storage (8 to 9 log cfu/g); however, the numbers significantly decreased in the product held at ambient temperature (25 °C) (Dhewa et al., 2014).

1.6. The Influence of Probiotic Dairy Products Obtained with *L. plantarum* on Human Health

Milk contains all the growth elements needed for probiotics, making dairy products a standout among typical probiotic carriers. Additionally, dairy products including cheese, yoghurt, kefir and frozen yoghurt, which are regularly supplemented with probiotics. It should come as no surprise that various species, including *L. plantarum, L. acidophilus, L. delbrueckii, L. brevis, L. rhamnosus, L. casei, and L. helveticus*, have been shown to be beneficial and are employed as starters or non-starters to aid in dairy products fermentation and preservation, as well as the generation of fragrance compounds and bacteriocins which expand their responsibilities to biotechnology uses (Abdelazez et al., 2018). Acetate (volatile) and lactate (nonvolatile) organic acids are balanced by the bacteria to provide food certain tastes and flavors. Different strains or recombinants of *Lactobacillus plantarum* in dairy products can help to restore the balance of the luxuriant flora in the intestines, inhibit a variety of harmful microbes, and may even be used as vaccine delivery systems (Zago et al., 2011). Interest in creating new foods with probiotic microbes has increased due to their health advantages. Probiotics thereby lessen the symptoms of lactose intolerance, prevent many types of bowel illness, and improve the balance of intestinal microbes (Lomer et al., 2008).

In our case, *L. plantarum* may positively affect human health as a probiotic by modulating the immune system, lowering cholesterol, maintaining a healthy gut flora, and lowering the risk of tumours. More importantly, *L. plantarum* produces lactic acid, antibacterial bioactive substances, and additional exopolysaccharides to show their antagonistic potential against the activities of intestinal pathogenic pathogens (De Vries et al., 2006). Therefore, strains of *L. plantarum* were utilized as fortifiers in the food business, notably in the dairy sector. Additionally, bacteriocins were created. PlnA and the two-peptide bacteriocins PlnJK, PlnEF, and plantaricin NC8 are examples of plantaricins produced by *L. plantarum*. Some of these plantaricins have antibacterial activity against the most common Gram-positive and Gram-negative foodborne pathogens, including *Listeria monocytogenes, Salmonella enterica, Escherichia coli, Staphylococcus aureus,* and others that can contaminate dairy products and lead to severe human illnesses (Jiang et al., 2016), including infectious endocarditis, gastroenteritis, maternofetal infections, meningoencephalitis, etc. (Field et al., 2016).

One study released by Hütt et al.,2015, demonstrated that three weeks of consuming the probiotic strain *L. plantarum TENSIA* in cheese or yoghurt decreased both systolic and diastolic blood pressure despite the food matrix, baseline levels of blood pressure and body mass index, confirming the role of the probiotic strain functional properties in reducing the risk of cardiovascular disease.

Additionally, *L. plantarum*, in particular, exhibits several advantageous properties as an anti-cancer, anticoagulant, antiviral, immunological modulator, anti-inflammatory, anti-diabetic, and antioxida. Moreover, it demonstrates free radical scavenging action (Kassayova et al., 2014). Kefir and yogurt extracts (Biffi et al., 1997), as well as fermented milk (Chen et al., 2007), containing five different probiotic species, all suppressed the proliferation of the MCF-7 breast cancer cell line. A mouse syngeneic model involving subcutaneous injection of the 4T1 tumoral cell line has been employed in a number of animal investigations (Rachid et al.,2006; de Moreno de LeBlanc et al., 2005; de Moreno de LeBlanc et al., 2007; Yazdi et al., 2010;). In these studies, *L. helveticus*-fermented milk and kefir (de Moreno de LeBlanc et al., 2005; de Moreno de LeBlanc et al., 2007) were able to inhibit the formation of breast tumors when given cyclically for 28 days following tumor induction. Long-term chemopreventive research, however, is still absent.

They also positively overall health effects for illnesses including psoriasis, allergies, and neurological system disorders (Kim et al., 2015). According to some research, *L. plantarum* strains are transported via fermented milk, which has a higher bacterial load when consumed. A daily therapeutic dosage of 10^8–10^9 CFU/g is advised because the probiotic bacteria may be reduced during passage through the GI system (Shah, 2000). Because of its resistance to GI tract simulating conditions, lack of hemolytic activity, susceptibility to antibiotics, and antagonistic effects against test pathogens, *L. plantarum* strain GCC_19M1 obtained from fermented, unpasteurised milk may be a potential probiotic bacteria. The study of Nath et al. (2020) supports the widespread opinion of the locals in the Cachar area of Assam, India, that drinking fermented raw milk helps digestion, eases constipation, and promotes overall health. The findings demonstrated that *L. plantarum strain GCC_19M1* has significant probiotic potential, and its presence in fermented raw milk products may act as a robust functional probiotic meal. Nevertheless, further, in vivo research is required to fully explain its potential for enhancing human health in real-world settings.

Conclusion

Dairy products and probiotic microorganisms have a long-standing association. Yoghurt is one dairy product that can deliver a suitable food carrier to introduce probiotics into the digestive system. *L. plantarum* strains have been well-compliant with probiotic needs for a long time and have been integrated into human diet and culture. The importance of this species as a leading probiotic candidate is further projected by the fact that numerous strains of *L. plantarum* have demonstrated health qualities throughout the gut-heart-brain axis, spanning elements of gut health, metabolic diseases, and mental health. This probiotic strain, found in the fermented food system, can contribute to/warrant boosting health and well-being and lowering danger to the consumer while also minimizing the need for pharmaceutical substances. Furthermore, *L. plantarum* has shown favourable characteristics for its usage as auxiliary culture in the cheese industry, fulfilling the dual function of being a probiotic and secondary starter cultures. Utilizing certain strains had both a technical and probiotic impact; it helped standardize cheese quality and had valuable health benefits at the gut mucosa in vivo.

References

[1] Abushelaibi, A., Al-Mahadin, S., El-Tarabily, K., Shah, N. P., Ayyash, M., (2017). Characterization of potential probiotic lactic acid bacteria isolated from camel milk. *LWT- Food Science and Technology*. 79, 316–325.

[2] Aadinath, Ghosh, T., Amaladhas, P. H., Anandharamakrishnan, C. Dried Dairy Products and Their Trends in the Global Market. *Handbook of Drying for Dairy Products*. 1-15. Ist ed, Edited by Anandharamakrishnan, C.-John Wiley & Sons Ltd. (2017).

[3] Agagündüz, D., Yılmaz, B., Sahin, T. O., Günesliol, B. E., Ayten, S., Russo, P., Spano, G., Rocha, J. M., Bartkiene, E., Özogul, F., (2021). Dairy Lactic Acid Bacteria and Their Potential Function in Dietetics: The Food–Gut-Health Axis. *Foods*, 10, 3099.

[4] Abdelazez, A., Muhammad, Z., Zhang, Q. X., Zhu, Z. T., Abdelmotaal, H., Sami, R., Meng, X. C., (2018). Production of a Functional Frozen Yoghurt Fortified with Bifidobacterium spp. *BioMed research international*, 6438528, 1-10.

[5] Ale, E. C, Perezlindo, M. J, Pavón, Y. Peralta, G. H., Costa, S., Sabbag, N., Bergamini, C., Reinheimer, J. A., Binetti, A. G., (2016). Technological, rheological and sensory characterizations of a yoghurt containing an exopolysaccharide extract from *Lactobacillus fermentum Lf2*, a new food additive. *Food Res Int*, 90:259–267.

[6] Ayyash, M., Abu-Jdayil, B., Hamed, F., Shaker, R., (2018). Rheological, textural, microstructural and sensory impact of exopolysaccharide producing *Lactobacillus plantarum* isolated from camel milk on low-fat akawi cheese. *LWT Food Sci Technol* 87,423–431.

[7] Bao, Y., Zhang, Y., Li, H., Liu, Y., Wang, S., Dong, X., Su, F., Yao, G., Sun, T., Zhang, H., (2012b). In vitro screen of *Lactobacillus plantarum* as probiotic bacteria and their fermented characteristics in soymilk. *Ann. Microbiol.* 62, 1311–1320.

[8] Bartkiene, E., Ruzauskas, M., Krungleviciute, V., Zavistanaviciute, P., Bernatoniene, J., Jakstas, V., Ivanauskas, L., Zadeike, D., Klupsaite, D., Viskelis, P., Bendoraitiene, J., Navikaite-Snipaitiene, V., Juodeikiene, G., (2017a). Development of antimicrobial gummy candies with addition of bovine colostrum, essential oils and probiotics. *International journal of food science & technology*, 1–9.

[9] Behera, S. S., Ray, R. C., Zdolec, N., (2018). *Lactobacillus plantarum* with Functional Properties: An Approach to Increase Safety and Shelf-Life of Fermented Foods. *BioMed Research International, 9361614,*1-18.

[10] Biffi A., Coradini D., Larsen R., Riva L. and Di Fronzo G., (1997). Antiproliferative effect of fermented milk on the growth of a human breast cancer cell line. *Nutr Cancer,* 28, 93-99.

[11] Burns, P., Cuffia, F., Milesi, M., Vinderola, G., Meinardi, C., Sabbag, N., Hynes, E., (2012).Technological and probiotic role of adjunct cultures of non-starter lactobacilli in soft cheeses. *Food Microbiology*, 30, 45-50.

[12] Cardoso, T., Marques, C., Dagostin, J. L. A., & Masson, M. L. (2019). Lactobionic acid as a potential food ingredient: Recent studies and applications. *Journal of Food Science*, 84, 1672–1681.

[13] Casarotti, S. N., Monteiro, D. A., Moretti, M. M. S., Penna, A. L. B., (2014). Influence of the combination of probiotic cultures during fermentation and storage of fermented milk. *Food Res. Int.*, 59,67–75.

[14] Champagne, C. P., Raymond, Y., Pouliot, Y., Gauthier, S. F., Lessard, M., (2014). Effect of bovine colostrum, cheese whey, and spray-dried porcine plasma on the in vitro growth of probiotic bacteria and Escherichia coli. *Can J Microbiol*, 60, 287-295.

[15] Chaucheyras-Durand, F., Durand, H., (2010). Probiotics in animal nutrition and health. *Benef Microbes,* 1(1), 3–9.

[16] Chen, K. N., Chen, M. J., Liu, J. R., Lin, C. W., Chiu, H. Y., (2005). Optimization of incorporated prebiotics as coating materials for probiotic microencapsulation. *Journal of food science*, 70 (5), M260-M266.

[17] Chen C., Hing M. C., Kubow, S., (2007). Kefir extracts suppress in vitroproliferation of estrogen-dependent human breast cancer cells but not normal mammary epithelial cells. *J Med Food*,10: 416-422.

[18] Ciocia, F., Mcsweeney, P., Piraino, P., Parente, E., (2013). Use of dairy and non-dairy *Lactobacillus plantarum, Lactobacillus paraplantarum* and *Lactobacillus pentosus* strains as adjuncts in cheddar cheese. *Dairy Sci. & Technol.*, 93,623–640.

[19] Cizeikiene, D., Juodeikiene, G., Paskevicius, A., Bartkiene, E., (2013). Antimicrobial activity of lactic acid bacteria against pathogenic and spoilage

microorganisms isolated from food and their control in wheat bread. *Food Control*, 31, 539–545.

[20] Cory, H., Passarelli, S., Szeto, J., Tamez, M., Mattei, J., (2018). The role of polyphenols in human health and food systems: A mini-review. *Front Nutr.* 5:87.

[21] Dallagnol, A. M., Pescum, M., De Valdez, G. F., Rollán, G., (2013). Fermentation of quinoa and wheat slurries by *Lactobacillus plantarum* CRL 778: proteolytic activity. *Appl Microbiol Biotechnol*, 97,3129–3140.

[22] Dan, T., Chen, H., Li, T., Tian, J., Ren, W., Zhang, H., Sun, T., (2019). Influence of *Lactobacillus plantarum P-8* on Fermented Milk Flavor and Storage Stability. *Frontiers in Microbiology, 9, 3133.*

[23] Daneshi, M., Ehsani, R. M., Razavi, H. S., Labbafi, M., (2013). Effect of refrigerated storage on the probiotic survival and sensory properties of milk/carrot juice mix drink. *Electronic Journal of Biotechnology*, 6, 1-12.

[24] Desai, K. G. H. and Park, H. J., (2005). Recent developments in microencapsulation of food ingredients. *Drying Technology*, 23, 1361-1394.

[25] De Moreno de LeBlanc A., Matar C., LeBlanc N., Perdigón G., (2005). Effects of milk fermented by *Lactobacillus helveticus* R389 on a murine breast cancer model. *Breast Cancer Res*, 7, R477-R486.

[26] De Moreno de LeBlanc, A., Matar, C., Farnworth, E., Perdigón G, (2007). Study of immune cells involved in the antitumor effect of kefir in a murine breast cancer model. *J Dairy Sci*, 90, 1920-1928.

[27] De Souza, A. H. P., Costa, G. A. N., Da Silva Miglioranza, L. H., Furlaneto-Maia, L., De Oliveira, A. F., (2013). Microbiological, physical, chemical and sensory characteristics of milk fermented with *Lactobacillus plantarum. Acta Scientiarum. Health Sciences, 35, 125-131.*

[28] De Vries, M. C., Vaughan,E. E., Kleerebezem, M., De Vos, W. M., (2006). *Lactobacillus plantarum* - Survival, functional and potential probiotic properties in the human intestinal tract. *Int. Dairy J.*,16,1018–1028.

[29] Dhewa, T., Pant, S., Mishra, V., (2014). Development of freeze dried synbiotic formulation using a probiotic strain of *Lactobacillus plantarum. J Food Sci Technol*, 51(1),83–89.

[30] Dos Santos, K. M. O., Vieira, A. D. S., Buriti, F. C. A., Do Nascimento, J. C. F., De Melo, M. E. S., Bruno, L. M., De Fátima Borges, M., Costa Rocha, C. R., De Souza Lopes, A. C., De Melo Franco, B. D. G., Todorov, S. D., (2015). Artisanal Coalho cheeses as source of beneficial *Lactobacillus plantarum and Lactobacillus rhamnosus* strains. *Dairy Sci. & Technol.*, 95, 209–230.

[31] Duan, C., Li, S., Zhao, Z., Wang, C., Zhao,Y., Yang, G., Niu, C., Gao, L., Liu, X., Zhao, L., (2019). Proteolytic Activity of *Lactobacillus plantarum* Strains in Cheddar Cheese as Adjunct Cultures. *Journal of Food Protection*, 82,12, 2108–2118.

[32] El-Sayed, H. S., Salama, H. H., El-Sayed, S. M., (2015). Production of synbiotic ice cream. *International Journal ChemTech Res*, 1(7), 138–147.

[33] Field, D., O'Connor, R., Cotter, P. D., Ross, R. P. and Hill, C., (2016). In vitro activities of nisin and nisin derivatives alone and in combination with antibiotics against Staphylococcus biofilms. *Frontiers in microbiology*, 7, 508(1-11).

[34] Fonseca, H. C., Duarte, E. R., Santos Souza,L. C. A., Alves Mariano, E. G., Dos Santos Pires, A. C., Santos Lima,T., Pinto, M. S., (2020). Growth, viability, and post-acidification of *Lactobacillus plantarum* in bovine transition milk. *Rev Mex Cienc Pecu*, 11(2), 539-552.

[35] Gadhiya, D., Patel, A., Prajapati, J. B., (2015). Current Trend and Future Prospective of Functional Probiotic Milk Chocolates and Related Products--a Review. *Czech Journal of Food Science*, 33, (4).

[36] Georgieva, R., Iliev, I., Haertlé, T., Chobert, J. M., Ivanova, I., Danova, S., (2009). Technological properties of candidate probiotic *Lactobacillus plantarum* strains. *Int. Dairy J.*, 19, 696–702.

[37] Gómez, J. V, Tarazona, A., Mateo-Castro, R., Gimeno-Adelantado, J. V., Jiménez, M., Mateo, E. M., (2018). Selected plant essential oils and their main active components, a promising approach to inhibit aflatoxigenic fungi and aflatoxin production in food. *Food Addit Contam: Part A* 35, 1581–1595.

[38] Granato, D., Branco, G. F., Cruz, A. C., Faria, J. de A. F., Shah, N. P. (2010). Probiotic dairy products as functional foods. *Comp. Rev, Food Sci. Food Safety.* 9, 455- 470.

[39] Hammam, A. R., Elfaruk, M. S., Ahmed, M. E. and Sunkesula, V., (2020). Characteristics and technological aspects of the Egyptian cheeses. *Int. J. Curr. Microbiol. Appl. Sci.* 9, 3338–3354.

[40] Hanafi, F. N. A., Kamaruding, N. A., Shaharuddin, S., (2022). Influence of coconut residue dietary fiber on physicochemical, probiotic (*Lactobacillus plantarum* ATCC 8014) survivability and sensory attributes of probiotic ice cream. *LWT - Food Science and Technology*, 154, 112725.

[41] Hegab, O. W., Abdel-Latif, E. F., Zaki, H. M. B. A., Ashraf, A. M., (2021). Fundamental role of *Lactobacillus plantarum* and inulin in improving safety and quality of Karish cheese. *Open Veterinary Journal*, 11(3), 356–363.

[42] Huang, C. M., Chia, P., Lim, C. S., Nai, J., Ding, D. Y., Seow, P., Chan, E. W., (2017). Synthesis and characterisation of Carboxymethyl cellulose from various agricultural wastes. *Cellulose Chemistry & Technology*, 51(7–8), 665–672.

[43] Hulak, N., Maksimovi, A. Z., Kai, A., Skelin, A., Fuka, M. M. (2016). Indigenous strains of lactobacillus isolated from the istrian cheese as potential starter cultures. *Mljekarstvo*, 66, 4, 282–292.

[44] Hütt, P., Songisepp, E., Rätsep, M., Mahlapuu, R., Kilk, K., Mikelsaar, M., (2015). Impact of probiotic Lactobacillus plantarum TENSIA in different dairy products on anthropometric and blood biochemical indices of healthy adults. *Beneficial Microbes*, 6(3), 233-243.

[45] Kacho, A. T., (2019). Industrial and Economic Importance of a Bacterium *Lactobacillus Plantarum*: A Review. *International Journal of Research Studies in Biosciences.* 7(6), 13-19.

[46] Kassayova, M., Bobrov, N., Strojný, L., Kiskova, T., Mikeš, J., Demečková, V., Orendáš, P., Bojkova, B., Péč, M., Kubatka, P., Bomba, A., (2014). Preventive effects of probiotic bacteria *Lactobacillus plantarum* and dietary fiber in chemically-induced mammary carcinogenesis. *Anticancer research*, 34(9), 4969-4975.

[47] Kaushik, J. K., Kumar, A., Duary, R. K., Mohanty, A. K., Grover, S., Batish, V. K., (2009). Functional and Probiotic Attributes of an Indigenous Isolate of *Lactobacillus plantarum.*

[48] Kim, H., Kim, H. R., Jeong, B. J., Lee, S. S., Kim, T. R., Jeong, J. H., Lee, M., Lee, S., Lee, J. S., Chung, D. K., (2015). Effects of oral intake of kimchiderived Lactobacillus plantarum K8 lysates on skin moisturizing. *Journal of Microbiology and Biotechnology*, 25(1), 74–80.

[49] Isa, J. K., Razavi, S. H., (2017). Characterization of *Lactobacillus plantarum* as a Potential Probiotic In vitro and Use of a Dairy Product (Yogurt) as Food Carrier. *Applied Food Biotechnology*, 4 ,1,11-18.

[50] Ivens, K. O., Baumert, J. L., Hutkins, R. L., Taylor, S. L., (2017). Effect of proteolysis during Cheddar cheese aging on the detection of milk protein residues by ELISA *J. Dairy Sci.,* 100,1629–1639.

[51] Jang, H. J., Jung, J., Yu, H. S., Lee, N. K., Paik, H. D., (2018). Evaluation of the Quality of Yogurt Using Ginseng Extract Powder and Probiotic *Lactobacillus plantarum* NK181. *Korean J. Food Sci. An.,* 38 (6),1160-1167.

[52] Jia, F. F., Zhang, L. J., Pang, X. H, Gu, X. X., Abdelazez, A., Liang, Y., Sun, S. R., Meng, X. C., (2017). Complete genome sequence of bacteriocin-producing Lactobacillus plantarum KLDS1. 0391, a probiotic strain with gastrointestinal tract resistance and adhesion to the intestinal epithelial cells," *Genomics,* 109, 5-6,432–437.

[53] Jiang, H., Li, P., Gu, Q., (2016). Heterologous expression and purification of plantaricin NC8, a two-peptide bacteriocin against salmonella spp. From lactobacillus plantarum ZJ316. *Protein expression and purification*, 127,28-34.

[54] Jouki, M., Khazaei, N., Ghasemlou, M., HadiNezhad, M., (2013). Effect of glycerol concentration on edible film production from cress seed carbohydrate gum. *Carbohydrate Polymers*, 96, 39–46.

[55] Landete, J. M, Plaza-Vinuesa, L., Montenegro, C., Santamarıa, L., Reveron, I., De las Rivas, B., Munoz, R., (2021). The use of *Lactobacillus plantarum* esterase genes: a biotechnological strategy to increase the bioavailability of dietary phenolic compounds in lactic acid bacteria. *International journal of food sciences and nutrition,* 72, 8, 1035–1045.

[56] Lang, F., Wen, J., Wu, Z., Pan, D., Wang, L., (2022). Evaluation of probiotic yoghurt by the mixed culture with *Lactobacillus plantarum* A3. *Food Science and Human Wellness,* 11, 323-33.

[57] Langa, S., Van den Bulck, E., Peirot´en, A., Gaya, P., Schols, H. A., Arqu´es, J. L. (2019). Application of lactobacilli and prebiotic oligosaccharides for the development of a synbiotic semi-hard cheese. *Lwt,* 114, 108361.

[58] Li, C., Song, J., Kwok, L. Y., Wang, J., Dong, Y., Yu, H., Hou, Q., Zhang, H., Chen, Y., (2017). Influence of *Lactobacillus plantarum* on yogurt fermentation properties and subsequent changes during post-fermentation storage. *J. Dairy Sci.,* 100, 2512–25.

[59] Li, C., Song, J., Kwok, L., Wang, J., Dong, Y., Yu, H., Hou, Q., Zhang, H., Chen,Y., (2017). Influence of *Lactobacillus plantarum* on yogurt fermentation properties and subsequent changes during postfermentation storage. *J. Dairy Sci.*, 100, 2512–2525.

[60] Lomer, M. C, Parkes, G. C, Sanderson, J. D, (2008). Lactose intolerance in clinical practice–myths and realities. *Alimentary pharmacology & therapeutics*, 27(2),93-103.

[61] Lucey, J. A. (2002). Formation and physical properties of milk protein gels. *Journal Dairy Science*, 85, 281–294.

[62] Marchiani, R., Bertolino, M., Ghirardello, D., Mcsweeney, P. L., Zeppa, G., (2016). Physicochemical and nutritional qualities of grape pomace powder-fortified semi-hard cheeses. *J. Food Sci. Technol.,* 53,1585–1596.

[63] Meidistria, T. R., Sembiring, L., Rahayu, E. S., Haedar, N., Dwyana, Z., (2020). Survival of *Lactobacillus plantarum dad 13* in probiotic cheese making. *IOP Conf. Series: Earth and Environmental Science*, 575, 012020.

[64] Nag, A., Han, K. S., Singh, H., (2011). Microencapsulation of probiotic bacteria using pH-induced gelation of sodium caseinate and gellan gum. *International Dairy Journal*, 21, 247-253.

[65] Nagpal, R., Yadav, H., Puniya, A. K., Singh, K., Jain, S., Marotta, F. (2007). Potential of probiotics and prebiotics for synbiotic functional dairy foods: an overview. *Int J Prob Preb*, 2, 75–84.

[66] Nahed A. A. E. and Amany M. E., (2020). Quality of Probiotic Gouda Cheese as a Functional Food. *J. Sus. Agric. Sci.* 46, 4, 89-97.

[67] Nath, S., Sikidar, J., Roy, M., Deb, B., (2020). In vitro screening of probiotic properties of Lactobacillus plantarum isolated from fermented milk product. *Food Quality and Safety*, 4, 213–223.

[68] Nishimura, M., Ohkawara, T., Tetsuka, K., Kawasaki, Y., Nakagawa, R., Satoh, H., Sato, Y., Nishihira, J., (2016). Effects of yogurt containing Lactobacillus plantarum HOKKAIDO on immune function and stress markers. *Journal of Traditional and Complementary Medicine*, 6, 275-280.

[69] Ngamsomchat, A., Kaewkod, T., Konkit, M., Tragoolpua, Y., Bovonsombut, S., Chitov, T. (2022). Characterisation of *Lactobacillus plantarum* of Dairy-Product Origin for Probiotic Chèvre Cheese Production. *Foods*, 11, 934.

[70] Nuraida, L., (2015). A review: Health-promoting lactic acid bacteria in traditional Indonesian fermented foods. *Food Sci. Hum. Wellness*, 4, 47–55.

[71] Ołdak, A., Zielinska, D., Rzepkowska, A., Kołozyn-Krajewska, D., (2017). Comparison of antibacterial activity of *Lactobacillus plantarum* strains isolated from two different kinds of regional cheeses from Poland: oscypek and korycinski cheese. *BioMed Research International,* 6820369, 1-10.

[72] Omar, S. R., Omar, S. N., (2018). Effect of microencapsulated lactobacillus plantarum on the rheological and sensorial properties of synbiotic ice cream. *International Journal of Current Research,* 10 (11), 75273-75278.

[73] Rachid, M., Matar, C., Duarte, J., Perdigón, G., (2006). Effect of milk fermented with a *Lactobacillus helveticus R389(+)* proteolytic strain on the immune system and on the growth of 4T1 breast cancer cells in mice. *Immunol Med Microbiol*, 47, 242-253.

[74] Saez-Orviz, S., Puertas, C. , Marcet, I., Rendueles, M., Díaz, M., (2020). Bioactive synbiotic coatings with lactobionic acid and Lactobacillus plantarum CECT 9567 in

the production and characterization of a new functional dairy product. *Journal of Functional Foods* 75, 104263.

[75] Shah, N. P. (2000). Probiotic bacteria: selective enumeration and survival in dairy foods. *Journal of Dairy Science*, 83(4), 894–907.

[76] Silva, L. A., Lopes Neto, J. H. P., Cardarelli, H. R., (2019). Exopolysaccharides produced by Lactobacillus plantarum: technological properties, biological activity, and potential application in the food industry. *Annals of Microbiology*, 69, 321–328.

[77] Stoyanova, S., Geuns, J., Hideg, E., Van Den Ende, W. (2010) The food additives inulin and stevioside counteract oxidative stress. *Int J Food Sci Nutr.* doi:10.3109/09637486.2010.523416.

[78] Parvez, S., Malik, K. A., Ah Kang, S. and Kim, H. Y. (2006). Probiotics and their fermented food products are beneficial for health. *Journal of Applied Microbiology*, 100 (6), 1171-1185.

[79] Pavli, F., Kovaiou, I., Apostolakopoulou, G., Kapetanakou, A., Skandamis, P., Nychas, G. J. E., Chorianopoulos, N., (2017). Alginate-based edible films delivering probiotic bacteria to sliced ham pretreated with high pressure processing. *International Journal of Molecular Sciences*, 18(9).

[80] Pereira de Souza, A. H., Costa, G. A. N., Miglioranza, L. H. S., Furlaneto-Maia, L., De Oliveira, A. F., (2013). Microbiological, physical, chemical and sensory characteristics of milk fermented with *Lactobacillus plantarum. Acta Scientiarum. Health Sciences*, 35, 1, 125-131.

[81] Pisano, M. B., Viale, S., Conti, S., Fadda, M. E., Deplano, M., Melis, M. P., Deiana, M., Cosentino, S., (2014). Preliminary evaluation of probiotic properties of Lactobacillus strains isolated from Sardinian dairy products. *BioMed Research International*, 286390, 1-9.

[82] Quigley, L., O'Sullivan, O., Stanton C., Beresford, T. P., Ross, R. P., Fitzgerald, G. F., Cotter, P. D., (2013). "The complex microbiota of raw milk," *FEMS Microbiology Reviews,* vol. 37, 5, 664–698.

[83] Rasovic, M. B., Mayrhofer, S., Martinovic, A., Dürr, K., Domig, K. J. (2017). Lactococci of local origin as potential starter cultures for traditional montenegrin cheese production. *Food Technol. Biotechnol*, 55, 55–66.

[84] Ricci, A., Allende, A., Bolton D., Chemaly, M., Davies, R., Girones, R., Koutsoumanis, K., Herman, L., Lindqvist, R., Nørrung, B., Robertson, L., Ru, G., Sanaa, M., Simmons, M., Skandamis, P., Snary, M., Speybroeck, N., Ter Kuile, B., Threlfall, J., Wahlstrom, H., Cocconcelli, P. S., Klein, G., Peixe, L., Maradona, M. P., Querol, A., Suarez, J. E., Sundh, I., Vlak, J., Correia, S., Escamez, P. S. F., (2017). Update of the list of QPS-recommended biological agents intentionally added to food or feed as notified to EFSA 5: suitability of taxonomic units notified to EFSA until September 2016. *EFSA Journal*, 15, 3, 2017.

[85] Rodrıguez, H., Curiel, J. A, Landete, J. M, de las Rivas, B., Lopez de Felipe, F, Gomez-Cordoves, C., Mancheno, J. M, Munoz, R., (2009). Food phenolics and lactic acid bacteria. *Int J Food Microbiol.* 132(2-3),79–90.

[86] Sabet-Sarvestani, N., Eskandari, M. H., Hosseini, S. M. H., Niakousari, M., Gahruie, H. H., Khalesi, M., (2021). Production of synbiotic ice cream using *Lactobacillus*

casei/Lactobacillus plantarum and fructooligosaccharides. *J Food Process Preserv.*, 45:e15423.

[87] Selma, N. V, Espin, J. C, Tomas-Barberan, F. A., (2009). Interaction between phenolics and gut microbiota role in human health. *J Agr Food Chem.* 57, 6585–6501.

[88] Tee, W. F., Nazaruddin, R., Tan, Y. N., Ayob, M. K., (2014). Effects of encapsulation on the viability of potential probiotic *Lactobacillus plantarum* exposed to high acidity condition and presence of bile salts. *Food Science and Technology International*, 20(6), 399-404.

[89] Tremonte, P., Pannella, G., Succi, M., Tipaldi, L., Sturchio, M., Coppola, R., Luongo, D., Sorrentino, E., (2017). Antimicrobial activity of *Lactobacillus plantarum* strains isolated from different environments: A preliminary study. *Int. Food Res. J.*, 24, 852–9.

[90] Tripathi, M. K., Giri, S. K., (2014). Probiotic functional foods: Survival of probiotics during processing and storage. *J Funct Foods*, 9(1), 225–241.

[91] Turchi, B., Torracca B., Fratini, F., Mancini, S., Pedonese, F., Nuvoloni, R., Galiero, A., Montalbano, B., Cerri, D., (2017). *Lactobacillus plantarum* and *Streptococcus thermophilus* as starter cultures for a donkey milk fermented beverage. *International Journal of Food Microbiology*, 256, 1, 54–61.

[92] Utami, T., Harmayani, E., Rahayu, E. S., (2016). Survival of *Lactobacillus plantarum* Dad 13 during Spray Drying and Its Application for Yoghurt Fermentation. *Int. Res. J. Biol. Sci.*, 5, 16–22.

[93] Zago, M., Fornasari, M. E., Carminati, D., Burns, P., Suàrez, V., Vinderola, G., Giraffa, G., (2011). Characterization and probiotic potential of *Lactobacillus plantarum* strains isolated from cheeses. *Food Microbiology*, 28(5), 1033-1040.

[94] Zhang, W., Sun, Z., Bilige, M., Zhang, H., (2015). Complete genome sequence of probiotic *Lactobacillus plantarum* P-8 with antibacterial activity. *J. Biotechnol.* 193, 41–42.

[95] Zhang, S. S., Xu, Z. S., Qin, L. H., Kong, J., (2020) Low-sugar yogurt making by the co-cultivation of *Lactobacillus plantarum* WCFS1 with yogurt starter cultures. *J. Dairy Sci.*, 103,3045–3054.

[96] Shariati, Z., Jouki, M., Rafiei, F., (2019). Flavored functional drinking yogurt (Doogh) formulated with Lactobacillus plantarum LS5, cress seed gum, and coriander leaves extract. *Food Sci Nutr.*, 8, 894–902.

[97] Vukasovic, T. Functional foods in line with young consumers: Challenges in the market place in Slovenia. In: *Developing New Functional Food and Nutraceutical products.* Edited by Bagchi, D. and Nair, S.1st ed., Academic Press. Cambridge (2017).

[98] Wang, J., Zhao, X., Yang, Y., Zhao, A., Yang, Z., (2015b) Characterization and bioactivities of an exopolysaccharide produced by *Lactobacillus plantarum* YW32. *Int J Biol Macromol* 74,119–126.

[99] Yazdi M. H., Dallal M. M. S., Hassan Z. M., Holakuyee M., Amiri S. A., Abolhassani M. and Mahdavi M, (2010). Oral administration of Lactobacillus acidophilus induces IL12 production in spleen cell culture of BALB/c mice bearing transplanted breast tumour. *Br J Nutr*, 104, 227-232.

[100] Yılmaz, C., Gökmen, V., (2017). Formation of Tyramine in Yoghurt during Fermentation – Interaction between Yoghurt Starter Bacteria and *Lactobacillus plantarum. Food Research International,* S0963-9969 (17) 30163-1.

[101] Zamani, N., Fazeli, M. R., Sepahi, A. A., Shariatmadari, F., (2022). A new probiotic Lactobacillus plantarum strain isolated from traditional dairy together with nanochitosan particles shows the synergistic effect on aflatoxin B1 detoxification. *Archives of Microbiology*, 204-624.

Chapter 7

Lactobacillus plantarum and Its Role in Meat Products Manufacturing

Rafael Sepúlveda Fonsêca Trevisan Passos
Camila Cristina Avelar de Sousa
Thiago da Matta Pires Cruz
Juliana Sant'Ana Falcão Leite
Maurício Costa Alves da Silva
and Carlos Pasqualin Cavalheiro*
Laboratório de Inspeção e Tecnologia de Carnes e Derivados (LabCarne), Universidade Federal da Bahia, Salvador, Brazil

Abstract

Consumers are pushing the food industry for functional and healthier products, increasing the demand for new products. Probiotics can be incorporated into several food matrices, such as meat and meat products, which have rich nutrient content as protein, minerals, water, and provide an environment capable of supporting microbial life and growth. Meat and meat products are highly consumed worldwide and can be presented in raw, cooked, fermented products. *Lactobacillus plantarum* is a lactic acid bacterium with high probiotic potential, which can provide health benefits as antidiabetic, anti-obesity, anti-inflammatory, and antioxidant properties to consumers. However, applying probiotic *L. plantarum* can be a hard task due to various factors such as strain selection, its behavior during meat processing, the intrinsic characteristics of meat products, and the probiotic survival rate on final products. Furthermore, the heat

---

* Corresponding Author's Email: carlos.cavalheiro@ufba.br.

In: Lactobacillus plantarum and Its Role in Human Health
Editors: Maria Simona Chiş, Adriana Paucean
ISBN: 979-8-89113-696-0

treatment that some types of meat products undergo can make it harder to use *L. plantarum* in cooked meat products. Thus, the incorporation of *L. plantarum* on different meat products has been studied. The application of *L. plantarum* in fermented products is easier because no thermal processing is used. However, to be successfully incorporated in raw and cooked meat products, *L. plantarum* needs to undergo auxiliary technologies such as encapsulation. Then, the incorporation of probiotic microorganisms as free cells or in encapsulated forms is an alternative for use in meat products. Then, we are aiming to analyze recent studies about the incorporation of this microorganism in meat products reformulation, focusing on their impact on technological, nutritional, microbiological, sensory properties and health benefits to consumers.

Keywords: cooked meat products, fermented meat products, fresh meat products, functional meat products, *Lactobacillus* spp., meat reformulation

1. Introduction

Fermented meat products are traditional products from different parts of the world, including European and African countries (Mokoena et al., 2016; Franciosa et al., 2018). Their origin can be traced to empirical methods of meat preservation in the post-Paleolithic past (Blaiotta et al., 2017). Fermentation is a biochemical process carried out by different microorganisms that leads to the degradation of non-digestible carbohydrates and enriches essential amino acids, minerals, and vitamins, affecting the nutritional quality and digestibility of fermented foods (Giri et al., 2018). In addition, these products have sensory characteristics that are desirable to consumers and therefore have a higher market value. Moreover, the acidifying effect of fermenting microorganisms and the production of bactericidal substances such as bacteriocins extend the shelf life of fermented products (Munekata et al., 2021).

Among the microorganisms involved in fermentation processes, there are several bacterial genera associated with fermentative processes in foods. The main genera include *Lactobacillus*, which is commonly found in fermented dairy products and lactic acid fermented foods such as pickles; *Streptococcus*, which is found in fermented dairy products such as yoghurt and cheese; *Bifidobacterium* and *Enterococcus*, which can be isolated from various foods such as salami, ham, yoghurt, cheese, pasteurized milk, and olives (Cavalheiro et al., 2021; Souza et al., 2021; Sun et al., 2023). In addition to their role in the fermentation process, bacteria of these genera may also serve as probiotics.

Probiotic microorganisms are microorganisms that have health benefits for consumers when consumed regularly in appropriate amounts. To be considered probiotic, a microorganism must meet certain safety, functional, and technological criteria. In terms of safety, the preferred probiotics are of human origin, are isolated from healthy gastrointestinal tracts, are nonpathogenic, and do not possess antimicrobial resistance genes. Functional requirements include tolerance to human gastric acid and bile, adhesion to surfaces, and colonization of the human gastrointestinal tract. Technologically, probiotics must remain viable in the product during processing and storage while exhibiting good sensory properties (Binda et al., 2020).

Foods enriched with probiotic microorganisms are considered functional because they have beneficial health effects on consumers when consumed in appropriate concentrations. To act as probiotics, the microorganisms must be consumed at a concentration of 6 to 7 log CFU/g in 100 grams of food (Nulkaekul et al., 2012). With the increasing global interest in healthier, more natural, and functional foods, the industry demand for research and development of these novel products is also increasing.

Among microorganisms with probiotic potential, *Lactobacillus plantarum*, a gram-positive and acidic lactic acid bacterium (LAB), is widely used in the production of fermented foods such as cheese, fermented milk, and yogurt (Li et al., 2017; Dan et al., 2019; Ngamsomchat et al., 2022). In meat products, it is mainly used for sausages, dry-fermented sausages, salami, and other products, playing a key role especially in sensory aspects such as texture and flavor (Yoo et al., 2015; Blaiotta et al., 2017; Ge et al., 2019). *L. plantarum* is also an important acidifier due to lactic acid production (Śmietana et al., 2023). In addition, it can produce bacteriocins, which are proteins or protein complexes with bactericidal activity against mostly closely related species (Todorov, 2009).

Studies have shown that *L. plantarum* strains have beneficial effects on human health. Modulation of the immune system, reduction of harmful bacteria and growth promotion of beneficial microorganisms, lowering cholesterol levels, anti-inflammatory and antioxidant properties, and improvement of skin barrier function are some of the effects of *L. plantarum* (Boyle & Tang, 2006; Ha et al., 2006; Lee et al., 2015; Qiu et al., 2018; Wang et al., 2019). Due to these health benefits, *L. plantarum* has been increasingly recognized in recent years as a probiotic strain that should be added to meat products (Yang et al. 2022).

Global meat consumption has increased significantly in recent decades and is expected to reach 465 million tons by 2050 (FAO, 2018). In addition, the demand for fermented meat products is also increasing. Moreover, fermented meat products are the main matrix for the application of probiotic microorganisms such as *L. plantarum*, but they can also be added to raw and cooked products (Trabelsi et al., 2019).

However, for *L. plantarum* to be consumed as a probiotic in meat products, it must be present at the appropriate concentration at the time of consumption. Although *L. plantarum* is sensitive to high temperatures, its addition to meat products is challenging, especially for meat products that require cooking before consumption. It is known that the cooking process kills bacteria, reducing the microbiota in the meat product and negating its probiotic effect. Subsequently, strategies can be developed for the effective use of these strains in cooked meat products. Cavalheiro et al. (2015) reported in their review the different strategies for the use of probiotics (including *L. plantarum* strains) in meat products.

In order to expand the choice of meat products enriched with probiotics, investments and research efforts are directed toward evaluating the viability of these microorganisms in different meat formulations. Therefore, it is critical for the food industry to understand the role of *L. plantarum* in the production of meat products to ensure the safety and quality of these products. In this chapter, we will investigate the feasibility of adding *L. plantarum* in various forms to meat products. In addition, we will investigate the effects of the addition of these microorganisms on the physical, chemical, microbiological, and sensory properties of various meat products.

2. *Lactobacillus Plantarum* in Raw Meat Products

Some possibilities of *L. plantarum* application under different strategies in meat products are shown in Table 1. During storage of meat products, especially raw meat, biochemical reactions, and microbial growth occur due to their biological properties and chemical composition, such as saturated and unsaturated lipids, proteins, carbohydrates, vitamins, and pigments, leading to their deterioration (Pateiro et al., 2018). This changes the sensory characteristics of the product and, consequently, its acceptability to the consumer. In this way, *L. plantarum* can be used as a form of bio preservation to maintain safety and microbiological quality and extend the shelf life of meat products due to its metabolites such as bacteriocins, organic acids, hydrogen peroxide, and enzymes (da Costa, Voloski, Mondadori, Duval, & Fiorentini, 2019).

Table 1. Addition of *L. plantarum* in meat products under different delivery strategies

	Meat product	Delivery strategy	Main results	Reference
Raw	Beef patties	Free cells and encapsulated	Addition of probiotics maintained the lightness and redness parameters during storage period. Lipid oxidation was lower in treatments with probiotic addition as free cells. Acidification on beef patties with probiotic addition.	Trevisan et al. (2022)
	Ground beef	Free cells	Reduction in lipid oxidation of ground beef with probiotic inoculation. Increase on lightness values during storage period.	Trabelsi et al. (2019)
	Fresh beef sausage	Free cells	*Salmonella enterica* reduction during storage period (from inoculated at 5 log CFU/g to 1.5 log CFU/g on the 5th day of storage).	Ben Slima et al. (2017)
Cooked	Beef patties	Encapsulated	Encapsulated probiotics were viable even after cooking treatment. No significative impact on the sensorial aspects of probiotic beef patties.	de Marins et al. (2022)
	Cooked sausage	Free cells	Better microbiological quality after three weeks of storage associated with good sensory acceptance.	Łaszkiewicz et al. (2021)
	Cooked chorizo	Free cells	Among 10 isolates of LAB from meat products, *L. plantarum* was the most promising to be used as bio preservation of cooked meat products	Lucumi-Baguero et al. (2021)
	Sucuk	Encapsulated	Probiotic strain survived the heat treatment at 70°C with only 1 log reduction in viable cell number.	Bilenler et al. (2017)
Fermented	Dry-sausages	Encapsulated	Chorizo sausages had adequate levels of *L. plantarum* counts even after 60 days of chilled storage.	Cavalheiro et al. (2020)

Table 1. (Continued)

	Meat product	Delivery strategy	Main results	Reference
Fermented	Dry-fermented sausages	Free cells	Good physicochemical, microbiological, and sensory aspects. The *L. plantarum* strain was a promising probiotic adjunct culture to be used in association with starter culture to develop functional dry-fermented sausages	Pavli et al. (2020)
	Chorizo	Encapsulated	Adequate sensory scores were achieved on treatments with *L. plantarum* addition. The encapsulation of probiotic in alginate beads proved to be a better alternative for the incorporation of probiotics in chorizo sausages because the physico-chemical characteristics of the meat products were adequate and exhibited the highest probiotic counts throughout ripening.	Cavalheiro et al. (2019)
	Dry-fermented sausages	Free cells	No differences on sensory properties among treatments with *L. plantarum* addition at different concentrations and control. The probiotic strains had potential to be a starter culture to produce dry-fermented meat products.	Ge et al. (2019)
	Fermented meat patties	Free cells	Inoculated *L. plantarum* had great antimicrobial activity against many pathogenic bacteria. In addition, improved the oxidative stability of meat product.	Hashemi et al. (2018)
	Beef sausage	Free cells	The myristic and arachidic acid content of the sausages with probiotics addition was significantly lower than that of the controls.	Arief et al. (2016)

As these are raw meat products, the viability of *L. plantarum* as a probiotic during storage is important due to its bioprotectant activity. However, for products that need to be cooked before consumption, the viability of probiotics can be expected to be affected by heat treatment. Thus, the encapsulation technique is an alternative for better survival of probiotic bacteria, resulting in reduced lipid oxidation, pH, color, and texture, and increased microbiological quality (Etchepare et al., 2016a; Etchepare et al., 2016b). According to Aryani et al. (2016), the inactivation temperature of *L. plantarum* is between 55 °C and 63 °C. Thus, a cooking temperature of 72 °C would lead to inactivation of the probiotic cells, resulting in the loss of probiotic potential in the food. This presents a challenge for the introduction of *L. plantarum* into cooked meat products, especially in the form of free cells. For this reason, there are few studies on this topic.

Regarding the reduction of lipid oxidation, Trabelsi et al. (2019) considered that *L. plantarum* TN8, when applied as free cells to ground beef at different concentrations (7 log CFU/g; 8 log CFU/g and 9 log CFU/g), was able to retard lipid oxidation as measured by thiobarbituric acid reactive substances (TBARS). However, the different concentrations of *L. plantarum* did not significantly affect the reduction of lipid oxidation, with TBARS values of 1.50 mg MDA/kg for the 7 log CFU/g treatment, 1.59 mg MDA/kg for the 8 log CFU/g treatment, and 1.83 mg MDA/kg for the 9 log CFU/g treatment. In the study conducted by Ben Slima et al. (2017), the application of *L. plantarum* strain TN8 as free cells at concentrations of 7 log CFU/g and 8 log CFU/g in combination with nitrite (50 mg/kg) was found to be effective in reducing lipid oxidation in beef sausages. In addition, this probiotic strain was found to exhibit similar antioxidant effects to nitrite, which is an important antioxidant in the processed meat industry. Therefore, it is possible to change the composition of these products by reducing the number of synthetic antioxidants and increasing their natural attractiveness, which is highly desirable for consumers. The antioxidant effect of probiotic strains is related to the prevention of the formation of primary and secondary oxidation products development (Danuta & Zbigniew, 2012). According to Trabelsi et al. (2019), the antioxidant effect of probiotic strains is related to their antimicrobial effect, as the reduction of bacterial load also reduces endogenous lipases and bacterial lipolytic enzymes. These enzymes are responsible for the release of free fatty acids, and the synthesis of these free fatty acids are the main precursors of volatile compounds that cause lipid oxidation. In addition, *L. plantarum* can hydrolyze sarcoplasmic proteins, such as myoglobin. Ferrylmyoglobin is known to be an effective agent contributing to lipid oxidation in meat products (Danuta & Zbigniew, 2012). Trevisan et al. (2022) used *L. plantarum* ATCC 7469 in beef patties, either as free cells or encapsulated in alginate beads. Regarding lipid oxidation, the encapsulation strategy had a strong effect on TBARS levels. In this study, TBARS values ranged from 0.360 to 0.801 mg MDA/kg and were lower in treatments with the addition of free probiotic strains.

Regarding pH, it is expected that the addition of *L. plantarum* contributes to the acidification of meat products. This acidification is caused by the production of lactic acid, which has been shown to have beneficial effects on certain meat products, such as sausages. Specifically, acidification of meat products can inhibit the growth of pathogenic bacteria and improve sensory characteristics in terms of tenderness and flavor (Ben Slima et al., 2017). These results suggest that the addition of *L. plantarum* to meat products could have important implications for product safety and quality in the meat industry. During cold storage (4 °C), beef treated with *L. plantarum* (109 CFU/g) showed significantly lower pH than control samples (5.41 and 6.01, respectively) (Trabelsi et al., 2019). Trevisan et al. (2022) observed that even in alginate beads, the metabolism of the encapsulated probiotic strains was intense, and the lactic acid produced was able to pass through the capsules into the meat matrix, lowering the pH of beef patties from 5.66 at the beginning of the storage period to 5.34 on the third day.

Color is one of the most important parameters evaluated by consumers of meat products. Generally, products are expected to have a more reddish color, represented by high values of a^* in instrumental color analysis. However, it is known that during the storage period, a decrease in the red content can be expected due to spoilage processes (Passos et al., 2022). According to Trabelsi et al. (2019), no differences in color parameters were observed between ground beef treated with *L. plantarum* TN8 and the control sample at the beginning of processing. However, the treatments with the inoculated probiotic strain showed an increase in a^* value after 4 days of storage. Regarding lightness, the application of *L. plantarum* in ground beef increased the L^* value on the 7th day of storage, and in beef sausages, no significant effect was observed (Ben Slima et al., 2017; Trabelsi et al., 2019). In addition, it is important to emphasize that small differences in instrumental color values are usually not perceived by consumers. In the study conducted by Ben Slima et al. (2017), it was observed that beef sausage samples maintained an acceptable appearance throughout the storage period, despite having lower L^* and a^* values compared to the initial storage phase. For the beef patties, the whitish color of the alginate beads used in the encapsulation of *L. plantarum* did not affect the L^* parameter. At the end of the storage period (10th day), the beef patties treated with free or encapsulated *L. plantarum* had a higher L^* parameter compared to the control. It can also be concluded that the presence of *L. plantarum* in beef patties has a protective effect on color stability when changes in the *a** parameter were observed. Although a decrease in this parameter was observed at the end of the study period in all treatments, this decrease was more pronounced in the control treatment.

Bacteria of the genus *Lactobacillus* are considered safe for consumption (GRAS), and for them to exert a probiotic effect, their numbers in the meat product are expected to remain stable or to increase during the storage period and to have a concentration between 106 and 107 log CFU/g per 100 g of product consumed. When counting lactic acid bacteria (LAB) in meat products treated with *L. plantarum*, the number is expected to increase. This was observed in the study by Trabelsi et al. (2017) where LAB showed 14.29 log CFU/g on the 10th day of storage in ground beef originally inoculated with 9 log CFU/g *L. plantarum*. In their study, Trevisan et al. (2022) reported that selective counts of *L. plantarum* using LPSM (*Lactobacillus plantarum* selective medium) agar on day 0 of cold storage were 9.47 log CFU/g for the encapsulated treatment, 10.26 CFU/g for the free cell treatment, and 3.88 CFU/g for the control treatment. This suggests that *L. plantarum* may be present in the natural microbiota of meat, albeit in insufficient amounts to exert its probiotic potential. At the conclusion of the storage studied period, Trevisan et al. (2022) observed that only the treatment with encapsulated probiotic retained a satisfactory level of probiotic viability, measuring 8.06 log CFU/g.

In terms of spoilage microorganisms, meat products to which probiotic bacteria such as *L. plantarum* have been added are expected to have a decrease in the total number of psychrotrophic bacteria (PTC). In their study, Trabelsi et al. (2019) found that treatment with *L. plantarum* at a concentration of 9 log CFU/g resulted in a reduction of 4.2 log CFU/g compared to control samples. When probiotic bacteria are used in meat products, an increase in mesophilic aerobic bacteria is expected. This was observed in the study by Trevisan et al. (2022), in which the bacterial counts on day 0 of cold storage for treatments with the addition of *L. plantarum* ranged from 10.43 to 10.48 log CFU/g, while the bacterial counts for the control group were 5.67 log CFU/g. It is important to note that although the generally accepted limit for mesophilic aerobic microorganisms is 10^6 CFU/g, this limit should not be applied to foods inoculated with beneficial microorganisms. The *Enterobacteriaceae* counts of the samples with the probiotic strain were significantly lower compared to the control sample. At the end of storage, the number of *Enterobacteriaceae* in the sample inoculated with 9 log CFU/g *L. plantarum* was 1.2 log CFU/g. In the work of Ben Slima et al. (2017), incorporation of *L. plantarum* in beef sausages initially with 5 log CFU/g reduced *Salmonella enterica* by 1.5 log

CFU/g on day 5 of storage, and by the end of the study, *S. enterica* counts ranged from 2.6 to 2.7 log CFU/g. This suggests that the use of *L. plantarum* in meat products may also help to reduce the burden of spoilage and pathogenic microorganisms.

L. plantarum can produce a small antibacterial compound (2-(2-1 mino-1-hydroxyethoxy) ethyl 2-methylpropanoate) that has been reported to inhibit spoilage and pathogenic bacteria such as *Listeria monocytogenes*, *Staphylococcus aureus*, *Salmonella* Typhi, *Escherichia coli*, *Cronobacter sakazakii*, and *Pseudomonas aeruginosa* in zones of inhibition ranging from 16.1 mm to 24.4 mm (Yi et al., 2020). Therefore, the addition of probiotic bacteria, especially *L. plantarum*, can serve as a natural bioprotectant for meat products.

2.1. *Lactobacillus Plantarum* in Cooked Meat Products

One of the most important points for the use of probiotics in food is based on their ability to survive in different and extreme conditions and produce bioactive compounds that also act against other pathogenic bacteria. In this context, the thermostability of probiotics is necessary to be used as starter cultures and to ensure the biological preservation and safety of food (Akbar, Ali & Anal, 2016; Prabhurajeshwar & Chandrakanth, 2018).

Łaszkiewicz et al. (2021) used the strain *L. plantarum* SCH1 at a concentration of 10^7 CFU/g in free form in cooked sausage made from mechanically separated poultry meat (MSPM). In the preparation of the product, the authors used hot smoke (56-65°C) for 50 min, followed by steam cooking (70-72°C) until the internal temperature of the sausages reached 70°C. In this study, the authors reported that the low sugar content in MSPM affected the low production of secondary metabolites from *L. plantarum*, including lactic acid. This justifies the similarity of pH values in the control group and in the group with probiotics addition. As for microbial quality, on the first day of storage there was no difference in the number of lactic acid bacteria (LAB), with a result of less than 1 log CFU/g. However, on the third day of storage, counts showed statistical differences, with counts of 5.92 log CFU/g in the treatment with the addition of *L. plantarum* compared to the control with 5.23 log CFU/g. Although, these counts suggest that thermal processes used in the production of sausages reduce the initial *L. plantarum* load of the product. Because meat products made from MSM must be cooked during the manufacturing process, the use of probiotic bacteria, mainly in the form of free cells, may not be effective. According to de Marins et al. (2022), *L. plantarum* added to beef patties as free cells (7 log CFU/g) is also ineffective because probiotic strains are inactivated to less than 3 log CFU/g during the cooking process.

According to Bilenler et al. (2017), the alginate-starch-based encapsulation technique improved the stability of microcapsules containing *L. plantarum* under adverse conditions. The authors found that the viability of probiotics was reduced to only 1 log CFU/g after heating treatment at 70 °C. The results indicated that encapsulation has the potential to protect probiotics during the cooking process and expand opportunities for the development of probiotic-enriched foods that are not affected by high-temperature processing. In another study by Cavalheiro et al. (2018), it was found that *L. plantarum strains*, when encapsulated in alginate beads, were able to resist after heating treatments.

In their study, Lucumi-Baguero et al. (2021) isolated LAB strains from different meat products, one of which was identified as *L. plantarum* (MW073312). The isolated strains had a positive effect on inhibiting pathogenic bacteria and were then tested as biopreservative in cooked chorizo sausages. Of the isolated strains, most were able to withstand 15 min at 50°C, but none of them maintained viability at 60°C and 80°C, which is consistent with Aryani et al. (2016) and Todotov et al. (2017) that there is inactivation of probiotic cells and loss of probiotic potential in foods at high temperatures, suggesting that the addition of probiotics in the form of free cells in cooked meat products may not be the best alternative.

According to de Marins et al. (2022), it is possible to produce functional beef patties with the addition of encapsulated *L. plantarum*. In this study, *L. plantarum* was encapsulated with alginate and xanthan gum and added to beef patties at a concentration of 7 log CFU/g as a pure strain and in combination with two other probiotic microorganisms (*Bifidobacterium animalis* spp. *lactis* and *Lactobacillus acidophilus*). Regarding the viability of the probiotics, it was found that the number of *L. plantarum* was higher in the treatments where the probiotics were used in combination with other strains at days 0, 15 and 30 of storage, while the number of pure *L. plantarum* was higher, reaching 9.75 log CFU/g in raw and 8.26 log CFU/g in cooked beef patties at the end of storage. During the storage period, the concentration of *L. plantarum* increased in the beef patties. Moreover, the concentration of probiotics after cooking treatment indicated that the product still contained enough probiotics for consumption. Thus, encapsulation of *L. plantarum* was effective in protecting the viability of probiotics during the cooking treatment of beef patties.

In terms of consumer acceptance and other sensory aspects, the addition of encapsulated *L. plantarum* had no effect on beef patties, and ratings for color, flavor, texture, and overall acceptability ranged from "moderately good" to "very good" (de Marins et al., 2022). It is well known that consumers consider appearance as one of the most important acceptance criteria when purchasing a meat product, as well as taste and tenderness, which are important sensory aspects (Garmyn, 2020). Therefore, it is critical that the addition of probiotic bacteria to meat products, either as free cells or in encapsulated form, does not negatively impact sensory attributes. It is crucial that consumers have a pleasant sensation when consuming probiotic meat products with added *L. plantarum*, in addition to the nutritional and health aspects.

2.2. *Lactobacillus Plantarum* in Fermented Meat Products

In the fermentation of meat products, LAB is the main bacterial group used. This group improves the safety and sensory properties of fermented meat products. In addition, they provide rapid acidification by producing lactic acid during the fermentation of meat products such as salami and chorizo (Ba et al., 2018; Kamiloğlu et al., 2020). Among the species of LAB, *L. plantarum* stands out in terms of its applicability as a starter culture in various types of fermented foods, especially in fermented sausages, but there are few studies on how the fermentation conditions or under which fermentation temperature conditions the inoculated *L. plantarum* could improve the technological and properties of the products (Sun et al., 2016; Ba et al., 2018).

It is known that in dry-fermented meat products, an adequate number of LAB is desirable both during maturation and storage to control the growth of pathogenic bacteria and increase the efficiency of sausage production (Cenci-Goga et al., 2008). During the maturation of chorizo sausages treated with different strategies of *L. plantarum* incorporation (free cells and encapsulated with alginate beads, emulsion, and double emulsion), the number of LAB was above 7 log CFU/g, which is justified by the addition of *L. plantarum* during the chorizo manufacturing process. However, when the probiotic was ingested in the form of free cells, 8.81 log CFU/g were detected, which is higher than in chorizos with encapsulated probiotic in emulsion and double emulsion forms (Cavalheiro et al., 2019). It is known that the microbiota of meat can initiate the fermentation process, but this is not indicated due to the irregular meat fermentation. In addition, it is noteworthy that the content of *L. plantarum* was maintained in sufficient numbers throughout the storage period. In this regard, it was possible to maintain selective *L. plantarum* counts to 8.34 log CFU/g after 60 days of refrigerated storage when this strain was applied in alginate beads to chorizo sausages (Cavalheiro et al., 2020). Other *L. plantarum* strains isolated from artisanal fermented sausages have a good ability to grow in acidic environments, and when inoculated onto other meat products, these strains showed exceptional adaptability and significant antimicrobial activity that prevented the growth of pathogenic bacteria (Sawitzki et al., 2007; Sawitzki et al., 2009).

Instead of antimicrobial activity, *L. plantarum* strains have also been used in meat and meat products for their antioxidant activity. In their study, Hashemi et al. (2018) inoculated *L. plantarum* at a concentration of 10^5 CFU/g and evaluated the antimicrobial and antioxidant activities during fermentation of ground beef patties. The authors found that *L. plantarum* exhibited good antimicrobial activity against a wide range of pathogenic bacteria. In addition, the inoculated LAB improved the oxidative stability of the fermented beef patties. Other studies have also shown that probiotics can be useful as natural antioxidants and are a good alternative to synthetic antioxidants that are detrimental to health (Mishra et al. 2015). The use of synthetic antioxidants in fermented meat products is a common practice to extend their shelf life and avoid lipid oxidation (D' Amore et al., 2020). However, the use of synthetic antioxidants has several drawbacks, such as safety concerns and consumer preference for natural ingredients. The most used synthetic antioxidants in fermented meat products are butylated hydroxyanisole (BHA), butylated hydroxytoluene (BHT), and propyl gallate (PG). These compounds have been shown to cause adverse health effects, including cancer, and are therefore subject to established consumption limits in various countries (Ribeiro et al., 2019). For example, the European Union has set a limit of 150 mg/kg for BHA and BHT in meat products, while the United States allows up to 200 mg/kg for these compounds in meat products (EU, 2010; FDA, 2018). Despite their effectiveness in preventing oxidation, the use of synthetic antioxidants in fermented meat products remains controversial, and the alternative of natural antioxidants is being explored as a potential replacement. Therefore, the use of probiotic bacteria as natural antioxidants in fermented meat products has been investigated.

In addition, the fatty acid quality of meat products with added *L. plantarum* has also been studied. Arief et al. (2016) evaluated the fatty acid profile of dry-fermented sausages with *L. plantarum* IIA-2C12 addition. Probiotic inoculation promoted dry-fermented sausages with lower levels of saturated fatty acids such as myristic (C14:0) and arachidic acid (C20:0) than the control treatment, likely due to the lipolytic activity of the probiotic strains. In this context, improving the fatty acid quality of meat products is the key for the manufacturing healthier products. High consumption of saturated fat has been associated with cardiovascular disease, colon cancer, and type 2 diabetes. Therefore, the use of probiotic meat products low in saturated fat may have a positive impact on consumer health.

The use of *L. plantarum* may influence the sensory aspects of fermented meat products. According to Cavalheiro et al. (2019), inoculation of *L. plantarum* in different presentation forms had an impact on the acceptability of chorizo sausages. In general, control samples (without *L. plantarum* inoculation) had higher values for the attribute of overall acceptability. However, treatments with probiotic supplement encapsulated in alginate beads and single and double emulsions also obtained good results in sensory analysis. Figure 1 shows the manufacturing process of chorizo sausages with encapsulated *L. plantarum* cells. One can see the direct addition of alginate beads onto the meat matrix (Figure 1A) and after the homogenization process (Figure 1B). After the filling process and before the fermentation and maturation steps, the control (Figure 1C) and the treatment with *L. plantarum* in alginate beads (Figure 1D) are quite different based on the visual perception of the beads in the sausages. Thus, the perception of alginate globules on the final product may be a disadvantage for sensory perception by consumers.

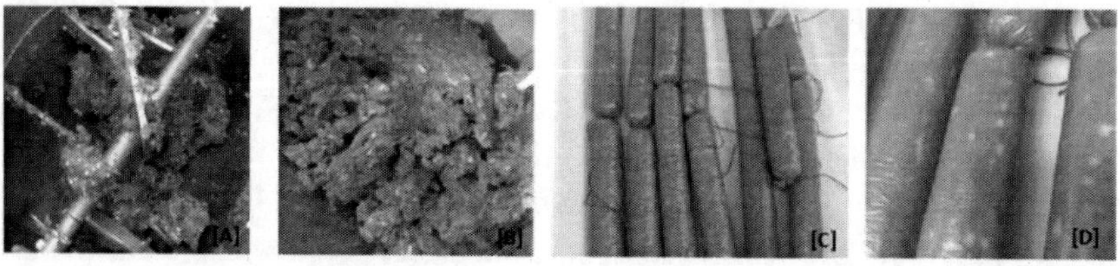

Figure 1. Manufacturing process of chorizo sausages with encapsulated *L. plantarum* cells. [A]: Addition of alginate beads with *L. plantarum* on the meat matrix; [B]: Meat matrix with the incorporation of *L. plantarum* encapsulated in alginate beads; [C]: Control chorizo sausages with no probiotic addition; [D]: Chorizo sausages with encapsulated *L. plantarum* in alginate beads. Courtesy of Dr. Carlos Pasqualin Cavalheiro.

However, after the fermentation and ripening steps of chorizo sausages with *L. plantarum* addition, it was found that the probiotic delivery system had no significant effect on the sensory characteristics of the dry-fermented sausages (Cavalheiro et al., 2019). Figure 2 shows that there is no difference between the visual aspects of the different chorizo sausages, even in the treatments with addition of *L. plantarum* in alginate beads (Figure 2C) compared to the control (Figure 2A) or other delivery systems.

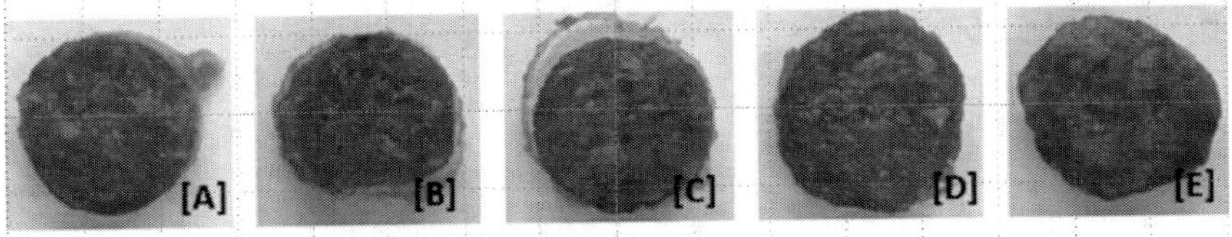

Figure 2. Effect of different strategies of *L. plantarum* incorporation on visual aspect of chorizo sausages after ripening process. [A]: Control; [B]: *L. plantarum* addition as free cells; [C]: *L. plantarum* encapsulated in alginate beads; [D]: *L. plantarum* encapsulated in simple emulsion; [E]: *L. plantarum* encapsulated in double emulsion. Courtesy of Dr. Carlos Pasqualin Cavalheiro.

Other studies also found little or no difference between control sausages and fermented sausages inoculated with *L. plantarum*. According to Ge et al. (2019), there were no significant differences between treatments in color, texture, aroma, odor, taste, salty, and sour. In addition, Pavli et al. (2020) conducted sensory evaluation of dry-fermented sausages on days 22 (end of ripening/beginning of storage), 48, 74, 100, 128, 152, and 182 of storage at 4 and 12°C. The authors found that the control sample and the samples with *L. plantarum* had few differences, mainly in the attributes of redness, raw odor, and sour taste, with the sour taste being slightly more intense in the probiotic samples, but not perceived as unpleasant by the subjects. In the same study, the temperature used affected the characteristics of paleness, odor, taste, and appearance, while storage time significantly affected all sensory characteristics except smoke odor. In general, the authors found that the overall assessment was similar between the control and the probiotic dry-fermented sausages. However, the addition of *L. plantarum* to the sausages retained better sensory characteristics at the end of the storage period (day 182), as evidenced by higher scores than the control sausages.

The addition of *L. plantarum* in the form of free cells did not affect the immediate composition of the dry-fermented sausages. Studies revealed no differences in moisture, protein, ash, and fat content between control sausages and treatments with direct addition of *L. plantarum* (Cavalheiro et al., 2019). However, encapsulation *of L. plantarum* in single and double emulsion had effects on the fat content of dry-fermented sausages due to the amounts of oil used in the emulsion encapsulation technique. However, the effects of the encapsulation process on the dry-fermented sausages ingredients composition depend more on the used raw materials than on the strain used.

Conclusion, Opportunities and Future Challenges

The growing interest in the use of *L. plantarum* in meat products provides an alternative for consumers who desire healthier and functional meat products. In this context, the use of *L. plantarum* in the reformulation of meat products is useful as it can provide healthier properties to new functional meat products. As we know, probiotics are often incorporated into fermented meat products because their technological processing characteristics favor the addition and growth of this group of microorganisms. However, *L. plantarum* can also be added to meat products that undergo a cooking process.

The use of encapsulation processes such as alginate beads and emulsification showed to be effective in protecting *L. plantarum* during cooking, which could otherwise affect cell viability if used as free cells. However, further studies are needed to optimize the procedures for encapsulating and incorporating *L. plantarum* into these products.

The antioxidant and antimicrobial activity of *L. plantarum* is another positive factor for its use as a probiotic microorganism in various meat products. In this context, the addition of *L. plantarum* as an antioxidant could replace the conventional synthetic antioxidants. However, further research in this area is needed.

Moreover, the addition of *L. plantarum* has no significant effect on the sensory aspects of meat products. Regarding nutritional aspects, the consumption of probiotics (such as *L. plantarum*) has been shown to have beneficial effects on human health and should therefore be promoted.

References

[1] Akbar, A., Ali, I., & Anal, A. K. (2016). Industrial Perspectives of Lactic Acid Bacteria for Biopreservation and food safety. *The Journal of Animal & Plant Sciences*, 26, 938–948. Available from ISSN: 1018-7081.

[2] Arief, I. I., Afiyah, D. N., Wulandari, Z., & Budiman, C. (2016). Physicochemical Properties, Fatty Acid Profiles, and Sensory Characteristics of Fermented Beef

Sausage by Probiotics *Lactobacillus plantarum* IIA-2C12 or *Lactobacillus acidophilus* IIA-2B4. *Journal of food science*, 81 11, M2761-M2769. Available from https://doi.org/10.1111/1750-3841.13509.

[3] Aryani, D. C., den Bersten, H. M. W., & Zwietering, M. H. (2016). Quantifying variability in growth and thermal inactivation kinetics of *Lactobacillus plantarum. Applied and Environmental Microbiology*, v. 82(16), p. 4896-4908. Available from https://doi.org/10.1128/AEM.00277-16.

[4] Ba, H. V., Seo, H., Seong, P., Kang, S. M., Kim, Y., Cho, S., Park, B., Ham, J., & Kim, J. (2018). *Lactobacillus plantarum* (KACC 92189) as a Potential Probiotic Starter Culture for Quality Improvement of Fermented Sausages. *Korean Journal for Food Science of Animal Resources*, 38, 189 - 202. Available from https://doi.org/10.5851/kosfa.2018.38.1.189.

[5] Ben Slima, S., Ktari, N., Trabelsi I., Triki, M., Feki-tounsi, M., Moussa, H., Makni, I., Herrero, A., Jiménez-Colmenero, F., Ruiz-Capillas, C., & Ben Salah, R. (2017). Effect of partial replacement of nitrite with a novel probiotic *Lactobacillus plantarum* TN8 on color, physico-chemical, texture and microbiological properties of beef sausages. *LWT*, v. 86, p. 219-226. Available from https://doi.org/10.1016/j.lwt.2017.07.058.

[6] Bilenler, T., Karabulut, I., & Candogan, K. (2017). Effects of encapsulated starter cultures on microbial and physicochemical properties of traditionally produced and heat treated sausages (sucuks). *LWT*, 75, 425-433. Available from https://doi.org/10.1016/j.lwt.2016.09.003.

[7] Binda, S., Hill, C., Johansen, E., Obis, D., Pot, B., Sanders, M. E., Tremblay, A., & Ouwehand, A. C. (2020). Criteria to Qualify Microorganisms as "Probiotic" in Foods and Dietary Supplements. *Frontiers in Microbiology*, 11:662. Available from https://doi.org/10.3389/fmicb.2020.01662.

[8] Blaiotta, G., Muru, N., Di Cerbo, A., Romano, R., & Aponte, M. (2017). Production of probiotic bovine salami using *Lactobacillus plantarum* 299v as adjunct. *Journal of the Science of Food and Agriculture*, 98(6), 2285-2294. Available from https://doi.org/10.1002/jsfa.8717.

[9] Boyle, R. J., & Tang, M. L. K. (2006). The role of probiotics in the management of allergic disease. *Clinical & Experimental Allergy*, 36, 568-576. Available from https://doi.org/10.1111/j.1365-2222.2006.02472.x.

[10] Cavalheiro, C. P., Ruiz-Capillas, C., Herrero, A. M., Jiménez-Colmenero, F., de Menezes, C. R., & Fries. L. L. M. (2015). Application of probiotic delivery systems in meat products. *Trends in Food Science and Technology, 46,* 120 – 131. Available from: http://dx.doi.org/10.1016/j.tifs.2015.09.004 .

[11] Cavalheiro, C. P., Ruiz-Capillas, C., Herrero, A. M., Jiménez-Colmenero, F., de Menezes, C. R., & Fries, L. L. M. (2018). Survival of probiotic *Lactobacillus plantarum* and *Enterococcus faecium* in alginate beads during stress treatments. *Nutrition and Food Science, 49(2)*, 273 – 283. Available from: https://doi.org/10.1108/NFS-05-2018-0132.

[12] Cavalheiro, C. P., Ruiz-Capillas, C., Herrero, A. M., Jiménez-Colmenero, F., Pintado, T., de Menezes, C. R., & Fries, L. L. M. (2019). Effect of different strategies of *Lactobacillus plantarum* incorporation in chorizo sausages. *Journal of*

the Science of Food and Agriculture, 99, 6706-6712. Available from https://doi.org/10.1002/jsfa.9952.

[13] Cavalheiro, C. P., Ruiz-Capillas, C., Herrero, A. M., Jiménez-Colmenero, F., Pintado, T., de Menezes, C. R., & Fries, L. L. M. (2020). Effect of encapsulated *Lactobacillus plantarum* as probiotic on dry-sausages during chilled storage. *International Journal of Food Science and Technology, 55(12),* 3613-3621. Available from: https://doi.org/ 10.1111/ijfs.14695.

[14] Cavalheiro, C. P., Ruiz-Capillas, C., Herrero, A. M., & Pintado, T. (2021). Dry-fermented sausages inoculated with *Enterococcus faecium* CECT 410 as free cells or in alginate beads. *LWT – Food Science and Technology* 139, 110561. Available from https://doi.org/10.1016/j.lwt.2020.110561.

[15] Cenci-Goga, B. T., Ranucci, D., Miraglia, D., & Cioffi, A. (2008). Use of starter cultures of dairy origin in the production of Salame nostrano, an Italy dry-cured sausage. *Meat Science*, v. 78, 381–390. Available from https://doi.org/10.1016/ j.meatsci.2007.07.001.

[16] da Costa, R. J., Voloski, F. L. S., Mondadori, R. G., Duval, E. H., & Fiorentini, A. M. (2019). Preservation of meat products with Bacteriocins produced by lactic acid bacteria isolated from meat: A review. *Journal of Food Quality*, 2019, p. 1–12. Available from https://doi.org/10.1155/2019/4726510.

[17] D'Amore, T., Di Taranto, A., Berardi, G., Vita, V., Chiaravalle, A. E., & Iammarino, M. (2020). Sulfites in meat: Occurrence, activity, toxicity, regulation, and detection. A comprehensive review. *Comprehensive Reviews in Food Science and Food Safety*, 19(5). Available from https://doi.org/ 10.1111/1541-4337.12607.

[18] Dan, T., Chen, H., Li, T., Tian, J., Ren, W., Zhang, H., & Sun, T. (2019). Influence of *Lactobacillus plantarum* P-8 on fermented milk flavor and storage stability. *Frontiers in Microbiology*, 9:3133. Available from https://doi.org/10.3389/ fmicb.2018.03.

[19] Danuta, K. K., & Zbigniew, J. D. (2012). Probiotic meat products and human nutrition: A review. *Process Biochemistry*, 47, p. 1761-1772. Available from https://doi.org/10.1016/j.procbio.2012.09.017.

[20] Etchepare, M. A., Raddatz, G. C., Cichoski, A. J., Flores, E. M. M., Barin, J. S., Zepka, L. Q., JACOB-Lopes, E., Grosso, C. R. F., & Menezes, C. R. (2016a). Effect of resistant starch (Hi-maize) on the survival of *Lactobacillus acidophilus* microencapsulated with sodium alginate. *Journal of Functional Foods*, v. 21, p. 321– 329. Available from https://doi.org/10.1016/j.jff.2015.12.025.

[21] Etchepare, M. A., Raddatz, G. C., Flores, E. M. M., Zepka, L. Q., Jacob-Lopes, E., Barin, J. S., Grosso, C. R. F., & Menezes, C. R. (2016b). Effect of resistant starch and chitosan on survival of *Lactobacillus acidophilus* microencapsulated with sodium alginate. *LWT – Food Science and Technology*, v. 65, p. 511-517. Available from https://doi.org/10.1016/j.lwt.2015.08.039.

[22] European Commission. Commission Regulation (EU) No 1129/2011 of 11 November 2011 amending Annex II to Regulation (EC) No 1333/2008 of the European Parliament and of the Council by establishing a Union list of food additives [Online]. 2011 [cited 2023 April 01]. Available from https://eur-lex.europa.eu/legal-content/EN/TXT/?uri=CELEX:32011R1129.

[23] FAO. (2018). The future of food and agriculture: Alternative pathways to 2050. [online]. 2018 [cited 2023 April 01]. Available from http://www.fao.org/3/a-i6583e.pdf.

[24] Franciosa, I., Alessandria, V., Dolci, P., Rantsiou, K., & Cocolin, L. (2018). Sausage fermentation and starter cultures in the era of molecular biology methods. *International Journal of Food Microbiology*, 279, 26-32. Available from https://doi.org/10.1016/j.ijfoodmicro.2018.04.038.

[25] Garmyn, A. (2020). Consumer preferences and acceptance of meat products. *Foods*, 9, 708. Available from http://dx.doi.org/10.3390/foods9060708.

[26] Ge, Q., Pei, H., Liu, R., Chen, L., Gao, X., Gu, Y., Hou, Q., Yin, Y., Yu, H., Wu, M., Zhang, W., & Zhou, G. (2019). Effects of *Lactobacillus plantarum* NJAU-01 from Jinhua ham on the quality of dry-cured fermented sausage. *LWT – Food Science and Technology*, 101, 513-528. Available from https://doi.org/10.1016/j.lwt.2018.11.081.

[27] Giri, S. S., Sen, S. S., Saha, S., Sukumaran, V., & Park, S. C. (2018). Use of potential probiotic, *Lactobacillus plantarum* L7, for the preparation of a rice-based fermented beverage. *Frontiers in Microbiology*, 9:473. Available from https://doi.org/10.3389/fmicb.2018.00473.

[28] Ha, C. G., Cho, J. K., Lee, C. H., Chai, Y. G., Ha, Y. A., & Shin, S. H. (2006). Cholesterol lowering effect of *Lactobacillus plantarum* isolated from human feces. *Journal of Microbiology and Biotechnology* 16(8):1201-1209. Available from ISSN: 1017-7825.

[29] Hashemi, S. M. B., Raeisi, S., Zanardi, E., Paciulli, M., & Chiavaro, E. (2018). Antimicrobial And Antioxidant Activities of Fermented Meat Patty with *Lactobacillus* Strains. *Italian Journal of Food Science*, 30(2), 268+. Available from https://doi.org/10.14674/IJFS-993.

[30] Kamiloğlu, A., Kaban, G., & Kaya, M. (2020). Technological properties of autochthonous *Lactobacillus plantarum* strains isolated from sucuk (Turkish dry-fermented sausage). *Brazilian Journal of Microbiology*, 51, 1279–1287. Available from https://doi.org/10.1007/s42770-020-00262-9.

[31] Łaszkiewicz, B., Szymański, P., Zielińska, D., & Krajewska, D. -K. (2021). Application of *Lactiplantibacillus plantarum* SCH1 for the bioconservation of Cooked Sausage made from mechanically separated poultry meat. *Applied Sciences*, 11, 1576. Available from https://doi.org/10.3390/app11041576.

[32] Lee, D. E., Huh, C. S., Ra, J., Choi, I. D., Jeong, J. W., Kim, S. H., Ryu, J. H., Seo, Y. K., Koh, J. S., Lee, J. H., Sim, J. H., & Ahn, Y. T. (2015). Clinical Evidence of Effects of *Lactobacillus plantarum* HY7714 on Skin Aging: A Randomized, Double Blind, Placebo-Controlled Study. *Journal of Microbiology and Biotechnology*, 25(12), 2160-2166. Available from https://doi.org/10.4014/jmb.1509.09021.

[33] Li, C., Song, J., Kwok, L., Wang, J., Dong, Y., Yu, H., Hou, Q., Zhang, H., & Chen, Y. (2017). Influence of *Lactobacillus plantarum* on fermentation properties and subsequent changes during postfermentation storage. *Journal of Dairy Science*, 100(4), 2512-2525. Available from https://doi.org/10.3168/jds.2016-11864.

[34] Lucumi-Banguero, R. S., Ramírez-Toro, C., & Bolívar, G. A. (2021). Potential Use of Lactic Acid Bacteria with Pathogen Inhibitory Capacity as a Biopreservative

Agent for Chorizo. *Processes*, 9, 1582. Available from https://doi.org/10.3390/pr9091582.

[35] de Marins, A. R., de Campos, T. A. F., Batista, A. F. P., Correa, V. G., Peralta, R. M., Mikcha, J. M. G., Gomes, R. G., & Feihrmann, A. C. (2022). Effect of the addition of encapsulated *Lactiplantibacillus plantarum* Lp-115, *Bifidobacterium animalis spp. lactis* Bb-12, and *Lactobacillus acidophilus* La-5 to cooked burger. *LWT – Food Science and Technology,* 155, 112946. Available from https://doi.org/10.1016/j.lwt.2021.112946.

[36] Mishra, V., Shah, C., Mokashe, N., Chavan, R., Yadav, H., & Prajapati, J. (2015). Probiotics as potential antioxidants: a systematic review. *Journal of agricultural and food chemistry*, 63(14), 3615-3626. Available from https://doi.org/10.1021/jf506326t.

[37] Mokoena, M. P., Mutanda, T., & Olaniran, A. O. (2016). Perspectives on the probiotic potential of lactic acid bacteria from African traditional fermented foods and beverages. *Food Nutrition & Research*, 60. Available from https://doi.org/10.3402/fnr.v60.29630.

[38] Munekata, P. E., Pateiro, M., Tomasevic, I., Domínguez, R., Barretto, A. C. S., Santos, E. M., & Lorenzo, J. M. (2021). Functional fermented meat products with probiotics – A review. *Journal of Applied Microbiology*, 133, 91-103. Available from https://doi.org/10.1111/jam.15337.

[39] Ngamsomchat, A., Kaewkod, T., Konkit, M., Tragoolpua, Y., Bovonsombut, S., & Chitov, T. (2022). Characterization of *Lactobacillus plantarum* of dairy-product origin for probiotic Chèvre Cheese production. *Foods*, 11, 934. Available from https://doi.org/10.3390/foods11070934.

[40] Passos, R. S. F. T., Barreto, B. G., Leite, J. S. F., Trevisan, A. B., de Souza, C. O., da Silva, M. C. A., & Cavalheiro, C. P. (2022). Green tea extract as natural preservative in chicken patties: Effects on physicochemical, microbiological, and sensory properties. *Food Processing and Preservation*, 46, e16224. Available from https://doi.org/10.1111/jfpp.16224.

[41] Pateiro, M., Barba, F. J., Domínguez, R., Sant'Ana, A. S., Khaneghah, A. M., Gavahian, M., & Lorenzo, J. M. (2018). Essential oils as natural additives to prevent oxidation reactions in meat and meat products: A review. *Food Research International*, 113, 156–166. Available from https://doi.org/10.1016/j.foodres.2018.07.014.

[42] Pavli, F. G., Argyri, A. A., Chorianopolous, N. G., Nychas, G.-J. E., & Tassou, C. T. (2020). Effect of *Lactobacillus plantarum* L125 strain with probiotic potential on physicochemical, microbiological and sensorial characteristics of dry-fermented sausages. *LWT – Food Science and Technology*, 118, 108810. Available from https://doi.org/10.1016/j.lwt.2019.108810.

[43] Prabhurajeshwar, C., & Chandrakanth, K. (2018). Evaluation of antimicrobial properties and their substances against pathogenic bacteria in-vitro by probiotic Lactobacilli strains isolated from commercial yoghurt. *Clinical Nutrition Experimental*, 23, 97–115. Available from https://doi.org/10.1016/j.yclnex.2018.10.001.

[44] Qiu, L., Tao, X., Xiong, H., Yu, J., & Wei, H. (2018). *Lactobacillus plantarum* ZDY04 exhibits a strain-specific property of lowering TMAO via the modulation of gut microbiota in mice. *Food & function*, 15;9(8):4299-4309. Available from https://doi.org/10.1039/c8fo00349a.

[45] Ribeiro, J. S., Santos, M. J. M. C., Silva, L. K. R., Pereira, L. C. L., Santos, I. A., Lannes, S. C. S., & Silva, M. V. (2019). Natural antioxidants used in meat products: A brief review. *Meat Science*, 148, 181-188. Available from https://doi.org/10.1016/j.meatsci.2018.10.016.

[46] Sawitzki, M. C., Fiorentini, A. M., Brod, F. C. A., Tagliari, C., Bertol, T. M., Arisi, A. C. M., Sant'Anna, E. S. (2007). Phenotypic characterization and species-specific PCR of promising starter culture strains of *Lactobacillus plantarum* isolated from naturally fermented sausages. *Brazilian Journal of Microbiology*, 38: 547-552. Available from https://doi.org/10.1590/S1517-83822007000300031.

[47] Sawitzki, M. C., Fiorentini, A. M., Bertol, T. M., Sant'Anna, E. S. (2009). *Lactobacillus plantarum* strains isolated from naturally fermented sausages and their technological properties for application as starter cultures. *Ciência e Tecnologia de Alimentos*, 29(2), 340-345. Available from https://doi.org/10.1590/S0101-20612009000200016.

[48] Śmietana, N., Śmietana, P., Drozlowska, E., & Łopusiewicz, Ł. (2023). The Influence of Lactic Acid Bacteria Fermentation on the Bioactivity of Crayfish (*Faxonius limosus*) Meat. *Fermentation*, 9(1), 66. Available from https://doi.org/10.3390/fermentation9010066.

[49] de Souza, E. L. (2021). Insights into the current evidence on the effects of essential oils toward beneficial microorganisms in foods with a special emphasis to lactic acid bacteria – A review. *Trends in Food Science & Technology*, 114, 333-341. Available from https://doi.org/10.1016/j.tifs.2021.06.011.

[50] Sun, Q., Chen, Q., Li, F., Zheng, D.M., & Kong, B. (2016). Biogenic amine inhibition and quality protection of Harbin dry sausages by inoculation with *Staphylococcus xylosus* and *Lactobacillus plantarum*. *Food Control*, 68, 358-366. Available from https://doi.org/10.1016/j.foodcont.2016.04.021.

[51] Sun, X., Qi, X., Han, Y., Guo, Z., Cui, C., & Lin, C. (2023). Characteristics of changes in volatile organic compounds and microbial communities during the storage of pickles. *Food Chemistry*, 409, 135285. Available from https://doi.org/10.1016/j.foodchem.2022.135285.

[52] Todorov, S. D. (2009). Bacteriocins from *Lactobacillus plantarum* – Production, genetic organization, and mode of action. *Brazilian Journal of Microbiology*, 40, 209-221. Available from https://doi.org/10.1590/S1517-83822009000200001.

[53] Todorov, S. D., Stojanovski, S., Iliev, I., Moncheva, P., Nero, L. A., & Ivanova, I. V. (2017). Technology and safety assessment for lactic acid bacteria isolated from traditional Bulgarian fermented meat product "lukanka." *Brazilian Journal of Microbiology, 48*, 576-586. Available from https://doi.org/10.1016/j.bjm.2017.02.005.

[54] Trabelsi, I., Ben Slima, S., Ktari, N., Triki, M., Abdehedi, R., Abaza, W., Moussa, H., Abdeslam, A., & Ben Salah, R. (2019). Incorporation of probiotic strain in raw minced beef meat: Study of textural modification, lipid and protein oxidation and

color parameters during refrigerated storage. *Meat Science*, v. 154, p. 29- 36. Available from https://doi.org/10.1016/j.meatsci.2019.04.005.

[55] Trevisan, A. B., dos Santos, M. C., Leite, J. S. F., Barreto, B. G., Passos, R. S. F. T., Franke, C. R., da Silva, M. C. A., & Cavalheiro, C. P. (2022). Encapsulation of probiotics and their application in beef patties. *Acta Scientiarum Polonorum Technologia Alimentaria*, v. 21(3), p. 281-291. Available from https://doi.org/10.17306/J.AFS.2022.1038.

[56] U.S. Food and Drug Administration (FDA). (2018). Code of Federal Regulations Title 21: *Food and Drugs* [Online]. 2018 [cited 2023 April 01] Available from https://www.accessdata.fda.gov/scripts/cdrh/cfdocs/cfcfr/CFRSearch.cfm?fr=182.3173.

[57] Wang, Q., Sun, Q., Qi, R., Wang, J., Qiu, X., Liu, Z., & Huang, J. (2019). Effects of *Lactobacillus plantarum* on the intestinal morphology, intestinal barrier function and microbiota composition of suckling piglets. *Journal of Animal Physiology and Animal Nutrition*, 103(6):1908-1918. Available from https://doi.org/10.1111/jpn.13198.

[58] Woraprayote, W., Pumpuang, L., Tosukhowong, A., Roytrakul, S., Perez, R. H., Zendo, T., Sonomoto, K., Benjakul, S., & Visessanguan, W. (2015). Two putatively novel bacteriocins active against Gram-negative food borne pathogens produced by *Weissella hellenica* BCC 7293. *Food Control*, 55, 176-184. Available from https://doi.org/10.1016/j.foodcont.2015.02.036.

[59] Yang, S., Deng, C., Li, Y., Li, W., Wu, Q., Sun, Z., Cao, Z., & Lin, Q. (2022). Complete genome sequence of *Lactiplantibacillus plantarum* ST, a potential probiotic strain with antibacterial Properties. *Journal of Animal Science and Technology*, 64(1), 183-186. Available from https://doi.org/10.5187/jast.2022.e7.

[60] Yi, L., Qi, T., Hong, Y., Deng, L., & Zeng, K. (2020). Screening of bacteriocin-producing lactic acid bacteria in Chinese homemade pickle and dry-cured meat, and bacteriocin identification by genome sequencing. *LWT – Food Science and Technology*, 125, 109177. Available from https://doi.org/10.1016/j.lwt.2020.109177.

[61] Yoo, S. A., Na, S. E., Seo, S. H., & Son, H. S. (2015). Characterization of fermented sausages using *Lactobacillus plantarum* MLK 14-2 as starter culture. *Journal of the Korean Society for Applied Biological Chemistry*, 58, 349-358. Available from https://doi.org/10.1007/s13765-015-0052-8.

Chapter 8

Lactobacillus plantarum in Cereals, Fruits and Vegetables

Elena Suzana Biriş-Dorhoi[1]
Mihaela Mihai[1]
and Delia Michiu[2,*]

[1]Department of Food Science, Faculty of Food Science and Technology, University of Agricultural Sciences and Veterinary Medicine, Cluj-Napoca, Romania
[2]Department of Food Engineering, Faculty of Food Science and Technology, University of Agricultural Sciences and Veterinary Medicine, Cluj-Napoca, Romania

Abstract

Lactobacillus plantarum is a species of lactic acid bacteria serving many useful purposes in the food industry. This versatile species can be found in many sources. As such, this chapter is a comprehensive literature review on the isolation and use of *L. plantarum* in cereals, fruits and vegetables. The literature overview yielded many scientific articles from various fields: identification from fermented beverages, raw fruits, cereals, fermented dough and vegetables (including fermented vegetable foods or juices). Fermented foods have gained increasingly more ground because they are known to increase food shelf life, influence its flavour and taste and increase food nutritional value. A small part of the literature presented the possibility of using fresh fruit salad as a vector for *Lactobacillus plantarum*. In some fruit juices the species was found to be more available, such as orange, pineapple and grapefruit. Additionally, some research provides isolates found in different fruits (such as Peruvian Amazonian fruits). *Lactobacillus plantarum* grows differently

[*] Corresponding Author's Email: elena.biris@usamvcluj.ro.

In: Lactobacillus plantarum and Its Role in Human Health
Editors: Maria Simona Chiş, Adriana Paucean
ISBN: 979-8-89113-696-0

depending on the food type it is used in. The species was also used as probiotic bacteria in the development of fruit powders. In the case of cereals, studies were conducted to test the availability of the bacteria. The species was found to be able to grow during quinoa sourdough fermentation or fermented durum wheat dough, where an increase in sensorial properties and compounds beneficial for human health was also revealed. Moreover, *Lactobacillus plantarum* was used in a fermented vegetable–fruit beverage with an increase in its antioxidant activity. Korean kimchi was revealed to have antimutagenic activity (specifically because of Lactobacillus plantarum). Future studies are needed in order to get an in-depth understanding of the species' growth in different fruits, cereals and vegetables and how it can be of further use in the food industry.

Keywords: silage production, fermented foods, beverages, cereals, fruits, vegetables, *Lactobacillus plantarum*

1. Introduction

In recent times, humans have become more and more conscious about their health, diet and general well-being. The COVID pandemic led, in a way, to a change in food patterns and consumer desires. In a study conducted in six countries – France, Germany, Mexico, Spain, the UK, and the US, consumers were asked how COVID changed their diet. Respondents agreed that a new trend has emerged and that it is not likely they would return to their old habits. The conclusion was that diet has changed during and after COVID (Zinklar, 2023). A diet which perfectly suits a person and adds beneficial elements is paramount and nature has all the elements we need in order to promote human health. The search for natural and beneficial elements is becoming more and more apparent. Species of lactic acid bacteria, such as *Lactobacillus plantarum* (*L. plantarum*), were found to have multiple uses in achieving a balanced diet. Some strains are found in the human microbiota, but many are found in sources such as fruits, vegetables and cereals. Some of these species, like *L. plantarum*, can be used as probiotics to improve gut health (Gaggia et al., 2011; Guan et al., 2021).

This chapter provides a comprehensive literature review on the isolation and use of *L. plantarum* in cereals, fruits and vegetables. It takes into account its role in fermented beverages, fermented foods, possibilities of isolation from various sources and its bioactive potential. The articles reviewed span over the last 30 years, in order to assess progress and to identify the starting point of interest regarding *L. plantarum*, its uses and potential benefits. The strains can have different types of bioactive potential. It can be used as a probiotic, as a culture starter or food preserver. The interest in *Lactobacillus plantarum* is clearly not new. Articles that study its potential in fermentation date back to 1992 and the early 2000s (Aukrust and Blom, 1992; Charalampopoulos et al., 2002; Lu et al., 2003).

To begin with, a probiotic is defined as a living organism which brings health benefits to its host (FAO and WHO, 2022). The use of probiotics is an interesting trend in the world, one which can help improve human health. Seddick et al. (2017) analysed literature in which the species' potential as a probiotic was studied. Several health benefits were discussed, including lower cholesterol, diarrhea prevention, a positive effect on inflammatory bowel disease and irritable bowel syndrome, among others. The same conclusions were observed in a study by Abdelazez et al. (2018).

Fermented foods draw more attention due to the potential health benefits they provide. Fermentation refers to a biotechnological process that uses different microorganisms to transform raw food matrices into complex foods or feeds (El-Sheika, 2022). This process is also one of the oldest methods for food preservation. El -Sheikha (2022) also agrees that fermented foods are a new trend in the food industry that promotes healthy food and lifestyles and can improve human life and health. After the COVID pandemic, new trends emerged in consumer preference, options and interests. In another study, several strains were isolated from Ukrainian traditional fermented foods and were analysed regarding their cellular fatty acids (Garmasheva et al., 2015).

Moreover, it has been proven that *L. plantarum* contributed to organoleptic properties, flavour, and texture when used as a starter culture in food fermentation (Todorov and Gombossy De Melo Franco, 2010). The addition of *L. plantarum* reduces spoilage risks and improves sensory characteristic which can influence flavour biogenesis (Fleming et al., 1985; Sabatini et al., 2008).

An effect of the species is the antimicrobial one, as pointed out by different studies. For instance, Bukhari et al. (2020) studied *L. plantarum* antimicrobial potential. Rice-rinsed water was used for isolation of *Lactobacillus plantarum* strains. The isolate was then used for testing against *Aspergillus flavus* and *Aspergillus fumigatus* successfully (Bukhari et al., 2020). Other studies continued the same trend, showing the clear antifungal and antimicrobial potential of several strains of *L. plantarum*. Another source of lactic acid bacteria strains in raw bee pollen using gene sequencing.

Amongst them, *Lactobacillus plantarum* was also isolated (Belhad et al., 2014). It was thus proven that sources for *Lactobacillus plantarum* can be, therefore, vegetables, fruits, cereals and fermented foods.

Lactobacillus plantarum was also identified from fermented beverages, such as kombucha and braga. The kombucha beverage naturally contains this species. Pei et al., (2020) isolated from kombucha a bacteriocin produced by *L. plantarum* which has effects against both Gram+ and Gram- bacteria. An interesting element noted in the literature study was that many traditional, fermented foods made from fruits, vegetables or cereals were the starting point for research. These are listed in the table below (Table 1):

Table 1. Summary of traditional foods used for the study *of L. plantarum*

Traditional foods	Country	Effect	Reference
Jangri batter	India	Probiotic	Lavanya et al., 2023
Akamu, kunu-zaki	Nigeria	Starter culture	Nwachukwu et al., 2010
Injera	Ethiopia	Probiotic/ health promoting	Tamene et al., 2019
Yellow Zabol Kashk	Iran	Probiotic	Saboktakin-Rizi, et al., 2021
Ogi	Nigeria	Production of exopolysaccharide	Adesulu-Danhundi et al., 2018
Persian pickles	Iran	Fermentation	Dallal et al., 2017
Inziangsang, Gundruk, sinki and khalpi	India	Presence of the species	Tamang et al., 2005
Raabadi	India	Probiotic potential	Yadav et al., 2016
Dua muoi' and 'ca muoi'	Vietnam	Isolation of the species	Nguyen et al., 2013
Jinangshui	China	Presence of the species	Jun et al., 2018
Stinky xiancaigeng	China	Phennyllactic acid	Zhang et al., 2022
Kombucha	China	Bactericin	Pei et al., 2020
Kimchi	Corea	Antimutagenic activity	Park and Ree, 2001
Sausages	Spain	Probiotic	Rubio et al., 2013
Sea buckthorn juice	Finland	Starter culture	Markkinen et al., 2021
Braga	Romania	Probiotic	Anghelescu et al., 2019
Sourdough	Europe, America, Australia	Probiotic	Pontonia and Rizello, 2019
Pastirma	Turkey	Probiotic	Aksu, Erdemir, and Cakici (2016)

Taking everything into account, the species is considered extremely useful and necessary in the food industry, as the studies and results speak for themselves.

In the next part, the sources of the species are described in detail for fruits, vegetables and cereals as well as its bioactive potential and use in the food industry.

2. *Lactobacillus plantarum* in Fruits

Lactobacillus plantarum can have multiple effects, such as probiotic, antimicrobial or antimutagenic (see Table 1) ones. In the case of fruits, *Lactobacillus plantarum* can be used in fruit matrices and can be extracted from fruit matrices. For instance, the species was used in fruit powders to improve the quality and obtain a functional food product. *L. plantarum* can be also isolated from fruit byproducts with a potential use as probiotic (de Albuquerque et al., 2018). This reveals its major usefulness for the food industry.

2.1. *Lactobacillus plantarum* in Fruits

Barache et al. (2020) concluded that some strains of *L. plantarum* found in blackberrys, fresh figs and prickly pears in Algeria possess important beneficial bioactive compounds. Strains of *Lactobacillus plantarum* were grown and stored in cherry, pineapple, carrot, and tomato juices to improve their fermentation and to be able to add more information to the field. They suggested the species be used as a highly successful starter for some of the matrices (Filannino et al., 2014).

The same species (*L. plantarum)* presented 3 isolates when researching the papaya fruits (Fessard and Remize, 2019) and was encapsulated in order to add quality in food products. The strain isolated from papaya was successfully tested against *Enterococcus faecalis* and *Listeria innocua* (Todorov et al., 2011). The species was proven to have probiotic activity, adding a plus to the product where it is used (Todorov et al., 2012). Salads made from fresh fruits including pineapple, banana, papaya, mango and apple were found to have the potential to be used as vectors for Lactobacillus plantarum and are considered an option for functional food benefits (while also being cost effective) (Martins et al., 2017; Abubakr and Al-Adiwish, 2017). In kiwifruit, the species also potentiated the existing antioxidant effect (Zhou et al., 2020). Notably, some fruits have a natural *Lactobacillus plantarum* content. A study was performed where lactic acid bacteria were isolated from fresh fruits, including guava, dragon fruit, papaya, peach, grape, banana, ginger, pear, star fruit and melon and then tested against *Colletotrichum glosporioeides* for their antifungal effect. This fungus can appear in chilli seeds and can produce damage that can disturb the agri-food chain (Elmabrok et al., 2013). A similar study was conducted but this time against another pathogen, *Trichothecium roseum*, which causes the muskmelon fruit to rot (Lv et al., 2018). The results were similar, meaning the species of lactic acid bacteria presented antifungal effects. *Prunus mahaleb*, a seldom unused fruit, is currently being rediscovered due to its bioactive potential. When fermented with *L. plantarum* and *S. cerevisiae* the juice became a functional one with many bioactive components (Gerardi et al., 2019).

A strain of the species isolated from the pulp of *Mangifera indica* L., and from industrial fruit pulp-processing byproducts of *Malphigia glactic* acid bacteria, *M. indica*, *Annona muricata* and *Fragaria ananassa* were tested as possible probiotics with a cholesterol decreasing capacity (da Costa et al., 2019). According to the study, the strains used were able to modulate biochemical parameters. This suggests that, in the future, for the management of metabolic diseases we will be able to use probiotics. *L. plantarum* was also isolated from fresh strawberry and tested against mold producing microorganisms (Chen et al., 2020). The species can also be found in amazonian fruits including casho (*Anacardiun occidentale*), huito (*Genipa americana*), aguajillo (*Mauritiella aculeate*), ungurahui (*Oenocarpus bataua)*, maracuya (*Passiflora edulis*) and many others (Sanchez et al., 2019). Regarding other fruits, the lactic acid bacteria was added in pineapple residue and a better preservation was observed. It also improved fermentation and the possibility of future additions (Lin et al., 2022). Additionally, the cactus pear fruit, or prickly pear, (*Opuntia ficus-indica*) is known to have a pleasant taste and healthy nutrients. Juices from this fruit are susceptible to microbial spoilage and this is where Lactobacillus plantarum makes a difference, by being able to protect against this specific spoilage (Veron et al., 2017).

In yellow passion fruit, the species was similarly inoculated and the probiotic potential was observed. There was also a change in color and sweetness although the aroma did not undergo any change (Lascano et al., 2020).

Different fruits such as banana, strawberry, kiwi, mango and pineapple were used as food matrices to test the viability of a *L. plantarum* strain, which depended on temperature and time. After 37 days, when the matrices were stored at room temperature, no viable cells were detected but after the same period of time, but with storage temperature at 40°C, viable cells were detected (Ribeiro et al., 2014).

2.2. *Lactobacillus plantarum* in Wine and Cider

Lactobacillus plantarum was also studied in wine samples (Sestelo et al., 2004; Tremonte et al., 2017). The prevalence suggested that the species has an important role in the turning of wine as Pinot Noir and Merlot (Valdens et al., 2015). The species is also considered to have an important impact on wine quality (Kantor et al., 2014). In addition, the lactic acid bacteria species was isolated from grape must, where it was found to present antimicrobial activity (Rojo Bezares et al., 2007). Some strains from *L. plantarum*, which were isolated from Apulian wines, were tested in order to select suitable starters (Berbegal et al., 2016).

Li et al. (2021) fermented apple juice with *L. plantarum* in order for the juice to show antioxidant activity and nutritional benefits (non-alcoholic). The apple cultivar greatly influences the fermentation performance of the species when added to a mixture of lactic acid bacteria, with *L. acidophilus* and *L. fermentum* (Peng et al., 2021). For cider, Chen et al. (2023) analysed the flavour when fermented with *L. plantarum*. When the cider is inoculated with *L. plantarum* (mixed) an improvement of flavor was observed because of their higher contents of volatiles such as esters and higher alcohols as well as higher contents of non-volatile compounds, in the form of organic acids and polyphenols when compared with the single culture of *S. cerevisiae*.

2.3. *Lactobacillus plantarum* in Cocoa Beans

In cocoa beans, the species was found to be prevalent in the beginning stage of fermentation (Ghana fruits) (Camu 2007; Lefeber 2011; Schwendimann et al., 2015). A different strain of *L. plantarum* with probiotic potential was isolated from different stages of cocoa bean fermentation (Ramos et al., 2013). However, it should be noted that the content of this species is different depending on its geographic origins (Bortolini et al., 2016).

2.4. *Lactobacillus plantarum* in Juices

Borges et al. (2016) obtained powders enriched with the lactic bacteria species and recommend its use in fruit juices (banana, strawberry and apple). Also, there are matrices that naturally contain the species. According to this study, there are elements that can affect the survival of a probiotic culture (in our case *L. plantarum*), depending on food processing stages and storage conditions. The study used different drying techniques (hot air and spray-drying) to obtain the best method for the species' survival. The powder can be stored at 4°, but also at room temperature when in a controlled and low humidity environment.

A mathematical model was developed to assess the possibility of *L. plantarum* use and survival rate. The species was also used in various fruit juices. From these tested juices the cells from the lactic acid bacteria survived the best in orange, grapefruit, blackcurrant, pineapple and lemon juices. In other types of juices, such as cranberry and pomegranate juices, the cells decreased rapidly which implies that the species is not suitable for fermentation and development in those particular cases (Nualkaekul and Charalampopoulos, 2011). However, according to Mousavi et al. (2011) the species can be used successfully as a fermentation starter and further as probiotic in pomegranate juice. Mantzourani et al., (2019) corroborated the results by using the species as a starter for pomegranate juice with low alcohol content.

Traditional juices were also studied regarding *L. plantarum*. For Sohiong juice, lactic acid bacteria were used to develop juices enzymatically. The product quality of probiotic Sohiong juice powder was proven to be maintained for 36 days without refrigeration. This information suggests new possible ways to use lactic acid bacteria in the food industry (Kambhampati et al., 2020). In this way, fermented juices can meet demand for a new product with enhanced flavor, probiotic elements and beneficial health aspects (Voaides et al., 2022). These results were corroborated by another study (Vivek et al., 2021).

Fermented juices (such as blackberry and blueberry) with lactic acid bacteria were observed to have increased ABTS radical scavenging activity (Wu et al., 2021). Also, some strains were used for fermentation of blueberry juice and blackberry juice, which presented antioxidant capacity (Wu et al., 2021). Zhang et al. (2021) and Wen-Qiong et al. (2021) fermented blueberry juice with a strain of *L. plantarum,* proving that the addition was correlated with a higher phenolic content. The species did not only improve the antioxidant possibilities for certain juices or fruits, but it can also have an antifungal effect when combined with specific oils (thyme and cumin), according to Zamani-Zadeh et al. (2014). The same antioxidant activity was observed when the species was inoculated in beverages containing apples, pears, and carrots (Yang et al., 2018). Meng et al. (2022) studied the antioxidant effect of *Lactobacillus plantarum* in loquat juice. The species fermented well in the juice with a high phenolic content, amino acids, peptides and terpenoids.

Black grape juice inoculated with the lactic acid bacteria species presented a quantity of GABA acid in the amount of 117, 33 mg/l after 21 days in storage. Therefore, the species is important in producing probiotic juices (Rezaei et al., 2022). The species of lactic acid bacteria was also inoculated in fermented juices made from tropical fruits, such as guava, where the addition gave a rich antioxidant content, total phenolics, and short and medium chain fatty acids (Bhat et al., 2015).

In litchi juice *L. plantarum* was treated with different probiotics which had both positive and negative effects on powder quality (Kalita et al., 2018) and it was demonstrated that the species impacts the aroma profile of the juice in the positive manner, giving the industry a potential application (Wang et al., 2023). On noni juice the species presented a similar response (Cheng et al., 2021).

Moreover, in mango and sapota juices, the species was found to be able to survive and also to utilise fruit juices for their cell synthesis, this being revealed by a decrease in fruit sugars and pH and increase in acidity with a total phenolic content of 145 mg/ml in sapota juice and 60.24 mg/ml in mango juice, at 72 h (Kumar et al., 2015).

Another study suggested that inulin addition to the fermented juices with *Lactobacillus plantarum* presented the possibility of greater shelf life (Valero-Cases and Frutos, 2017).

When *L. plantarum* was added to coconut water to obtain a fermented beverage, this beverage is thought to be a novel functional beverage, due to its probiotic and beneficial health components (Kantachote et al., 2017).

3. *Lactobacillus plantarum* in Vegetables

L. plantarum can be used in different matrices (including Chinese pickled vegetables, raw vegetables or vegetable juices) and can be isolated and extracted from many sources (Cen et al., 2020). Its bioactive potential was studied in a great number of research articles such as Dogan et al., (2021), Cagno et al. (2010), Kim et al. (2019), Karasu et al. (2010) and many others.

For instance, Cagno et al. (2010) isolated and characterized 72 different isolates of *L. plantarum* from raw vegetables and fruits. The study presents a possible extraction and use of this lactic acid bacteria in the food industry, as it can be found in many matrices and added to a diverse list of matrices making it easy and affordable to use. Lactic acid bacteria species was isolated and tested from fresh vegetables such as cauliflower, gherkins, cluster beans, fenugreek, cow pea, bitter gourd, french beans, tomato, ridged gourd, cucumber and bottle gourd in order to asses its antioxidant activity. *L. plantarum* was proven to have a potent antioxidant activity and even an antibacterial one, against human pathogens (Priti et al., 2016; Junnarkar et al., 2019). The species was also isolated and used in a test that resulted in *Lactobacillus plantarum* exibiting a beneficial response against constipation in mice (Li et al., 2019).

In plant-based matrices the species was found to present good growth, while in animal-based matrices, such as unprocessed milk, the species presented poor growth (Makimattila et al., 2011). On the same pattern *Lactobacillus plantarum*, isolated from vegetables was demonstrated to have antimicrobial activity against *Escherichia coli*, *Salmonella typhi*, *Shigella dysenteriae*, *Bacillus anthracis* and *Staphylococcus aureus* (Amin et al., 2009).

3.1. *Lactobacillus plantarum* in Fermented Foods

Fermented foods present more and more interest for their beneficial health effects. The species was isolated from fermented vegetables, such as cucumber, olive and sauerkraut and tested as a probiotic (Karasu et al., 2010) and for its antioxidant activity (Li et al., 2012). The species of lactic acid bacteria was also isolated from pickled vegetables such as cabbage, sauerkraut, cucumber, in order to show that the species can be found and isolated from many matrices with usability in the food industry (Mäkimattila et al., 2011). Not only that, but a strain of *L. plantarum* isolated from sauerkraut was proven to have cholesterol-controlling capacity and was proposed for further use in functional foods (Yu et al., 2013). Isolated from pickled cabbage the strain of *L. plantarum* presented an increased proteolytic, acidific and GABA-producing activity in cheese (Karimian et al., 2020).

Lactobacillus plantarum was also isolated from the Korean traditional fermented vegetable, kimchi. The species was proven to possess a strong antimutagenic activity against various mutagens including MNNG, NQO, NPD and aflatoxin B1 (Park and Ree, 2001). Strains isolated from kimchi were evaluated for their antioxidant and immune-enhancing properties with the recommendation to be used as probiotic for people of old age (Yang et al., 2019). A strain of the species was identified and proven to have also antifungal potential against *Aspergillus flavus*, *A. fumigatus*, *A. petrakïi*, *A. ochraceus*, *A. nidulans*, *Epicoccum nigrum*, and *Cladosporium gossypiicola* (inhibiting the growth) (Yang and Chang, 2008; Park et al., 2014). Not only that, but it can also be used for lowering cholesterol (Choi and Chang, 2015) and presents the possibility of being used as a GABA-producing starter for probiotic production (Wang et al., 2021). Its antioxidant potential was studied in a research which isolated strains of the lactic acid bacteria in kimchi (Son et al., 2017).

The species of lactic acid bacteria was also isolated from other types of fermented food (such as pickled Chinese cabbage, pickled chili, pickled cabbage, pickled carrot, pickled leaf mustard, pickled cowpea, and pickled ginger) and assessed its antimicrobial activity successfully.

Fermented cucumber is another product the species was isolated from and used to improve other food and feed matrices. A plasmid from *L. plantarum* that was isolated from Chinese pickels was described by Pan et al. (2011). Also, a traditional Chinese fermented vegetable, Stinky xiancaigeng, was found to contain high concentrations of phenyllactic acid which is a known antimicrobial agent. The species that was found to produce this phenyllactic acid was *Lactobacillus plantarum* (Zhang et al., 2022). Bacteriocin production by the species was also studied by Hu et al., (2013) with plantaricin suggested as an antimicrobial capacity (from fermented Chinese vegetables). Rizello et al., (2014) also investigated the antimicrobial activity of the lactic acid bacteria species. The results suggest that the size of the inoculum was an important factor alongside substrate type (solid media was found to have better production of bacteriocins).

Dua muoi (mustard and beet fermentation) and ca muoi (eggplant fermentation) are types of popular traditional fermented vegetables of Vietnamese origin in which *Lactobacillus plantarum* was isolated (Nguyen et al., 2013). In Hainan, China, a study regarding the lactic acid bacteria content from fermented vegetables was performed. *Lactobacillus plantarum* was found in all samples and was the most abundant with a percentage of 32.31%

(Peng et al., 2018). The species was also found in a traditional food called Jinangshui (Jun et al., 2018).

In traditional Persian pickles the species was also found to be in high concentrations and is recognized as a probiotic. This finding brings an improvement for the pickling industry (Dallal et al., 2017).

The microbial content was assessed in Inziangsang (a fermented leafy vegetable product of Nagaland and Manipur in India), gundruk, sinki and khalpi, which are also traditional Indian fermented foods. The lactic acid bacteria species were present with a good content for *Lactobacillus plantarum* (Tamang et al., 2005). *Lactobacillus plantarum* isolated from pickled vegetables was found to alleviate constipation in mice (Li et al., 2019).

3.2. *Lactobacillus plantarum* and Olive Fermentation

Lactobacillus plantarum is also considered to be responsible for the fermentation of table olives, which are widely consumed wordlwide (Hurtado et al., 2012; Blana et al., 2014). Moreover, the species is thought to have a huge impact on flavor coumpounds, therefore it can change taste profiles (Sabatini et al., 2008). *Lactobacillus plantarum* strain B282, isolated from fermented table olives was screened in vitro for its probiotic potential. Afterwards, it was investigated as starter culture in green olives that were fermented in the traditional Spanish style (Blana et al., 2014). Two strains isolated from fermeneted olives have antimicrobial activity against Gram+ and Gram- bacteria. The same strains were suggested to be used as probiotics due to their responses to high bile salt concentration and low pH values (Mourad and Nour Eddine, 2006). *L. plantarum* strains presented free-radical scavenging ability in the fermentation process, reduced the oxidation of unsaturated fatty acids and also took to a recution in peroxide value (abadi Sherahi et al., 2018). Abouloifa et al. (2019) studied 14 antifungal Lactobacillus strains that were isolated from traditional fermenting Moroccan green olives. Their results showed that the strains obtained from Lactobacillus species (including *L. plantarum*) possess probiotic culture properties and they are suitable as starters and as biopreservative cultures in different areas such as agriculture, food, and pharmaceutical industries. Olives were fermented with *Lactobacillus plantarum* strain, at room temperature, for 120 days, using 2 different concentrations, namely, NaCl (2.4–13.6% w/v) and sucrose (0–0.82% w/v). The results suggeste species suitability for useas fermentation starter (Rosa et al., 2016).

Lactobacillus plantarum can and was used in order to obtain high-added-value peptides from the fermentation process by using tomato seed meal extract as a substrate known to possess antioxidant activity. The results show that the species uses tomato proteins and turns them into bioactive compounds (Mechmeche et al., 2017).

3.3. *Lactobacillus plantarum* in Vegetable Juices

In this respect, Karasu et al. (2010) studied the possibility for the lactic acid bacteria to be used in fermented vegetable beverages with great success. A strain of *L. plantarum* was proven to enhance the functional activities of vegetable sponge beverage without negatively affecting its sensory properties. In addition, the species presented antioxidant and anti-inflammatory activities (Jeong et al., 2022). The presence of this lactic acid bacteria species was also found in tomatoes and pickled white cabbage sampled from Reunion Island (Fessard and Remize, 2019). In tomato juice the species was used as a fermentation starter (Liu et al., 2018). As a starter culture strain *Lactobacillus plantarum* was proven to be adequate for vegetable fermentations, having better results compared to other species of lactic acid bacteria (Wouters et al., 2013).

Vegetables juices (including those obtained from carrots, endive, iceberg lettuce, garden rocket) acted as a substrate for the lactic acid bacteria species to be used as a fermentation starter and an antibacterial element against *Staphylococcus aureus* (Scolari et al., 2004). A strain of *L. plantarum* was isolated from carrot juice and modified in order to change the sensory qualities of the juice. The results showed a decrease of terpene flavor and an improvement in the sensory quality of the juice (Zhang et al., 2019). In juices made from vegetables like bitter gourd (*Momordica charantia)*, bottle gourd (*Lagenaria siceraria*) and carrot (*Daucus carota*) the species was studied in regard to growth pontential by using a model (Sharma and Mishra, 2014).

In carrot and beetroot juices the species presents an antioxidant activity in addition to its benefits as a probiotic (Malik et al., 2019). Therefore, the *L. plantarum* species was yet again proven to be useful in food as a probiotic (Liu et al., 2022). Chinese pickle juices are also abundant with microorganisms, from which *L. plantarum* was isolated. A bacteriocin from the isolated strain was found to have antimicrobial effect, especially against Gram- bacteria (Zhou et al., 2014).

3.4. *Lactobacillus plantarum* in Silage Production

The species was also isolated from corn silage (Tallon et al. 2003). Lactic acid bacteria were found to improve the fermentation of corn silage towards increasing the lactic acid concentration and decreasing the pH in the first stages of fermentation. The idea of using LAB species for silage fermentation resides in the fact that some species, such as *Lactobacillus plantarum*, are able to produce a needed quantity of acetic acid in order to improve aerobic stability and increase the pH (Xu et al., 2019). A strain of *L. plantarum* tested for silage production presented positive effects on protein preservation during ensiling, which then helped enhance ruminal in vitro microbial biomass production (Contreras-Govea et al., 2013). In a study performed by Xu et al. (2019) the species performed identically. Moreover, it increased the relative concentrations of pyrogallol and tetrahydrocorticosterone. It was also found to help degrade pesticides faster, such as chlorpyrifos and phorate during storage (Zhang et al., 2016). *L. plantarum* strains were found to be able to improve silage quality and ferment to produce a good amount of lactic acid. Not only that but *L. plantarum* presents important functional probiotic properties such as high tolerance to low pH, bile salts and is capable to produce extracellular enzymes (Arasu et al., 2014). Xi et al., (2021) studied the effect of L. plantarum addition in silage production and quality, with succesfull results including increased lactic acid content with decreased pH. Moreover, it reduced contents of acetic acid, propionic acid, and ammonia-N.

Several strains of *Lactobacillus plantarum* were tested against *Salmonella typhimurium* and proved to have an antimicrobial effect (Lapsiri et al., 2011). Another study corroborated these results with *Lactobacillus plantarum* isolated from cabbage, silage and cucumber and tested against many bacterial species in order to assess its antimicrobial potential. It was revealed that the species presented antimicrobial activity against *Staphylococcus aureus, Salmonella typhimurium and Escherichia coli*, with the highest inhibiting effect against *Salmonella typhimurium* (Darsanaki et al., 2012).

4. *Lactobacillus plantarum* in Cereals

In cereals, *Lactobacillus plantarum* is considered to present roles such as ease of fermentation (starter culture), addition of health benefits (can be used as probiotic) and sensory functions (taste, aroma etc.) (Oguntoyinbo and Narbad, 2015; Ferri et al., 2016).

When used for fermentations by *Lactobacillus plantarum* in order to obtain baked goods, it was found to have a higher potential in quinoa (9.8 log cfu/mL, 23.1 g/L) than in wheat (8.9 log cfu/mL, 13.9 g/L), while an antifungal activity was also observed (Dallagnol et al., 2013). *L. plantarum* strains were also used to obtain fermented oat foods in order to improve some nutritional and technological traits (Russo et al., 2016). When a *Lactobacillus plantarum* supplemented oat-fermented food was administrated to rats, a possibility for glucose and lipidic potential but also antioxidant effect was discovered (Alrhabi et al., 2022). The species was added to teff flour revealing the possibility for the creation of future probiotics (Alemneh et al., 2021). Another use of the species was in oat-based yogurt where antioxidant and antimicrobial potential is present (Lim, 2018). Isolated from cereal-based products a strain of the species was demonstrated to possess antifungal activity. Also, when the nutritional properties were analysed, an improvement was detected when the strain was used (Quattrini et al., 2018; Wronkowska et al., 2022).

4.1. *Lactobacillus plantarum* in Cereal-Based Beverages

Lactobacillus plantarum can be used for the enrichment of different beverages made from fermented cereals in order to help different populations from poorer areas of the world which have difficulties in leading a healthy lifestyle. In West Africa, this species can be used in this respect for both small and large-scale industrial cereal food production with enhanced health benefits (Oguntoyinbo and Narbad, 2015).

For instance, *Lactobacillus plantarum* isolated from spontaneously fermenting cereals was used in order to preserve nutritional factors in soy-fermented foods (Adeyemo and Onilude, 2013). The viability of the species was also assessed in barley, wheat and barley malt extracts as potentially probiotic. As such, the *Lactobacillus plantarum* strain was observed to survive much better in the malt extracts compared to barley and wheat extracts during refrigerated storage (Charalampopoulos, Pandiella, 2010).

The species can also be used in cereal substrates in order to change the aroma profile as suggested by Sameron et al. (2009). The study aimed to assess the volatile compounds for the oat, wheat, barley and malt substrate in which *Lactobacillus plantarum* was used.

Soy milk fermented with *Lactobacillus plantarum* was proven to possess pathogenic inhibition of foodborne pathogens (Savedboworn and Wanchaitanawong, 2015).

Spontaneous fermentation of cereals (maize, millet, sorghum) for the production of indigenous Nigerian foods, in particular akamu and kunu-zaki, were selected for the identification of lactic acid bacteria. *Lactobacillus plantarum* was found to be useful as a starter culture for the Nigerian foods, especially for akamu (Nwachukwu et al., 2010).

4.2. *Lactobacillus plantarum* in Fermented Cereal-Based Foods

Fermented cereals are widely used as foods with a strong probiotic potential. *Lactobacillus plantarum* was isolated from different sources (fruits, fresh and fermented vegetables, fermented cereals) and was screened for antimicrobial activity against food spoiling bacteria. The species was found to have antimicrobial activity against Staphylococcus aureus and presented great bacteriocin production (Grosu-Tudor et al., 2014).

Jangri batter is a fermented, cereal-based traditional Indian food from which *L. plantarum* was isolated in order to assess if the species can be used as a probiotic. The study confirmed that *Lactobacillus plantarum* can be used effectively as a probiotic, delivering viable cells after many hours and protecting against food-borne pathogens (Lavanya et al., 2023). Another Indian dish is raabadi, a fermented beverage made from barley and other ingredients. A study conducted in 2016 concluded that some strains of *L. plantarum* isolated from this beverage presented excellent probiotic potential (Yadav et al., 2016). Idli batter, an Indian traditional food, can be used as a source of L. plantarum with a probiotic potential (Ahire et al., 2021). Similar results were reported by Gupta and Tiwari (2014) when strains were isolated from dosa. *L. plantarum* isolated from Marcha of Sikkim beverage (made from rice, herbs and others) presented good antioxidant potential (Das and Goyal, 2015).

In Nigerian traditional fermented cereal gruel ogi, lactic acid bacteria were investigated on the basis of their capability to produce exopolysaccharides. They were found to have strong antioxidant potential with such values as 1.36 g/L and 2.18 g/L for the two exopolysaccharides investigated (Adesulu-Danhundi et al., 2018). These exopolysaccharides were also found to also have antimicrobial potential against *Pseudomonas aeruginosa, E. coli, Salmonella typhimurium* and *Staphylococcus aureus* (Liu et al., 2017).

In Iranian traditional food such as Yellow Zabol Kashk the species was isolated and characterised. The results suggested that it can be of further use as a probiotic due to its properties (Saboktakin-Rizi, et al., 2021).

In countries where food is scarce, such as Ethiopia, probiotic foods can help with different problems that occur due to the inefficient and ineffective manner that food is consumed. There, injera is widely consumed fermented flat bread. Folate-producing Lactobacillus plantarum could have a purpose in helping with congenital defects in fetuses or anaemia, which appear often (Tamene et al., 2019).

Conclusion

The present literature research offered a perspective in the practical use possibilities for *Lactobacillus plantarum*. The species can be found and isolated from many sources including vegetables, fruits and cereals. The multitude of uses in the food industry makes this species one of great importance, as shown by the attention granted by many scientists who studied its potential. There are articles which present the possibility of using the species as an alternative treatment for burns (with further need to study its implications and relevance) (Peral et al., 2009).

Lactobacillus plantarum is a novel and useful way to create probiotics in order to promote health, food and feed safety and even economic revenue. Studies are being carried out in order to create a larger array of possibilites for the species in the food industry. Different strains of the lactic acid bacteria possess different options for usage, from antimutagenic to antioxidant activity. There are many natural sources for the species. Regardless of the source, the species was proven to have excellent potential for the food industry, showing several activities with the aim of improving human health. Most of the strains were isolated from fermented foods. These fermented foods present as a new trend globally. Interestingly, some traditional fermented foods were the starting point for research. This relies on the fact that fermentation is an old preservation method which presents potential for the use of probiotics or as probiotics. Also, beverages obtained from either fruits, cereals or vegetables are used for *L. plantarum* isolation or they can be used as probiotic or fermentation starter.

References

Abadi Sherahi, M. H., Shahidi, F., Yazdi, F. T., Hashemi, S. M. B., Effect of *Lactobacillus plantarum* on olive and olive oil quality during fermentation process. *LWT*. 2018. 89: p. 572-580.

Abdelazez, A., Abdelmotaal, H., Zhu, Z. T., Fang-Fang, J., Sami, R., Zhang, L. J., Al-Tawaha, A. R., Meng, X. C., Potential benefits of *Lactobacillus plantarum* as probiotic and its advantages in human health and industrial applications: A review. *Advances in Environmental Biology*. 2018. 12 :1.

Abouloifa, H., Rokni, Y., Bellaouchi, R., Ghabbour, N., Karboune, S., Brasca, M., Asehraou, A., Characterization of probiotic properties of antifungal *Lactobacillus* strains isolated from traditional fermenting green olives. *Probiotics and antimicrobial proteins*. 2020. 12: p. 683-696.

Abubakr, M. A., Al-Adiwish, W. M., Isolation and identification of lactic acid bacteria from different fruits with proteolytic activity. *International Journal of Microbiology and Biotechnology*. 2017. 2: 2, p. 58-64.

Adesulu-Dahunsi, A.T., Jeyaram, K., Sanni, A. I. Banwo, K., Production of exopolysaccharide by strains of *Lactobacillus plantarum* YO175 and OF101 isolated from traditional fermented cereal beverage. *PeerJ*. 2018. 6.e5326.

Adeyemo, S. M., Onilude, A. A., Enzymatic reduction of anti-nutritional factors in fermenting soybeans by *Lactobacillus plantarum* isolates from fermenting cereals. *Nigerian Food Journal*. 2013. 31: 2, p. 84-90.

Ahire, J. J., Jakkamsetty, C., Kashikar, M. S., Lakshmi, S. G. Madempudi, R. S., In vitro evaluation of probiotic properties of *Lactobacillus plantarum* UBLP40 isolated from traditional indigenous fermented food. *Probiotics and antimicrobial proteins*. 2021. 13: 5, p. 1413-1424.

Aksu, M. I., Erdemir, E., Cakici, N., Changes in the physico-chemical and microbial quality during the production of pastirma cured with different levels of sodium nitrite. *Korean Journal for Food Science of Animal Resources*. 2016. 36: 5, p. 617–625.

Alemneh, S. T., Emire, S. A. Hitzmann, B., Teff-based probiotic functional beverage fermented with *Lactobacillus rhamnosus* and *Lactobacillus plantarum*. *Foods*. 2021. 10: 10, 2333.

Alharbi, H. F., Algonaiman, R. Barakat, H., Ameliorative and Antioxidative Potential of *Lactobacillus plantarum*-Fermented Oat (*Avena sativa*) and Fermented Oat Supplemented with Sidr Honey against Streptozotocin-Induced Type 2 Diabetes in Rats. *Antioxidants*. 2022. 11: 6, 1122.

Amin, M., Jorfi, M., Khosravi, A. D., Samarbafzadeh, A. R. Sheikh, A. F., Isolation and identification of *Lactobacillus casei* and *Lactobacillus plantarum* from plants by PCR and detection of their antibacterial activity. *Journal of Biological Sciences*. 2009. 9: 8, p. 810-814.

Angelescu, I. R., Zamfir, M., Stancu, M. M., Grosu-Tudor, S. S., Identification and probiotic properties of lactobacilli isolated from two different fermented beverages. *Annals of Microbiology*. 2019. 69: p. 1557-1565.

Arasu, M. V., Al-Dhabi, N. A., Ilavenil, S., Choi, K. C., Srigopalram, S., In vitro importance of probiotic *Lactobacillus plantarum* related to medical field. *Saudi journal of biological sciences*. 2016. 23: 1, p. 6–10.

Arasu, M. V., Jung, M. W., Kim, D. H., Ilavenil, S., Jane, M., Park, H. S., Choi, K. C., Enhancing nutritional quality of silage by fermentation with *Lactobacillus plantarum. Indian journal of microbiology*. 2014. 54: p. 396-402.

Aukrust, T., Blom, H., Transformation of *Lactobacillus* strains used in meat and vegetable fermentations. *Food Research International*. 1992. 25: 4, p. 253-261.

Barache, N., Ladjouzi, R., Belguesmia, Y., Bendali, F., Drider, D., Abundance of *Lactobacillus plantarum* strains with beneficial attributes in blackberries (*Rubus sp.),* fresh figs (*Ficus carica*), and prickly pears (*Opuntia ficus-indica*) grown and harvested in Algeria. *Probiotics and antimicrobial proteins*. 2020. 12, p. 1514-1523.

Belhadj, H., Harzallah, D., Bouamra, D., Khennouf, S., Dahamna, S., Ghadbane, M., Phenotypic and genotypic characterization of some lactic acid bacteria isolated from bee pollen: a preliminary study. *Bioscience of microbiota, food and health*. 2014. 33: 1, p. 11-23.

Berbegal, C., Peña, N., Russo, P., Grieco, F., Pardo, I., Ferrer, S., Spano, G., Capozzi, V., Technological properties of *Lactobacillus plantarum* strains isolated from grape must fermentation. *Food microbiology*. 2016. 57: p. 187-194.

Bhat, R., Suryanarayana, L. C., Chandrashekara, K. A., Krishnan, P., Kush, A., Ravikumar, P., *Lactobacillus plantarum* mediated fermentation of *Psidium guajava* L. fruit extract. *J Biosci Bioeng*. 2015. 119: 4, p. 430-432.

Blana, V. A., Grounta, A., Tassou, C. C., Nychas, G. J. E., Panagou, E. Z., Inoculated fermentation of green olives with potential probiotic *Lactobacillus pentosus* and *Lactobacillus plantarum* starter cultures isolated from industrially fermented olives. *Food microbiology*. 2014. 38 :p. 208-218.

Borges, S., Barbosa, J., Silva, J., Gomes, A. M., Pintado, M., Silva, C. L. M., Morais, A. M. M. B., Teixeira, P., A feasibility study of *Lactobacillus plantarum* in fruit powders after processing and storage. *International Journal of Food Science & Technology*. 2016. 51: 2, p. 381-388.

Bortolini, C., Patrone, V., Puglisi, E., Morelli, L., Detailed analyses of the bacterial populations in processed cocoa beans of different geographic origin, subject to varied fermentation conditions. *Int J Food Microbiol*. 2016. 236: p. 98-106.

Bukhari, S. A., Salman, M., Numan, M., Javed, M. R., Zubair, M., Mustafa, G., Characterization of antifungal metabolites produced by *Lactobacillus plantarum* and *Lactobacillus coryniformis* isolated from rice rinsed water. *Molecular Biology Reports*. 2020. 47: p. 1871-1881.

Camu, N., De Winter, T., Verbrugghe, K., Cleenwerck, I., Vandamme, P., Takrama, J.S., Vancanneyt, M., De Vuyst, L., Dynamics and biodiversity of populations of lactic acid bacteria and acetic acid bacteria involved in spontaneous heap fermentation of cocoa beans in Ghana. *Appl Environ Microbiol*. 2007. 73: 6, p. 1809-24.

Cen, S., Yin, R., Mao, B., Zhao, J., Zhang, H., Zhai, Q., Chen, W., Comparative genomics shows niche-specific variations of *Lactobacillus plantarum* strains isolated from human, *Drosophila melanogaster*, vegetable and dairy sources. *Food Bioscience*. 2020. 35: 100581.

Charalampopoulos, D., Pandiella, S. S., Survival of human derived *Lactobacillus plantarum* in fermented cereal extracts during refrigerated storage. *LWT-Food Science and Technology*. 2010. 43: 3, p. 431-435.

Charalampopoulos, D., Wang, R., Pandiella, S. S., Webb, C., Application of cereals and cereal components in functional foods: a review. *International journal of food microbiology*. 2002. 79: 1-2, p. 131-141.

Chen X., Lin M., Hu L., Xu T., Xiong D., Li L., Zhao Z., Research on the Effect of Simultaneous and Sequential Fermentation with *Saccharomyces cerevisiae* and *Lactobacillus plantarum* on Antioxidant Activity and Flavor of Apple Cider. *Fermentation*. 2023. 9: 2, 102.

Chen, C., Cao, Z., Li, J., Tao, C., Feng, Y., Han, Y., A novel endophytic strain of *Lactobacillus plantarum* CM-3 with antagonistic activity against *Botrytis cinerea* on strawberry fruit. *Biological Control*. 2020. 148: 104306.

Cheng, Y., Li, P., Hu, B., Xu, L., Liu, S., Yu, H., Guo, Y., Xie, Y., Yao, W., Qian, H., Correlation analysis reveals the intensified fermentation via *Lactobacillus plantarum* improved the flavor of fermented noni juice. *Food Bioscience*. 2021. 43: 101234.

Choi, E. A., Chang, H.C., Cholesterol-lowering effects of a putative probiotic strain *Lactobacillus plantarum* EM isolated from kimchi. *LWT-food Science and Technology*. 2015. 62: 1, p. 210-217.

Contreras-Govea, F. E., Muck, R. E., Broderick, G. A., Weimer, P. J., *Lactobacillus plantarum* effects on silage fermentation and in vitro microbial yield. *Animal feed science and technology*. 2013. 179: 1-4, p. 61-68.

da Costa, W. K. A., Brandão, L. R., Martino, M. E., Garcia, E. F., Alves, A. F., de Souza, E. L., de Souza Aquino, J., Saarela, M., Leulier, F., Vidal, H., Magnani, M., Qualification of tropical fruit-derived *Lactobacillus plantarum* strains as potential probiotics acting on blood glucose and total cholesterol levels in Wistar rats. *Food Research International*. 2019. 124: p. 109-117.

Dallagnol, A. M., Pescuma, M., De Valdez, G. F., Rollán, G., Fermentation of quinoa and wheat slurries by *Lactobacillus plantarum* CRL 778: proteolytic activity. *Applied microbiology and biotechnology*. 2013. 97: p. 3129-n3140.

Dallal, M. S., Zamaniahari, S., Davoodabadi, A., Hosseini, M., Rajabi, Z., Identification and characterization of probiotic lactic acid bacteria isolated from traditional persian pickled vegetables. *GMS hygiene and infection control*. 2017. 12.

Darsanaki, R. K., Rokhi, M. L., Aliabadi, M. A., Issazadeh, K., Antimicrobial activities of *Lactobacillus* strains isolated from fresh vegetables. *Middle-east journal of scientific research*. 2012. 11: 9, p. 1216-1219.

Das, D., Goyal, A., Antioxidant activity and γ-aminobutyric acid (GABA) producing ability of probiotic *Lactobacillus plantarum* DM5 isolated from Marcha of Sikkim. *LWT-food Science and Technology*. 2015. 61: 1, p. 263- 268.

de Albuquerque, T. M. R., Garcia, E. F., de Oliveira Araújo, A., Magnani, M., Saarela, M., de Souza, E. L., In vitro characterization of *Lactobacillus* strains isolated from fruit processing by-products as potential probiotics. *Probiotics and antimicrobial proteins*. 2018. 10: p. 704-716.

Dogan, K., Akman, P. K., Tornuk, F., Role of non-thermal treatments and fermentation with probiotic *Lactobacillus plantarum* on in vitro bioaccessibility of bioactives from vegetable juice. *J Sci Food Agric*. 2021. 101: 11, p. 4779- 4788.

El -Sheikha A. F., Why Fermented Foods are the Promising Food Trends in the Future?. *Curr Res Nutr Food Sci*. 2022. 10: 3.

Elmabrok, A., Hassan, Z., Hussin, K., Mokhtar, A., Antifungal Activity of *Lactobacillus Plantarum* Lactic acid bacteria-C5 and Lactic acid bacteria-G7 Isolated from Malaysian Fruits. *Acta Biologica Malaysiana*. 2013. 2: 1, p. 22-30.

FAO /WHO, Evaluation of Health and Nutritional Properties of Probiotics in Food Including Powder Milk with Live Bacteria; A Joint FAO/WHO Expert Consultation: Cordóba, Argentina. 2001.

Ferri, M., Serrazanetti, D. I., Tassoni, A., Baldissarri, M., Gianotti, A., Improving the functional and sensorial profile of cereal-based fermented foods by selecting *Lactobacillus plantarum* strains via a metabolomics approach. *Food research international*. 2016. 89: p. 1095- 1105.

Fessard, A., Remize, F., Genetic and technological characterization of lactic acid bacteria isolated from tropically grown fruits and vegetables. *International journal of food microbiology*. 2019. 301: p. 61-72.

Filannino, P., Cardinali, G., Rizzello, C. G., Buchin, S., De Angelis, M., Gobbetti, M., Di Cagno, R., Metabolic responses of *Lactobacillus plantarum* strains during fermentation and storage of vegetable and fruit juices. *Applied and environmental microbiology*. 2014. 80: 7, p. 2206- 2215.

Fleming, H.P., McFeeeters, R. F., Daeschel, M. A., The lactobacilli, pediococci and leuconostocs: vegetable products. In Bacterial starter cultures for foods; Gilliland, S. E.; Ed.; CRC Press. Inc.: New York . 1985. 97.

Gaggia, F., Di Gioia, D., Baffoni, L., Biavati, B., The role of protective and probiotic cultures in food and feed and their impact in food safety. *Trends in food science & technology*. 2011. 22: p. 58-66.

Garmasheva I., Vasyliuk O., Kovalenko N., Ostapchuk A., Oleschenko L., Intraspecies cellular fatty acids heterogeneity of *Lactobacillus plantarum* strains isolated from fermented foods in Ukraine. *Lett Appl Microbiol*. 2015. 61: 3, p. 283-92.

Gerardi, C., Tristezza, M., Giordano, L., Rampino, P., Perrotta, C., Baruzzi, F., Capozzi, V., Mita, G., Grieco, F., Exploitation of *Prunus mahaleb* fruit by fermentation with selected strains of *Lactobacillus plantarum* and *Saccharomyces cerevisiae*. *Food microbiology*. 2019. 84: 103262.

Grosu-Tudor, S. S., Stancu, M. M., Pelinescu, D., Zamfir, M., Characterization of some bacteriocins produced by lactic acid bacteria isolated from fermented foods. *World Journal of Microbiology and Biotechnology*. 2014. 30: p. 2459-2469.

Guan, Q., Xiong, T., Xie, M., Influence of probiotic fermented fruit and vegetables on human health and the related industrial development trend. *Engineering*. 2021. 7: 2, p. 212-218.

Gupta, A., Tiwari, S. K., Probiotic potential of *Lactobacillus plantarum* LD1 isolated from batter of Dosa, a South Indian fermented food. *Probiotics and antimicrobial proteins*. 2014. 6: p. 73-81.

Hu, M., Zhao, H., Zhang, C., Yu, J., Lu, Z., Purification and characterization of plantaricin 163, a novel bacteriocin produced by *Lactobacillus plantarum* 163 isolated from traditional Chinese fermented vegetables. *Journal of agricultural and food chemistry.*2013. 61: 47, p. 11676- 11682.

Hurtado, A., Reguant, C., Bordons, A., Rozès, N., Lactic acid bacteriafrom fermented table olives. *Food Microbiology*. 2012. 31: 1, p. 1-8.

Jiang, F., Cheng, H., Liu, D., Wei, C., An, W., Wang, Y., Sun, H., Song, E., Treatment of Whole-Plant Corn Silage with Lactic acid bacteria and Organic Acid Enhances Quality by Elevating Acid Content, reducing ph, and Inhibiting Undesirable Microorganisms. *Front. Microbiol. Sec. Food Microbiology*. 2020. 11 :p.1-10.

Jun, Z., Shuaishuai, W., Lihua, Z., Qilong, M., Xi, L., Mengyang, N., Tong, Z., Hongli, Z., Culture-dependent and-independent analysis of bacterial community structure in Jiangshui, a traditional Chinese fermented vegetable food. *LWT*. 2018. 96: p. 244-250.

Junnarkar, M., Pawar, S., Gaikwad, S., Mandal, A., Jass, J., Nawani, N., Probiotic potential of lactic acid bacteria from fresh vegetables: Application in food preservation. *Indian Journal of Experimental Biology*. 2019. 57: p. 825-838.

Kalita, D., Saikia, S., Gautam, G., Mukhopadhyay, R., Mahanta, C.L., Characteristics of synbiotic spray dried powder of litchi juice with *Lactobacillus plantarum* and different carrier materials. *LWT*. 2018. 87: p. 351-360.

Kantachote, D., Ratanaburee, A., Hayisama-ae, W., Sukhoom, A., Nunkaew, T., The use of potential probiotic *Lactobacillus plantarum* DW12 for producing a novel functional beverage from mature coconut water. *Journal of Functional Foods*. 2017. 32: p. 401-408.

Kántor, A., Kluz M., Puchalski C., Terentjeva M., Kačániová M., Identification of lactic acid bacteriaisolated from wine using real-time PCR. *J Environ Sci Health B*. 2016. 51: 1, p. 52-56.

Karasu, N., Şimşek, Ö., Çon, A. H., Technological and probiotic characteristics of *Lactobacillus plantarum* strains isolated from traditionally produced fermented vegetables. *Annals of microbiology*. 2010. 60: 2, p. 227- 234.

Karimian, E., Moayedi, A., Khomeiri, M., Aalami, M., Mahoonak, A. S., Application of high-GABA producing *Lactobacillus plantarum* isolated from traditional cabbage pickle in the production of functional fermented whey-based formulate. *Journal of Food Measurement and Characterization*. 2020. 14: p. 3408- 3416.

Kim, J., Choi, K. B., Park, J. H., Kim, K. H., Metabolite profile changes and increased antioxidative and antiinflammatory activities of mixed vegetables after fermentation by *Lactobacillus plantarum*. *PLoS One*. 2019. 14: 5, e0217180.

Kumar, B. V., Sreedharamurthy, M., Reddy, O. V. S., Probiotication of mango and sapota juices using *Lactobacillus plantarum* NCDC LP 20. *Nutrafoods*. 2015. 14: p. 97–106.

La Hens, V., D., Bravo-Ferrada, B. M., Delfederico, L., Caballero, A. C., Semorile, L.C., Lactic acid bacteria diversity in Patagonian wines. *Australian Journal of Grape and Wine Research*. 2015. 21: p. 49-56.

Lapsiri, W., Nitisinprasert, S., Wanchaitanawong, P., *Lactobacillus plantarum* strains from fermented vegetables as potential probiotics. *Agriculture and Natural Resources*. 2011. 45: 6, p. 1071- 1082.

Lascano, R. A., Gan, M. G. L. D., Sulabo, A. S. L., Santiago, D. M. O., Ancheta, L. B., Zubia, C. S., Physico-chemical properties, probiotic stability and sensory characteristics of *Lactobacillus plantarum* S20–supplemented passion fruit (*Passiflora edulis f. flavicarpa Deg.*) juice powder. *Food Research*. 2020. 4: 2, p. 320-326.

Lavanya, B. S., Sreejit, V., Preetha, R., *Lactobacillus plantarum* J9, a potential probiotic isolated from cereal/pulses based fermented batter for traditional Indian food and its microencapsulation. *J Food Sci Technol*. 2023. 60: p. 906– 915.

Lefeber, T., Gobert, W., Vrancken, G., Camu, N., De Vuyst, L., Dynamics and species diversity of communities of lactic acid bacteria and acetic acid bacteria during spontaneous cocoa bean fermentation in vessels. *Food Microbiology*. 2011. 28: 3, p. 457- 464.

Li, F., Zhou, H., Zhou, X., Yi, R., Mu, J., Zhao, X., Liu, W., *Lactobacillus plantarum* CQPC05 Isolated from Pickled Vegetables Inhibits Constipation in Mice. *Applied Sciences*. 2019. 9: 1, 159.

Li, H., Jintao H., Yaqin W., Xingnan W., Yichen R., Tianli Y., Zhouli W., Zhenpeng G., Study on the nutritional characteristics and antioxidant activity of dealcoholized sequentially fermented apple juice with *Saccharomyces cerevisiae* and *Lactobacillus plantarum* fermentation. *Food Chemistry*. 2021. 363: 130351.

Li, S., Zhao, Y., Zhang, L., Zhang, X., Huang, L., Li, D., Niu, C., Yang, Z., Wang, Q., Antioxidant activity of *Lactobacillus plantarum* strains isolated from traditional Chinese fermented foods. *Food chemistry*. 2012. 135: 3, p. 1914- 1919.

Lim, E. S., Preparation and functional properties of probiotic and oat-based synbiotic yogurts fermented with lactic acid bacteria. *Appl Biol Chem*. 2018. 61: p. 25– 37.

Liu, C., Xue, W. J., Ding, H., An, C., Ma, S. J., Liu, Y., Probiotic Potential of *Lactobacillus* Strains Isolated From Fermented Vegetables in Shaanxi, China. *Frontiers in Microbiology*. 2022. 12: 4168.

Liu, Y. W., Liong, M. T., Tsai, Y. C., New perspectives of *Lactobacillus plantarum* as a probiotic: The gut-heart-brain axis. *J Microbiol*. 2018. 56: 9,p. 601-613.

Liu, Y., Chen, H., Chen, W., Zhong, Q., Zhang, G., Chen, W., Beneficial Effects of Tomato Juice Fermented by *Lactobacillus plantarum* and *Lactobacillus casei*: Antioxidation, Antimicrobial Effect, and Volatile Profiles. *Molecules*. 2018. 23: 9, 2366.

Liu, Z., Zhang, Z., Qiu, L., Zhang, F., Xu, X., Wei, H., Tao, X., Characterization and bioactivities of the exopolysaccharide from a probiotic strain of *Lactobacillus plantarum* WLPL04. *Journal of Dairy Science*. 2017. 100: 9, p. 6895- 6905.

Lu, Z., Breidt Jr, F., Fleming, H. P., Altermann, E., Klaenhammer, T. R., Isolation and characterization of a *Lactobacillus plantarum* bacteriophage, ΦJL-1, from a cucumber fermentation. *International journal of food microbiology*. 2003. 84: 2, p. 225- 235.

Lv, X., Ma, H., Lin, Y., Bai, F., Ge, Y., Zhang, D., Li, J., Antifungal activity of *Lactobacillus plantarum* C10 against *Trichothecium roseum* and its application in promotion of defense responses in muskmelon (*Cucumis melo L.*) fruit. *Journal of food science and technology*. 2018. 55: p. 3703- 3711.

Mäkimattila, E., Kahala, M., Joutsjoki, V., Characterization and electrotransformation of *Lactobacillus plantarum* and *Lactobacillus paraplantarum* isolated from fermented vegetables. *World Journal of Microbiology and Biotechnology*. 2011. 27: p. 371- 379.

Malik, M., Bora, J., Sharma, V., Growth studies of potentially probiotic lactic acid bacteria (*Lactobacillus plantarum*, *Lactobacillus acidophilus*, and *Lactobacillus casei*) in carrot and beetroot juice substrates. *Journal of Food Processing and Preservation.* 2019. 43: 11,e14214.

Mantzourani, I., Kazakos, S., Terpou, A., Alexopoulos, A., Bezirtzoglou, E., Bekatorou, A., Plessas, S., Potential of the Probiotic *Lactobacillus plantarum* ATCC 14917 Strain to Produce Functional Fermented Pomegranate Juice. *Foods*. 2019. 8: 4.

Markkinen, N., Laaksonen, O., Yang, B., Impact of malolactic fermentation with *Lactobacillus plantarum* on volatile compounds of sea buckthorn juice. *European Food Research and Technology*. 2021. 247: 3, p. 719-736.

Martins, E. M. F., Ramos, A. M., Stringheta, P. C., Lago-Vanzela, E. S., Oliveira, P. M., Martins, M. L., Fresh cut fruit salads as a promising vehicle for *Lactobacillus acidophilus* and *Lactobacillus plantarum*. *International Food Research Journal*. 2017. 24: 5, p. 2185- 2192.

Mechmeche, M., Kachouri, F., Ksontini, H., Hamdi, M., Production of bioactive peptides from tomato seed isolate by *Lactobacillus plantarum* fermentation and enhancement of antioxidant activity. *Food Biotechnology*. 2017. 31: 2,p. 94- 113.

Meng, F. B., Lei, Y. T., Li, Q. Z., Li, Y. C., Deng, Y., Liu, D. Y., Effect of *Lactobacillus plantarum* and *Lactobacillus acidophilus* fermentation on antioxidant activity and metabolomic profiles of loquat juice. *LWT*. 2022. 171: 114104.

Mourad, K., Nour-Eddine, K., In vitro preselection criteria for probiotic *Lactobacillus plantarum* strains of fermented olives origin. *International Journal of Probiotics and Prebiotics*. 2006. 1: 1, 27.

Mousavi, Z. E., Mousavi, S. M., Razavi, S. H., Emam-Djomeh, Z., Kiani, H., Fermentation of pomegranate juice by probiotic lactic acid bacteria. *World Journal of Microbiology and Biotechnology*. 2011. 27: p. 123-128.

Nguyen, D. T. L., Van Hoorde, K., Cnockaert, M., De Brandt, E., Aerts, M., Vandamme, P., A description of the lactic acid bacteria microbiota associated with the production of traditional fermented vegetables in Vietnam. *International journal of food microbiology*. 2013. 163: 1, p. 19- 27.

Nwachukwu, E., Achi, O. K., Ijeoma, I. O., Lactic acid bacteriain fermentation of cereals for the production of indigenous Nigerian foods. *African Journal of Food Science and Technology*. 2010. 1: 2, p. 021-026.

Oguntoyinbo, F. A., Narbad, A., Multifunctional properties of *Lactobacillus plantarum* strains isolated from fermented cereal foods. *Journal of Functional Foods*. 2015. 17: p. 621- 631.

Pan, Q., Zhang, L., Li, J., Chen, T., Chen, W., Wang, G., Yin, J., Characterization of pLP18, a novel cryptic plasmid of *Lactobacillus plantarum* PC518 isolated from Chinese pickle. *Plasmid*. 2011. 65: 3, p. 204-209.

Park, H. D., Rhee, C. H., Antimutagenic activity of *Lactobacillus plantarum* K 21 lactic acid bacteria isolated from kimchi Korean fermented vegetables. *Biotechnology Letters*. 2001. 23: p. 1583– 1589.

Park, S. Y., Lee, J. W., Lim, S. D., The probiotic characteristics and GABA production of *Lactobacillus plantarum* K154 isolated from kimchi. *Food Sci Biotechnol*. 2014. 23: p. 1951– 1957.

Pei, J., Jin, W., Abd El-Aty, A.M., Baranenko, D.A., Gou, X., Zhang, H., Geng, J., Jiang, L., Chen, D., Yue, T., Isolation, purification, and structural identification of a new bacteriocin made by *Lactobacillus plantarum* found in conventional kombucha. *Food Control*. 2020. 110: 106923.

Peng, Q., Jiang, S., Chen, J., Ma, C., Huo, D., Shao, Y., Zhang, J., Unique microbial diversity and metabolic pathway features of fermented vegetables from Hainan, China. *Frontiers in Microbiology*. 2018. 9: 399.

Peng, W., Diaoqin M., Tianli Y., Zhouli W., Zhenpeng G., Effect of the apple cultivar on cloudy apple juice fermented by a mixture of *Lactobacillus acidophilus*, *Lactobacillus plantarum*, and *Lactobacillus fermentum*. *Food Chemistry*. 2021. 340: 127922.

Peral, M. C., Huaman Martinez, M. A., Valdez, J. C., Bacteriotherapy with *Lactobacillus plantarum* in burns. *International wound journal*. 2009. 6: 1, p. 73 -81.

Pontonia, E., Rizzello, C. G., Minor and ancient cereals: Exploitation of the nutritional potential through the use of selected starters and sourdough fermentation. In V. Preedy, R. Watson, & V. Patel (Eds.), Flour and Breads and Their Fortification in Health and Disease Prevention. Amsterdam, The Netherlands London, UK: *Elsevier IncAcademic Press*. 2019. p. 443–452.

Priti, K., Singh, S., Jaiswal, N., Chaurasia, S. N. S., Isolation and Identification of *Lactobacillus plantarum* from Vegetable Samples. *Food Biotechnology*. 2016. 30: 1, p. 49-62.

Quattrini, M., Bernardi, C., Stuknytė, M., Masotti, F., Passera, A., Ricci, G., Vallone, L., De Noni, I., Brasca, M., Fortina, M. G., Functional characterization of *Lactobacillus plantarum* ITEM 17215: A potential biocontrol agent of fungi with plant growth promoting traits, able to enhance the nutritional value of cereal products. *Food Research International*. 2018. 106 :p. 936- 944.

Ramos, C. L., Thorsen, L., Schwan, R. F., Jespersen, L., Strain-specific probiotics properties of *Lactobacillus fermentum*, *Lactobacillus plantarum* and *Lactobacillus brevis* isolates from Brazilian food products. *Food microbiology*. 2013. 36: 1, p. 22-29.

Rezaei, M., Sharifan, A., Bakhoda, H., Producing and analyzing gamma-aminobutyric acid containing probiotic black grape juice using *Lactobacillus plantarum* IBRC (10817) and *Lactobacillus brevis* IBRC (10818). *Measurement: Food*. 2022. 8: 100056.

Ribeiro, C., Freixo, R. J., Silva, J. G., Gibbs, P. A., Morais, A. M., Teixeira, P., Dried Fruit Matrices Incorporated with a Probiotic Strain of *Lactobacillus plantarum. International Journal of Food Studies*. 2014. 3: p. 69-73.

Rizzello, C. G., Filannino, P., Di Cagno, R., Calasso, M., Gobbetti, M., Quorum-sensing regulation of constitutive plantaricin by *Lactobacillus plantarum* strains under a model system for vegetables and fruits. *Applied and Environmental Microbiology*. 2014. 80: 2, p. 777- 787.

Rojo-Bezares, B., Sáenz, Y., Navarro, L., Zarazaga, M., Ruiz-Larrea, F., Torres, C., Coculture-inducible bacteriocin activity of *Lactobacillus plantarum* strain J23 isolated from grape must. *Food Microbiol*. 2007. 24: 5, p. 482- 491.

Rosa, A. D., da Silveira, S. M., Coutinho, E. F., Steffens, C., Cansian, R. L., Rigo, E., Backes, G. T., Green olive fermentation using spontaneous and *Lactobacillus plantarum* cultures. *Journal für Verbraucherschutz und Lebensmittelsicherheit*. 2016. 11: 3,p. 249- 257.

Roselló Prados, G., Characterization and improvement of plant-associated Lactobacillus plantarum. Novel biocontrol agent for fire blight disease, Universitat de Girona. *Departament d'Enginyeria Química, Agrària i Tecnologia Agroalimentària*, PhD Thesis. 2016.

Rubio, R., T. Aymerich, S. Bover-Cid, M. Dolors Guàrdia, J. Arnau, M. Garriga, Probiotic strains *Lactobacillus plantarum* 299V and *Lactobacillus rhamnosus* GG as starter cultures for fermented sausages. *LWT-Food Science and Technology*. 2013. 54: 1, p. 51- 56.

Russo, P., de Chiara, M. L. V., Capozzi, V., Arena, M. P., Amodio, M. L., Rascón, A., Dueñas, M. T., López, P., Spano, G., *Lactobacillus plantarum* strains for multifunctional oat-based foods. *LWT-Food Science and Technology*. 2016. 68: p. 288- 294.

Sabatini, N., Mucciarella, M. R., Marsilio, V., Volatile compounds in uninoculated and inoculated table olives with *Lactobacillus plantarum* (*Olea europaea L.*, cv. *Moresca and Kalamata). LWT - Food Science and Technology.*) 2008. 41: 10, p. 2017- 2022.

Saboktakin-Rizi, M., Alizadeh Behbahani, B., Hojjati, M., Noshad, M., Identification of *Lactobacillus plantarum* TW29-1 isolated from Iranian fermented cereal-dairy product (Yellow Zabol Kashk): probiotic characteristics, antimicrobial activity and safety evaluation. *Journal of Food Measurement and Characterization*. 2021. 15: 3, p. 2615 -2624.

Salmeron, I., Fuciños, P., Charalampopoulos, D., Pandiella, S. S., Volatile compounds produced by the probiotic strain *Lactobacillus plantarum* NCIMB 8826 in cereal-based substrates. *Food Chemistry*. 2009. 117: 2, p. 265- 271.

Sanchez, J., Vegas, C., Zavaleta, A. I., Esteve-Zarzoso, B., Predominance of Strains in Peruvian Amazonian Fruits. *Polish Journal of Microbiology*. 2019. 68: 1, p. 127- 137.

Savedboworn, W., Wanchaitanawong, P., Viability and probiotic properties of *Lactobacillus plantarum* TISTR 2075 in spray-dried fermented cereal extracts. *Maejo International Journal of Science and Technology*. 2015. 9: 3, 382.

Schwendimann, L., Kauf, P., Fieseler, L., Gantenbein-Demarchi, C., Schwenninger, S. M., Development of a quantitative PCR assay for rapid detection of *Lactobacillus plantarum* and *Lactobacillus fermentum* in cocoa bean fermentation. *Journal of microbiological methods*. 2015. 115: p. 94- 99.

Scolari, G., Vescovo, M., Zacconi, C., Bonadé, A., Influence of *Lactobacillus plantarum* on *Staphylococcus aureus* growth in a fresh vegetable model system. *European Food Research and Technology*. 2004. 218: p. 274- 277.

Seddik, H. A., Bendali, F., Gancel, F., Fliss, I., Spano, G., Drider, D., *Lactobacillus plantarum* and its probiotic and food potentialities. *Probiotics and Antimicrobial Proteins*. 2017. 9: p. 111- 122.

Sestelo, A. B. F., Poza, M., Villa, T. G., β-Glucosidase activity in a *Lactobacillus plantarum* wine strain. *World Journal of Microbiology and Biotechnology* . 2004. 20: p. 633- 637.

Sharma, V., Mishra, H. N., Unstructured kinetic modeling of growth and lactic acid production by *Lactobacillus plantarum* NCDC 414 during fermentation of vegetable juices. *LWT-Food Science and Technology*. 2014. 59: 2, p. 1123- 1128.

Son, S. H., Jeon, H. L., Jeon, E. B., Lee, N. K., Park, Y. S., Kang, D. K., Paik, H. D., Potential probiotic *Lactobacillus plantarum* Ln4 from kimchi: Evaluation of β-galactosidase and antioxidant activities. *LWT-Food Science and Technology*. 2017. 85: p. 181- 186.

Tallon, R., Bressollier, P., Urdaci, M.C., Isolation and characterization of two exopolysaccharides produced by *Lactobacillus plantarum* EP56. *Res Microbiol*. 2003. 154: 10, p. 705- 712.

Tamang, J. P., Tamang, B., Schillinger, U., Franz, C. M., Gores, M., Holzapfel, W. H., Identification of predominant lactic acid bacteria isolated from traditionally fermented vegetable products of the Eastern Himalayas. *International journal of food microbiology* . 2005. 105: 3, p. 347- 356.

Tamene, A., Baye, K., Kariluoto, S., Edelmann, M., Bationo, F., Leconte, N., Humblot, C., *Lactobacillus plantarum* P2R3FA Isolated from Traditional Cereal-Based Fermented Food Increase Folate Status in Deficient Rats. *Nutrients*. 2019. 11: 11, 2819.

Todorov, S. D., Franco, B. D. G. D. M., *Lactobacillus plantarum*: Characterization of the species and application in food production. *Food Reviews International*. 2010. 26: 3,p. 205- 229.

Todorov, S. D., Leblanc, J. G., Franco, B. D., Evaluation of the probiotic potential and effect of encapsulation on survival for *Lactobacillus plantarum* ST16Pa isolated from papaya. *World J Microbiol Biotechnol*. 2012. 28: 3, p. 973- 984.

Todorov, S. D., Prévost, H., Lebois, M., Dousset, X., LeBlanc, J. G., Franco, B. D., Bacteriocinogenic *Lactobacillus plantarum* ST16Pa isolated from papaya (*Carica papaya*)—From isolation to application: Characterization of a bacteriocin. *Food Research International*. 2011. 44: 5, p. 1351-1363.

Tremonte, P., Pannella, G., Succi, M., Tipaldi, L., Sturchio, M., Coppola, R., Luongo, D., Sorrentino, E., Antimicrobial activity of *Lactobacillus plantarum* strains isolated from different environments: a preliminary study. International *Food Research Journal*. 2017. 24: 2.

Valero-Cases, E., Frutos, M. J., Effect of Inulin on the Viability of *L. plantarum* during Storage and in Vitro Digestion and on Composition Parameters of Vegetable Fermented Juices. *Plant Foods Hum Nutr*. 2017. 72: p. 161– 167.

Verón, H. E., Di Risio, H. D., Isla, M. I., Torres, S., Isolation and selection of potential probiotic lactic acid bacteriafrom *Opuntia ficus-indica* fruits that grow in Northwest Argentina. *LWT*. 2017. 84: p. 231- 240.

Vivek, K., Mishra, S., Pradhan, R. C., Characterization of spray dried probiotic Sohiong fruit powder with *Lactobacillus plantarum*. *LWT*. 2020. 0117: 108699.

Vivek, K., Mishra, S., Pradhan, R. C., Optimization of spray drying conditions for developing nondairy based probiotic sohiong fruit powder. *International Journal of Fruit Science*. 2021, 21: 1, p. 193- 204.

Voaides, C., Boiu-Sicuia, O., Israel-Roming, F., Zamfir, M., Grosu-Tudor, S. S., Angelescu, I. R., Cornea, C. P., *Lactobacillus* Strains for Vegetable Juice Fermentation—Quality and Health Aspects. *Biomedicines*. 2022. 10: 2867.

Wang, D., Deng, Y., Chen, X., Wang, K., Zhao, L., Wang, Z., Liu, X., Hu, Z., Elucidating the effects of *Lactobacillus plantarum* fermentation on the aroma profiles of pasteurized litchi juice using multi-scale molecular sensory science. *Current Research in Food Science*. 2023. 6: 100481.

Wang, D., Wang, Y., Lan, H., Wang, K., Zhao, L., Hu, Z., Enhanced production of γ-aminobutyric acid in litchi juice fermented by *Lactobacillus plantarum* HU-C2W. *Food Bioscience*. 2021. 42: 101155.

Wang, Z., Wu, J., Tian, Z., Si, Y., Chen, H., Gan, J., The Mechanisms of the Potential Probiotic *Lactiplantibacillus plantarum* against Cardiovascular Disease and the Recent Developments in its Fermented Foods. *Foods*. 2022.1 :, 17, 2549.

Wen-Qiong, W., Jie-Long, Z., Qian, Y., Ji-Yang, Z., Mao-Lin, L., Rui-Xia, G., Yujun, H., Structural and compositional changes of whey protein and blueberry juice fermented using *Lactobacillus plantarum* or *Lactobacillus casei* during fermentation. *RSC advances*. 2021. 11: 42, p. 26291- 26302.

Wouters, D., Grosu-Tudor, S., Zamfir, M., De Vuyst, L., Applicability of *Lactobacillus plantarum* IMDO 788 as a starter culture to control vegetable fermentations. *Journal of the Science of Food and Agriculture*. 2013. 93: 13, p. 3352- 3361.

Wronkowska, M., Rostek, D., Lenkiewicz, M., Kurantowicz, E., Yaneva, T. G., Starowicz, M., Oat flour fermented by Lactobacillus strains– Kinetics of volatile compound formation and antioxidant capacity. *Journal of Cereal Science*. 2022. 103: 103392.

Wu, Y., Li, S., Tao, Y., Li, D., Han, Y., Show, P. L., Wen, G., Zhou, J., Fermentation of blueberry and blackberry juices using *Lactobacillus plantarum*, *Streptococcus thermophilus* and *Bifidobacterium bifidum*: Growth of probiotics, metabolism of phenolics, antioxidant capacity in vitro and sensory evaluation. *Food Chem*. 2021. 348; 129083.

Xu D., Ding W., Ke W., Li F., Zhang P., Guo X., Modulation of Metabolome and Bacterial Community in Whole Crop Corn Silage by Inoculating Homofermentative *Lactobacillus plantarum* and Heterofermentative *Lactobacillus buchneri*. *Front. Microbiol*. 2019. 9:3299.

Yadav, R., Puniya, A. K., Shukla, P., Probiotic properties of *Lactobacillus plantarum* RYPR1 from an indigenous fermented beverage Raabadi. *Frontiers in microbiology*. 2016. 7: 1683.

Yang, E., Chang, H., Antifungal activity of *Lactobacillus plantarum* isolated from kimchi. *Microbiol. Biotechnol. Lett.* 2008. 36: 4, p. 276- 284 .

Yang, S. J., Lee, J. E., Lim, S. M., Kim, Y. J., Lee, N. K., Paik, H. D., Antioxidant and immune-enhancing effects of probiotic *Lactobacillus plantarum* 200655 isolated from kimchi. *Food science and biotechnology*. 2018. 28: 2, p. 491– 499.

Yang, X., Zhou, J., Fan, L., Qin, Z., Chen, Q., Zhao, L., Antioxidant properties of a vegetable-fruit beverage fermented with two *Lactobacillus plantarum* strains. *Food Sci Biotechnol*. 2018. 27: 6, p. 1719- 1726.

Yu, Z., Zhang, X., Li, S., Li, C., Li, D., Yang, Z., Evaluation of probiotic properties of *Lactobacillus plantarum* strains isolated from Chinese sauerkraut. *World Journal of Microbiology and biotechnology*. 2013. 29: p. 489- 498.

Zamani-Zadeh, M., Sabihe, S. Z., Mahmoudm S. Z., Sayed, Amir, H. G., Integration of *Lactobacillus plantarum* A7 with thyme and cumin essential oils as a potential biocontrol tool for gray mold rot on strawberry fruit, Postharvest. *Biology and Technology*. 2014. 92: p. 149- 156.

Zhang, J., Zhang, C., Lei, P., Xin, X., Liu, D., Yi, H., Isolation, purification, identification, and discovery of the antibacterial mechanism of ld-phenyllactic acid produced by *Lactiplantibacillus plantarum* CXG9 isolated from a traditional Chinese fermented vegetable. *Food Control*. 2022. 132: 108490.

Zhang, X., Duan, W., Zou, J., Zhou, H., Liu, C., Yang, H., Flavor and antioxidant activity improvement of carrot juice by fermentation with *Lactobacillus plantarum* WZ-01. *Journal of Food Measurement and Characterization*. 2019. 13: p. 3366-3375.

Zhang, Y. H., Xu, D., Zhao, X. H., Song, Y., Liu, Y. L., Li, H. N., Biodegradation of two organophosphorus pesticides in whole corn silage as affected by the cultured *Lactobacillus plantarum*. *Biotech*. 2016. 6: p.1- 6.

Zhang, Y., Liu, W., Wei, Z., Yin, B., Man, C., Jiang, Y., Enhancement of functional characteristics of blueberry juice fermented by *Lactobacillus plantarum*. *LWT*. 2021. 139: 110590.

Zhou, F., Zhao, H., Bai, F., Piotr, D., Liu Y., Zhang, B., Purification and characterisation of the bacteriocin produced by *Lactobacillus plantarum*, isolated from Chinese pickle. *Czech J. Food Sci*. 2014. 32: p. 430-436.

Zhou, Y., Wang, R., Zhang, Y., Yang, Y., Sun, X., Zhang, Q., Yang, N., Biotransformation of phenolics and metabolites and the change in antioxidant activity in kiwifruit induced by *Lactobacillus plantarum* fermentation. *Journal of the Science of Food and Agriculture*. 2020. 100: 8, p. 3283- 3290.

Zi, X., Li, M., Chen, Y., Lv, R., Zhou, H., Tang, J., Effects of citric acid and *Lactobacillus plantarum* on silage quality and bacterial diversity of king grass silage. *Frontiers in Microbiology*. 2021. 12: 631096.

Zinklar, https://zinklar.com/54-of-consumers-have-changed-how-they-eat-and-drink/. Accesses on 25.05.2023.

Chapter 9

The Use of *Lactobacillus plantarum* in Sugar Confectionery and Chocolate-Based Products

Andreea Pușcaș
Alexandra Lazăr
and Vlad Mureșan*
Food Engineering Department, Faculty of Food Science and Technology,
University of Agricultural Sciences and Veterinary Medicine Cluj-Napoca,
Cluj-Napoca, Cluj, Romania

Abstract

In order to functionalize the confectionery group, which is considered a high energy food due to its rich amount of fat and sugar, various strains of *Lactobacillus plantarum* are included in products, and studies are performed to test their viability. Confectionery products are classified based on their main ingredients as sugar confectionery (I), chocolate (II), flour or milk based confectionery products (III). In this chapter, the sugar confectionery, including non-milk dairy and chocolate or chocolate-based products functionalized with *L. plantarum* are discussed. Various strains of *L. plantarum* can be added in their formulation, as raw ingredients, encapsulated, freeze-dried, or even cultivated during the product processing, taking into account some factors such as its thermosensitivity, H_2O_2 or CO_2 production during fermentations. The main ingredients of confectionery products, such as cocoa beans, oligosaccharides, molasses, also represent ideal food matrices for the isolation of novel strains of *L. plantarum*, for which reason the direct

* Coresponding Author's Email: vlad.muresan@usamvcluj.ro.

In: Lactobacillus plantarum and Its Role in Human Health
Editors: Maria Simona Chiș, Adriana Paucean
ISBN: 979-8-89113-696-0

development of lactobacillus (LAB) during the manufacturing of products can be considered.
Jellies, chewing candies or gummy candies containing some strains of *L. plantarum* were designed, because of LAB's antimicrobial activity and potential implication in hindering the occurence of dental caries , as influenced by high sugar content. In milk and dark chocolate and even in chocolate mousse, a high viability was revealed for *L. plantarum* included in encapsulated or powdered formabd good sensory acceptance of the products being reported, the incorporation methodologies being further discussed. In both dairy and non-dairy ice cream, the inclusion of probiotics, including *L. plantarum* is possible since the first class of products ensure its survival due to the presence of lactose and other milk sugars. *L. plantarum* 299v strain used in lyophilized form in a vegan ice cream formulation did not influence the sensory and functional properties of the product.
It is well known that products containing high levels of sugars evoke excessive plasma-glucose and insulin responses, which is why they are not recommended for consumption to those who are known to have conditions related to any type of diabetes. *L. plantarum* was proved to reduce blood glucose levels and inflammatory responses, so its inclusion to these group of products helps to solve a problem.
Besides their popularity among consumers, confectionery products possess the advantage of having a long shelf life, being a viable medium for the long-term delivery of probiotics.

Keywords: sugar confectionery, chocolate, isolation, products formulation, glucose response

1. Introduction

Confectionery products can be classified based on their main ingredients as sugar confectionery (boiled sweets, aerated confections, gelled candies, coatings, etc.), chocolate and chocolate-based products (dark chocolate, milk chocolate, ruby and white chocolate, but also chocolate mousse, compounds, etc.), and flour or milk based confectionery products (cakes, muffins, waffles, etc.) [1]. Since the World Health Organization (WHO) recommended the daily consumption of free sugars to be less than 10% of the total energy intake of a person to reduce the risk and prevalence of obesity and dental decay, the nutritional profile of confectionery products, which are high in sugar content, is mostly improved by means of using sugar replacers and bulking agents for reformulation purposes. WHO estimates that by 2025, approximately 167 million people will be overweight and might develop various stages of obesity [2], starting from childhood, therefore, improving the nutritional profile of confectionery products is a current challenge. Products containing high levels of sugars evoke excessive plasma-glucose and insulin responses, which limits their consumption by people who have conditions related to diabetes. Besides this, a new class of consumers, known as health-conscious consumers, are demanding functionalized confectionery products with natural and sustainable ingredients, which does not imply high energy for refining processes [3].

Various sugar replacers and sweeteners were studied as substitutes for sugar as an initiative to improve the nutritional quality of products and making them available for people with certain diseases. However, some sugar replacers, such as corn syrup, are commonly employed for economic reasons. To enrich the composition of some confectionery products with biologically active substances or simply to replace sugar with natural substances, juices or fruit and vegetable pastes have also been employed, leading to the development of marshmallows [4], Turkish delight [5], gummy jellies [6], etc. Other natural sugar substitutes such as inulin [7] or agave syrup were used for developing gummy jellies with suitable textural properties [8].

In chewing gum, polyols such as xylitol, sorbitol and mannitol are used instead of sucrose [9], while for sugar-free toffees, maltitol, isomalt and lactose-free whey powders can be employed. In hard-boiled candies, isomalt is suitable as sugar replacer [10]. The usage of multiple polyols is also successfully replacing sugar in chocolate with some implications and modification required for the main operations of chocolate manufacturing such as refining or tempering [11]. Dietary fibers (e.g., inulin), oligofructans, syrups or other natural sweeteners were explored for developing chocolate with less sugar content [12]. Chocolate, especially the dark and ruby type, are however perceived as healthier products by some consumers, due to their antioxidant potential, high content of polyphenols and flavonoids [13]. Dark chocolate is a source of copper [14], a product which hinders the development of cardio-metabolic disorders and demonstrates insulin resistances [15]. Milk chocolate is considered a source of Ca (Calcium) and proteins. Candies and gummies are well known confectionery products which could play a nutraceutical role when they are delivering vitamins, minerals or essential oils from their composition, the oral path for administration of these substances being a convenient one.

Besides vitamins, antioxidants and dietary fibers, prebiotic and probiotic microorganisms are also included in the matrix of confectionery products in order to functionalize them. Fructo-oligosaccharides (digestible β-($1 \rightarrow 2$)

linked fructo-oligosaccharides, excluding the sucrose) and galacto-oligosaccharides (indigestible) β-(1 → 3 or 6) linked disaccharides and α-galactosyllactose, excluding the lactose) are the two important groups of prebiotics encountered in confectionery products [16], but blends of the most common bulking agent, polydextrose and galacto-oligosaccharides can also ensure the viability of probiotics.

The preparation of probiotic confectionery products and their properties were previously discussed regarding the inclusion of lyophilized bacterial cultures of *Lactobacillus casei* and *L. paracasei* in wafers, chocolate-covered raisins, or biscuits [17], but also regarding the bacterial cultures of *Bacillus* strains used in manufacturing gummy bears or jelly beans [18]. Confectionery products are reported to be a good vehicle for *Lactobacillus* bacteria, because of the abundance of carbohydrates, the low water content and water activity but also limited oxygen permeability [17]. In this chapter, recent studies (<5 years) related to the addition of *L. plantarum* in sugar confectionery products, including non-milk dairy and chocolate or chocolate-based products and other confectionery products, is discussed. Moreover, the usage of ingredients specific to confectionery products for growing *L. plantarum* and its health related effects are revisited.

1.1. Sugar Confectionery Products

In addition to issues related to obesity and increase of the glycemic index, high sugar content in products, such as candies, gums and jellies, can cause caries and tooth decay. These issues form because bacteria from the mouth is fed with sucrose, leading to the formation of a bacterial plaquedue to their texture and serving. Probiotic bacteria were included in the formulation of these products, but in their sugar-free variant, due their antibacterial effect and high resistance to lyzozim, mechanical and antibiotic based removal techniques were reported to be inefficient and also leading to increased antibiotic resistance [19, 20]. Probiotics are possessing antimicrobial effects because they produce organic acids, hydrogen peroxide, bacteriolytic enzymes, ensuring the tolerance of the *L. plantarum* at low pH. For instance, chewing gum with *Lactobacillus reuteri* lead to the decrease of the plaque and *Streptococcus mutans* levels [21], as the last being the main cause of dental caries development. The effects of various strains of *L. plantarum* on the bacterial colonies from the oral cavity [20] were tested both in rats [22] and humans [23]. *L. plantarum* was delivered in a mixture with *Levilactobacillus brevis* in chewing gums, and during sensory analysis, the gums were not perceived as different in comparison to aplacebo reference in terms of global evaluation, texture rating and aftertaste g, but they were percieved slightly different in terms of taste.

Lactobacillus plantarum FB-T9, isolated from healthy human feces, exhibited a strong inhibitory effect on *Streptococcus mutans* in a study conducted on rats [20]. Regarding the dental plaque of the population who consumed probiotic gums twice per day for 6 weeks, positive effects on the dental plaque's health were correlated with *L. brevis* and not *L. plantarum* KABPTM-051. In another study, thymol (2-isopropyl-5-methylphenol), *L. plantarum* (ATCC 14917) cell-free supernatant, and cardamom (*Elettaria cardamomum*) essential oil and their nanoparticle's, were included in sugar free candy formulation, and the inhibiting effect against *S. mutans* was demonstrated [24]. These candies had low acceptance and scores in the sensory evaluation, except for the formulation containing cardamom essential oil, which was comparable with a reference in terms of oral sense. Isomalt and stevia were used as sweetening agent, and the inclusion of the biologically active substances (thymol or cardamom essential oil) was done after cooling the concentrated syrup to 50°C.

The antibacterial mechanism of *L. plantarum* is considered to be due to the acidic medium it provides, or some substances it might produce, however, this feature is strain dependent and needs to be further studied. The Fourier transform infrared spectroscopy (FTIR) spectra of the candies containing *L. plantarum* ATCC 14917, revealed peaks in the 1037 -1154 cm^{-1} region because of glycosidic bonds (=C–H), OH bonds and C–O bond, but also at 1772 cm^{-1}, peaks corresponding to the N-H linkages present in aminoacids or proteins, peaks specific for C=O anhydride group and for carbohydrates. The candy containing encapsulated probiotic bacteria presented solely one different peak, and this could have been only because of the encapsulation medium [24].

L. plantarum MBTU-HK1 alone or in symbiotic relationship with acacia gum, a prebiotic substance was evaluated *in vivo* in terms of safety and growth performances in a study conducted on minces, with the usage of biochemical, hematological, physiological, and immunological tests [22]. The growth of *L. plantarum* was stimulated by the acacia gum, a viability higher than 6 log CFU/g was detected in the gastrointestinal epithelial wall of the mice after 21 days. Acacia gum, known also as arabic gum, is commonly used in the confectionery industry because it has ability to prevent crystallization of sugar. Acacia gum is employed in manufacturing hard candies, chewing gum, cough drops and candy lozenges [25], lollipops or fruit candies, caramels, and aerated products such as marshmallows, products which require smooth surface and a creamy texture. In *vitro* studies demonstrated that *L. plantarum* MBTU-HK1, and other strains of *L. plantarum*, have the ability to assimilate cholesterol from the growth media [22]; demonstrating cholesterol lowering effects *in vitro* and *in vivo* studies, the effects strain dependency, the underlying mechanism (still under study), and the influence of other factors [26].

For candy manufacturing, the dispersed ingredients are cooked until caramelization, then the mass is kneaded, cooled by convection in tunnels or chambers, then molded, a stage where acids, flavoring and coloring agents are added. After the formation and final cooling, the water activity of the products are checked, and if within the desired values, the products are packed and stored.

L. plantarum Dad-13 (7.58×10^9 CFU/g) was mixed with skim milk powder and included in the formulation of a gummy candy, in which bovine gelatin was used as a gelling agent, resulting in the formation of a protein loaded hydrogel with an internal matrix developed due to the interaction of the ingredients. The study employed the supposition that the probiotics might be protected against degradative actions in the structure of the product [27]. The inclusion of the indigenous probiotic bacteria isolated from buffalo milk, was done after cooling the candy mixture to 40°C. However, the *in vitro* simulation of the gastrointestinal digestion of the gummy candy revealed a decrease of 44.26% reduction from the initial cells after the gastric phase, and an 88.13% reduction after the intestinal phase [27]. The shelf life prediction was modelled mathematically with the usage of Arrhenius equation, which estimated up to 90 days shelf life if the sample would be stored at 4°C, 34 days if samples they would be stored at 11°C. The products would still possessed a probiotic viability of 2.50×10^7CFU/g. In regard to the physicochemical parameters of the gummies, the value of some textural parameters such as gumminess, hardness and chewiness was increased during storage, along with the water activity, which was too high for this class of products (ranging between 0.81-0.82). However, storage can also be influenced by other factors such as packaging material and external humidity, which were not considered in this study, however, further studies could include these factors in their experimental designs.

Gelatin based gummies containing polysaccharides from mushroom as prebiotics, were inoculated with *L. plantarum* YC5 because of the resistance which it exhibited against the simulated gastrointestinal fluids and because of its interaction with the prebiotics. The survival rate of *L. plantarum* F-23 and

Cad-8 in the simulated gastric fluid was determined as 100.36% and 99.24%, respectively while that of *L. plantarum* YC-5 in the simulated intestinal fluid was 97.27%. Also, the YC-5 strain growth performance was higher in the media containing mushroom polysaccharides than in that containing glucose [28]. Priory, 25 strains of *L. plantarum* were analyzed in terms of hemolytic activity and antibiotic susceptibility, antioxidant and antimicrobial potential [28], revealing that the antioxidant potential ranged between 13.32 -16.26 mg Ascorbic Acid equivalents/L and that all the strain could inhibit gram-negative bacteria (such as *E. coli, Salmonella*) and gram-positive bacteria (*Staphylococcus aureus, E. faecalis*), with an average inhibition rate of 10–16 mm on the growth of indicator bacteria.

Berry by-products obtained from juice or wine processing are rich in polyphenols and anthocyanins, being commonly employed in manufacturing chewable, gummy or jelly candies bcause of some sustainability and nutritional, reasons. Blackcurrant and raspberries lyophilized by-products, milk permeate, lyophilized *L. plantarum* previously isolated from spontaneous fermented cereals, xylitol and gelatin, were used to design a healthier confectionary product [29]. Milk permeate is also a by-product resulting from the dairy industry, and its usage as substrate for LAB multiplication is known, being revealed to possess a protective role for the probiotic bacteria during the drying process of the jelly. Jellies with *L. plantarum* 135 and raspberry by-products exhibited the highest total polyphenolic content (TPC) of 147.16±0.13 mg 100 g $^{-1}$ d.m, while the lowest TPC was for the samples with *L. plantarum* 135 and blackcurrants, namely84.12±0.15 mg 100 g $^{-1}$ d.m. After 14 days of storage sample with *L. plantarum* 135 and raspberry had a viability of 7.53 ± 0.45 CFU/g, after 24 days their viability was decreased to 6.85 ± 0.46 CFU/g and presented high overall acceptability in a sensory evaluation [29].

Gelatin was employed in manufacturing gummies because of its quick gelling capacity at a low pH of 3.8, but also because it demonstrated protective capacities for bioactive compounds and prebiotics, increassing their solubility, but also the bio-availability or survival [30]. Gelatine is highly employed in the encapsulation techniques [31], forming complexes with alginates [32], caseins [31], carboxymethyl cellulose (CMC) [30], etc. However, gelatin exposure to high temperatures will degrade the compound, breaking the hydrogen bonds and exposing the probiotic cells to factors which might decrease their viability. Gelatin is less and less employed in manufacturing jellies, because of the consumer's negative perception on animal origin ingredients.

Pectin is a more commonly used gelling agent in confectionery, because of its ability to jellify quickly, being perceived as a natural compound obtained from vegetable sources. It is well known that the gelling capacity of the pectin is influenced by pH, the presence of the sugar and heating temperatures and the type of pectin, i.e., low (LMP) or high methoxyl (HMP).

Recently, apple sourced pectin (HMP), enforced with apple pomace, was explored in the formation of hydrogels, as carriers for probiotic compounds, including *L. plantarum* [33]. The gel formation was controlled with ultrasound (US) emissions, as well as US cavitation, which permitted the reduction of manufacturing temperatures from 80°C to 50°C, a temperature where the inoculation and viability of the probiotic bacteria are not altered. In these conditions the hydrogel presented higher firmness than the control. *L. plantarum* was immobilized in the hydrogel after ultrasonic treatment to reach a level of 10^8 CFU/g and an immobilization efficiency of 93%. In terms of pH resistance, after 4 h at a pH of 2.0, *L. plantarum* LUHS18 registered a decrease of 58.4- 43.7% in the viable cells out of the initial number and this strain were not revealed to be as resistant as desired. In regard to the viability during storage, it was revealed that *L. plantarum* could not be practically retained at 20°C for more than 7–14 days. Further studies should be carried on with LMP, since hydrogels with low methoxyl pectin can be developed at lower temperatures (35°C) by employing the high hydrostatic pressure technique [33].

1.2. Chocolate and Chocolate-Based Products

Chocolate with probiotics is not considered an innovative assortment among these class of products since studies started around 20 years ago [17]. When searching for available data regarding chocolate and probiotics in the web of science core collection, we identified increasing interest towards this topic and of the number of publications, which increased from 10 per year in 2016-2019 to 15-16 per year in 2021-2022. Some of the probiotic bacterias which were employed the most in these studies are LAB (*L. paracasei, L. acidophilus, L. rhamnosus, L. helveticus, and L. plantarum*) but also the *Enterococcus faecium* strain, *Bifidobacterium* and others. It was revealed that chocolate is a suitable food matrix for probiotic bacteria incorporation, since, after the chocolate mass is obtained, it only undergoes a few processing steps which do not impair probiotic bacteria viability. These steps are the refining process, where the presence of oxygen is limited and heating of the product is avoided, followed by conching, where a maximum temperature of 72°C is reached and the tempering step. During the tempering process, the maximal temperature involved is 50°C, after which the chocolate mass is cooled for the crystallization of the cocoa butter, this temperature being ideal for the inclusion of probiotic bacteria in chocolate products. Moreover, the protein or sugar from the chocolate composition are also affecting the viability of probiotics, both during and after the manufacturing process.

Melted dark chocolate (at 36–37°C) was inoculated with 8 log CFU/g of *L. plantarum* pellet and tempered for 10 minutes then poured into molds [34]. The pH of the chocolate was not influenced by this addition, while the viscosity was increased, which might lead to the inclusion of more air bubbles in the matrix and sensorial defects, including some related to taste [35]. *L. plantarum* presented a high survival rate, counting for 6 log CFU/g after 3 months storage at 4°C, and the refrigeration temperature was employed during the storage of the product, because it is preferred by the probiotic bacteria [34]. However, only if this content of probiotic bacteria reaches the ileum, it can be considered an efficient supplement [36], since the presence of the probiotic bacteria in a product does not guarantee its resistance throughout the gastrointestinal tract [37]. *L. plantarum* needs to resist the stomach conditions (pH of 2.5–3.5 and 0.3% bile salts) [38].

Chocolate is indicated to be handled and stored at temperatures higher than 6°C, a correct tempering ensuring good storage at 12-18°C, otherwise the low Temperature Bloom phenomenon can occur, and chocolate might become unappealing to consumers. For a dark chocolate, the highest flavonoid content and antioxidant potential was maintained during 45 days of storage at 4°C, instead of 22°C or 32°C [39]. While some studies stipulated that due to the presence of antioxidant compounds including polyphenols, chocolate is a better probiotic carrier, other recent studies concluded that the survivability of probiotics in dark chocolate during storage is strongly influenced by the strain and the inoculum procedure of the probiotic bacteria and is independent of the presence of these compounds [40]. Recently, *L. plantarum* LBP UFSC023 among other probiotic bacteria, was included in both milk and dark chocolate (70% cocoa), which were stored for 90 days. The viability in milk chocolate was higher than that registered in the dark chocolate, while the bio-accessibility of the phenolic compounds, flavonoids, and antioxidant compounds was higher in the latter. Changes in the pH of all the samples considered for the study were not registered [41].

It was found that lyophilized powder of *Lactobacillus plantarum* (previously freeze-dried at – 80°C for 48 h with cryo protective substances) presented a higher survivability in both artificial gastric and intestinal juice (1-3 h incubation) when it was incorporated in a chocolate paste. The inclusion of 1% probiotic bacteria was done after the 94% cacao mass was heated at 100°C for 1 h and cooled to 40°C, this strain being heat tolerant due to the proteins from its composition [42]. Then, it was subjected to a conching process for 4 h at 30 rpm. The survival rate after 60 days storage of the lyophilized powders was 93.0 log % for L. *plantarum* LRCC5193 and higher rate of 96.3% log was registered for *L. plantarum* KCTC3099, while in the chocolates higher rates of survival were determined (98.2 log % and 97.2 log% respectively). The research investigated the influence of storage temperature on the viability of the bacteria, revealing an 100-fold, decrease in viable cell counts, thus lower viability at 33°C in comparison to 20°C. *L. plantarum*-LRCC5193 isolated from Kimchi, a fermented vegetable, demonstrated a significantly higher degree of heat, acid, and bile acid tolerance compared to other lactic acid bacteria employed in the study [42].

Dark chocolates were fortified with *L. plantarum* strains used in spray dried encapsulated form [43], more specifically with the commercially available strain *Lactobacillus plantarum* 299v and with the *Lactobacillus plantarum* 564 strain isolated from artisanal Serbian white brined cheese, and stored during 360 days at room temperature. An amount of 1% g spray dried cells were added to the dark chocolate during the tempering process and the survival was up to 6 months for *Lactobacillus plantarum* 564 and for 9 months for the commercially available strain [43]. One possible advantage of enriching confectionery products with probiotic bacteria of L. *plantarum* type, is that this might resist to the high temperatures which are specific processing conditions for spray-drying, since previous study conducted on *L. plantarum* 564 cells revealed that spray drying at inlet air temperature of 170°C and outlet temperature of 80°C did not affect the bacterial preservation [44]. This is quite an elevated temperature, for which reason electro-hydrodynamic atomization can be considered a better process for delivering L. *plantarum*. However, due to the complex scaling process and high processing costs, it is worth exploring novel methods of increasing the viability of the probiotics which are directly suspended in chocolates.

Lactobacillus plantarum 299v *(L. p* 299v*)*, in microencapsulated form, was added as probiotic ingredients in a sugar free milk chocolate, along with *Lactobacillus acidophilus* La3 *(*DSMZ 17742*)*, the products also being functionalized with ω-3 PUFAs from fish oil [35]. The probiotics were included in the milk chocolate, containing sugar or sugar replacers, after the tempering phase, at a ratio of 1×10^{13} UFC/g [35]. For the sugar-free sample, isomalt and stevia were used as sweetening ingredients, the isomalt also reducing the water activity of the chocolate, because of its hygroscopic properties. While the inclusion of microencapsulated probiotics might increase the lightness of the product, the replacement of sugar is decreasing the parameter overall, in a sugar-free chocolate enriched with probiotics, a balance of the color parameters can be created. However, the usage of carbohydrates in designing the protective layer of the microcapsules can induce fat blooming, loss of shine and defects in chocolate products during storage [45]. Carbohydrates also affect the lipid crystallization during tempering, leading to an altered texture of the chocolates and increased apparent viscosity of the chocolate mass. Despite this, the changes in the products due to the inclusion of microencapsulated LAB were not perceived by the consumers, the overall acceptability of milk chocolate with sugar and probiotics, was statistically similar to that of the control, while the sample with probiotic and fish oil, received the lowest acceptability score [35]. In regard to the sugar free samples, the inclusion of probiotics did not influence the scores received for flavor, appearance, texture and overall acceptability of the samples with or without fish oil.

A complex encapsulation media was used for *L. plantarum* Mar 8 and KMar C2 which were spray dried at outlet temperature of 125°C with 10% skim milk and 3% cocoa butter fat. Cocoa butter is revealed to provide enhanced protection against processing factors during encapsulation, product development or storage, but also during digestion [46]. The powders resulting after spray drying were stored for 14 days and different percentages of the viability were registered for the samples, depending on their storage conditions. When the storage was done at 4°C, a 9% reduction of the viable cells occurred, when the storage temperature was between 27 – 30°C, 23% loss of the viability occurred, and for storage at 37°C the highest percentage of loss of viability (28%) was registered. However, the samples were still considered to posses probiotic potential (1.385 x 10^{10} CFU/g). The total cells accounted for 1.70 x 10^{9} CFU/g, after mixing the probiotics with chocolate and for 1.07 x 10^{9} CFU/g, after 14 days of storage. However, if the milk chocolate enriched with probiotics is containing stevia instead of sugar, higher survival rates can be obtained, independent of the storage temperature [46]. While maltodextrin is commonly used in addition to alginate for microencapsulation purposes, due to its prebiotic effect, in chocolate, this combination might lead to fat bloom due to the presence of carbohydrates, for which reason whey protein coated alginate beads are more recommended instead.

The inclusion of probiotic bacteria in aerated chocolate desserts was done so far mainly for biopreservation purposes, since contamination might occur from the ingredients such as egg yolks or cream, from the processing equipments and due to the gas included for aeration, or the water phase [47]. Chocolate mousse was shown to be an excellent vehicle for the delivery of *L. paracasei*, of which viability was not influenced by the presence of prebiotic substances such as inulin in the formulation, during 21 days storage The product presented good sensory acceptance. Chocolate mousses had a pH ≥6 and a water activity of 0.9, and the inclusion of *L. plantarum* D2,_isolated from mayonnaise in this matrix, was shown to be more effective in the presence of 1% citrus zest oils (lemon or grapefruit) essential [48]. *L plantarum* D2 was added in free or immobilized form in chocolate mousse and the viability of the free probiotic bacteria supplemented with lemon essential oil, was maintained during 20 days storage, registering a total count higher than 10^7 CFU/g. Also, the study revealled the antibacterial potential of the formulation against mesophilic aerobic and facultative anaerobic microorganisms, yeasts and molds, *E coli* and *S. Aureus*. The mousse with free cells of *L. plantarum* D2 was not evaluated positively in the sensory analysis, while the mousse with immobilized probiotic bacteria, or those with *L. plantarum* D2 and essential oil, were highly appreciated [48].

Based on the conducted studies, the effects of inoculating *L. plantarum* and the survival of the bacteria through chocolate manufacturing and digestion depend on various factors, including the strain of bacteria, chocolate formulation, processing conditions. However, chocolate remains a strong vehicle for the delivery or probiotic bacteria because its popularity among consumers, the sugar and amino acids it provides, but also due to the fact that it is able to neutralize the stomach acid [18] and ensure the delivery of the probiotics in the ileum.

1.3. Perspective Application of *L. plantarum* in Confectionery Products

Granola bar is a cereal bar which contains cereals and multi grains, chocolate chips or fruits, that are hold together by a sugar syrup, for which reason it belongs to the confectionery segment, being similar to groundnut chikki dessert, which is considered indian confectionery product, according to the Indian snacks and sweets/codex/FSSAI-2021 [49]. Currently several types of probiotic bacteria were included in this ready to eat product, such as the

Lacticaseibacillus rhamnosus R0011, *Lactobacillus acidophilus* and *Bifidobacterium animalis subsp. Lactis*, a strategy for their prolonged viability being the inclusion in chocolate chips, which is then added to the granola bar. However, they might be added directly, freely, or in immobilized or encapsulated form [50, 51].

The inclusion of *Lactobacillus plantarum* 299v in peanut butter containing dextrose (2%) and glycerol (2%), was done with the purpose of controlling biogenic amines quantity during the storage of the product [52] and to maintain their level under 10 μg/g in order to ensure the safety of the product. The addition of the probiotic bacteria was done after pasteurization of the sample at 70°C and cooling. Probiotics were dissolved in cold water and added to achieve a final concentration of 10^8 CFU/g, and the pH were adjusted to 6.8. After 6 weeks of storage at 37°C, *L. plantarum* survival was reduced, while after 12 weeks, in each storage protocol, (with storage temperature of 4°C, 25°C and 37°C) the reduction of the total counts occurred. The inclusion of *L. plantarum* led to lower reduction of the biogenic amines content, in comparison to the results obtained for *B. infantis* [52].

Exopolysaccharides (EPS) are complex molecules which are proven to be produced by *L. plantarum*, with applicability in confectionery products as texturizers and stabilizers. *L. plantarum* produces also other molecules of different structures, sizes and thus, and different technological functions could be obtained. These products can be classified as heteropolysaccharides or homopolysaccharides, depending on the saccharides type, linear or branched, depending also on their special arrangement [53]. They have been reported to improve viscosity and prevent sugar crystallization [54]. The EPS production is influenced by the sugar types present in the growing media, its grown being controlled when probiotic bacteria are fed with the right sugar type. For instance, *L. plantarum* LPC-1 increased EPS production when grown in media containing sucrose. Sucrose was found to be a better source of carbon in comparison to glucose for 6 strains of *L. plantarum* (NCDC 378, NCDC 373, NCDC 377, NCDC 382, UBLP-40, NCDC 20) [55].

Artificial intelligence was also employed in studying the optimal medium in which *Lactobacillus plantarum* produces EPS. The Plackett-Burman (PB) design method, artificial neural networks (ANN) and genetic algorithms (GA) revealed that a media containing lactose, casein hydrolysate and triammonium citrate would lead to a yield of 7.01 g/l [56].

EPS producing probiotic bacteria, was either directly inoculated in the formulation of an ice-cream, in a mixture with skimmed milk, or included as a lyophilized powder in order to deliver probiotic bacteria within this product

[57]. The direct inoculation was followed by a 4 hour fermentation conducted at 37°C, while the rest of the samples were aged and freezed directly after homogenization. Besides this, the EPS have other positive effects on human wellbeing, such as radical scavenging activity, anti-tumor, anti-bacteria, anti-mutagen effects or immune regulation [58]. The amount of viable counts decreased after each processing step, but were still higher than 6 log CFU/g, while in terms of formulation, the ice-cream with LAB included along with skimmed milk presented the highest viability after 4 weeks of storage. The products presented statistically significant differences for their pH (which was ranging between 6.06-6.60) and a textural attribute, the inclusion of probiotic bacteria decreasing the firmness, while the inclusion of activated *L. plantarum* YW11 led to increase in viscosity. This study also revealed that the impact of introducing probiotic bacteria in terms of flavor is reduced when lyophilized powder is used, rather than direct inoculation [57]. This is in accordance with the findings of Siti et al., who reported that ice cream containing free *L. plantarum* was less favored in terms of taste due to higher acidity, in comparison with the encapsulated form, while a symbiotic formulation was not accepted by the panelists [59]. *L. plantarum* isolated from cocoa beans on the 4th day of their fermentation process, was freeze dried (–40°C and 0.3 mPa) using a solution containing 6% (w/v) lactose and 6% (w/v) skimmed milk as cryoprotective agents emulsified with Tween 80 and vegetable oil.While no data regarding the total cell count in ice-cream is given by this article, information regarding the rheological properties, namely that the presence of probiotics enhanced the elastic modulus of the ice cream formulations and altered the melting properties, were revealed.

In another study, the influence of agricultural residues, namely of the coconut fiber, addition (0.01–0.03 g/mL) to a fermented probiotic ice-cream containing 1 mL of *L. plantarum* was assessed [60]. This ice cream was produced by using non-fat milk powder, milk fat, heavy cream, sugar, egg yolk, stabilizer, and maltodextrin, 1% of *L. plantarum* and different concentrations of coconut residue fiber (0.01–0.03 g/mL). Probiotic ice cream fermented with *L. plantarum* ATCC 8014 had a cell count of 7.55 log CFU/mL after fermentation and 8.1 log CFU/mL after storage, being increased due to the presence of 0.03 g/mL coconut fiber.

The growth parameters of *L. plantarum*, in presence of various amounts of royal jelly (0.001–10.0 mg/mL) was modelled with Gompertz model to evaluate the suitability for producing a Turkish desert similar to a pudding, called "Keskul," containing milk, egg, flour, starches and sugar. The dessert containing *L. plantarum* and 1% Royal jelly (RJ), presented probiotic properties (>6 log CFU/g), but decreased the pH of the food product for storage periods higher than 10 days [61], changed the appearance and color parameters assessed in the CIELAB color test. On manufacturing day, the rheological properties were not different of the reference, in terms of yield stress (τ_0) for any of the samples (probiotic with or without 1% RJ), while the consistency coefficient (K) from the Herschel–Bulkley model was higher for probiotic samples than for the reference, and increased during the storage period for the sample containing *L. plantarum* and 5% RJ. Also, in this sample, the growth of total LAB count occurred during storage [61], meaning RJ had a prebiotic effect on it, mainly due to the sugars, proteins and the B vitamins from its composition.

Polyols are carbohydrates with a chemical structure that partially resembles that of sugar and partially that of alcohol (hydrogenation of sugars) and are widely employed as sugar or fat replacers in confectionery products, being naturally found in a wide variety of fruits and vegetables or synthetized with the usage of various bacteria and enzymes. *Lactobacillus plantarum*, was reported to produce sorbitol from fructose-6-phosphate by reverting the sorbitol catabolic pathway in a mutant strain deficient for both L- and D-lactate dehydrogenase activities [62]. *Lactobacillus plantarum* NCIM 2912 was also employed in sorbitol production in 7.5 l lab scale bioreactor and submerged conditions, a scale up study predicting a maximum sorbitol yield (Yp/x) and productivity of 1.11 g xl^{-1} and 0.50 g xl^{-1} under submerged fermentation, respectively [63]. This is of high importance for the confectionery products, since polyols, including sorbitol, are highly employed in manufacturing sugar free chewing gum, candy, desserts, ice cream, antidiabetic foods, providing texture and acting as a humectant [64].

D-Tagatose is a novel food, as stated by the European Commission regulation 2470/2017 [65], and it is reported to be used as sweetener and prebiotic compound, in confectionery products. It is stated that if the level of D-Tagatose exceeds 15 g per serving, the foodstuffs should have mentioned on their label that 'excessive consumption may produce laxative effects'. *L. plantarum* WU14 was used as the D-tagatose biotransformation fermentation starter, the study revealing three fermentation kinetic models which governed the biotransformation of D-tagatose [66].

The main ingredients of confectionery products, such as sugar and its by-products, cocoa beans, oligosaccharides, also represent ideal food matrices for the isolation of novel strains of *L. plantarum.* Sugar cane molasses, which is considered a by-product of the sugar processing industry, was successfully used as media for the growth of *L. plantarum* strain Huil, isolated from fruits

(Genipa Americana), the results being 4.8-folds more effective in comparison to a reference [67], while for *Lactobacillus plantarum LMISM6* isolated from cassava waste-water, the medium was optimized with the addition of a nitrogen source, K_2HPO_4 and Tween 80 [68]. The usage of bagasse as supplementation for the growing medium is not as suitable as the molasses, because of the presence of aromatic inhibitors from its composition, which affect the productivity *L. plantarum* [69].

L. plantarum was grown on agar plates enriched with cocoa beans pulp, which undergo a four-day fermentation and the successful isolation of the strain was confirmed with morphological and biochemical tests and API 50 CHL ready to use inspection medium [34]. Yeasts and some other organisms seemed to be responsible for the preliminary changes during the fermentation of cocoa beans, including sugar hydrolysis to glucose and fructose, CO_2 production followed by ethanol production in a second phase, which is an exothermal process responsible also for the development of flavor compounds, in anaerobic and acidic conditions [70]. The third phase is an aerobic phase characterized by the production of some acids, including acetic and lactic acids and finally some undesirable acids such as gluconic acid [71]; the oxygen presence was ensured due to the pulp liquefaction by yeasts or supplementary enzymes and ensured the growth of bacteria, including some varieties of *Lactobacillus*. *L. plantarum* 15-HL demonstrated an antifungal effect during the fermentation of cocoa beans, without imparting their quality traits [72]. Other particularities of various strains of *L. plantarum* such as the *L. plantarum* 80 obtained from cocoa pulp simulation media was a gene responsible for its preference for fructose consumption [70].

A concentration of 4% of inulin or fructooligosaccharide were used as prebiotics in fermenting watermelon juice inoculated with *L. plantarum* ATCC 8014 on MRS agar for 6 hours under anaerobic incubation at 37°C but with no statistically significant effect on the proliferation rate [73]. A-Glucans (alpha-glucans) are polysaccharides of D-glucose monomers linked with glycosidic bonds of the alpha form and possess prebiotic properties, since it was revealed that they were able to enhance the viability of LAB added to a chocolate pudding [74].

Fructans are oligosaccharides and polysaccharides of fructose units, found in the cell walls of various plants such as chicory (*Cichorium intybus*), Jerusalem artichoke (*Helianthus tuberosus*), garlic (*Allium sativum*), onion (*Allium cepa*), asparagus (*Asparagus officinalis*) and agave, know to possess prebiotic properties, being consumed by gut microbiota, promoting human health through the production of short-chain fatty acids [75]. They are employed in the production of confectionery products such as low-calorie sweeteners, fat replacers, textural and viscosity modifiers [76] having positive influences on the glucose metabolism, combating obesity and overweight [77]. Gelatin gel systems, developed in acidic conditions of pH values of around ~3.5, with agave fructans or agave syrups instead of glucose and sucrose, were explored as prebiotic enriched media able to promote the growth of *L. plantarum*, as functional ingredients in the confectionery industry [75]. However, it was revealed that *L. plantarum* strains prefer glucose and sucrose as carbon sources, in comparison to other LAB which performed well in the fructans containing medium [75].

1.4. *L. plantarum* and Blood Glucose Levels, Obesity, Cholesterolemia

It is well known that products containing high levels of sugars evoke excessive plasma-glucose and insulin responses, for which reason they are not recommended for consumption to those who are known to have conditions related to any types of diabetes. Type 2 diabetes Mellitus (T2DM) is a common condition that causes the level of sugar (glucose) in the blood to become too high. Initially, there is a compensatory increase in insulin production (hyperinsulinemia), which keeps glucose levels normal or pre-diabetic [78]. However, the pancreas is unable to continue producing enough insulin, resulting in persistent hyperglycemia and a diabetes diagnosis. Hyperglycemia manifests itself first as an increase in postprandial blood glucose induced by cellular insulin resistance, followed by an increase in fasting glucose concentrations. The gut microbiota is proved to be involved in the etiology of diabetes, by influencing glucose homeostasis and insulin resistance in major metabolic organs such as liver, muscle and fat, as well as by affecting digestion of sugars and production of gut hormones that control this process [79, 80]. Prebiotics are digested by the gut microbiota in the distal intestine (ileum and colon) to produce short-chain fatty acids (SCFAs) and gases (carbon dioxide, hydrogen, and methane). SCFAs (acetate, propionate, butyrate) play a variety of biological activities, including water and electrolyte absorption, intraluminal pH reduction, cell proliferation and differentiation, and modulation of intestinal immunological and inflammatory processes. *L. plantarum* was proved to reduce the blood glucose levels, but also to reduce the inflammatory responses, for which reason its inclusion to confectionery products will improve their nutritional status.

Hetero polysaccharides, in the composition of *Lactobacillus plantarum H31*, obtained in the insulin-resistant HepG2 cell line, reduced -amylase and increased gene expression of GLUT-4 (insulin-regulated glucose transporter type 4), AKT-2, and activated protein kinase (AMPK). Through the insulin signaling system, these genes enhance glucose absorption in insulin-resistant cells. The PI3K/AKT signaling system regulates insulin effect in trapping blood glucose in cells (hepatocytes) via translocating GLUT-4 vesicles (vesicles cannot be translocated in T2DM, resulting in suppression of glucose intake) [81, 82].

Lactobacillus plantarum LRCC5310 and LRCC5314 (10^8 -10^{10} CFU/g) increased the expression of GLUT-4 and adiponectin, while decreasing the expression of pro inflammatory genes (interleukin-6 [IL-6], Ccl2, leptin), implying that oral administration of lactic acid bacteria can prevent a rise in blood glucose levels by normalizing metabolic gene expression and inhibiting inflammatory responses [83]. Besides successfully lowering blood glucose, it was revealed that the *L. plantarum* SCS2 strain may alleviate weight loss, correct insulin insufficiency, and minimize oxidative stress by enhancing antioxidant enzyme activity [84].

After supplementation with *L. plantarum* 299, lower systolic blood pressure was found, which might be due to decreased tissue insulin resistance coupled with lower blood leptin concentrations. Also, considerable decreases were found in fibrinogen, total and LDL-cholesterol concentrations, an increase of (high density lopoproteins) HDL cholesterol (10%) [85]. *L. plantarum* PH04, was also found to possess potential for reducing cholesterol levels[86]. It was proved that *L. plantarum* administration leads to a reduction in cardiovascular disease risk factors and could be useful as a protective agent in the primary prevention of atherosclerosis [85].

The strains MP2026 and MP2420 may be used in the development of probiotics intended to alleviate symptoms associated with gastrointestinal disorders caused by sugar malabsorption due to their ability to consume dietary sugars lactose and fructose, the absence of gas production, good adhesion, survival in gastrointestinal (GI) conditions, and susceptibility to clinically relevant antibiotics [87]. The *L. plantarum* KR6 strain is also fructose tolerant and consuming.

Conclusion

Confectionery products such as chewing candies, jellies or gummy candies, chocolates or chocolate containing products, peanut butter, were already studied in formulations containing some strains of *L. plantarum,* which was included because of its antimicrobial capacity, because confectionery products possess high carbohydrate content which could ensure their viability and because they represent important vehicles for the delivery of probiotic bacteria given their popularity among consumers. Sensory acceptance was commonly tested for the proposed food product formulations, along with the survival rates of the bacteria during storage. However, not all the confectionery products were proved to be excellent hosts for some strains of *L. plantarum.* In peanut butter containing dextrose (2%) and glycerol (2%), *L. plantarum* was added with the purpose of controlling biogenic amines quantity during the storage of the product, but the results were not as promising as expected probably because of the ingredients or processing conditions. While the growth of *L. plantarum* is stimulated by acacia gum and by mushroom polysaccharides in comparison with the media containing glucose, no influence was found in regard to the prebiotic activity of inulin or fructans. Also, in sugar free candies containing, thymol and cardamom essential oils and *L. plantarum* (ATCC 14917) cell-free supernatant, only the formulation containing cardamom essential oil was comparable with the reference in terms of oral sense, having high chance of acceptability from the consumers. For gelatin based products, in their sugar free variant, gummies containing lyophilized raspberry by products and *L. plantarum 135* isolated from spontaneous fermented cereals exhibited highest total polyphenolic content in 24 days storage, with overall high acceptability in a sensory evaluation [29]. In general, because probiotic confectionery products are designed for improving the nutritional profile of the products, these are proposed in sugar free formulation, with polyols and other natural sugar replacers such as inulin, agave syrup, honey, in their composition. *L. plantarum* strains grow better when they have glucose and sucrose as carbon sources, in comparison the fructans containing medium; while Huli strain, was positively influenced by the presence of sugar cane molasses, which is considered a by-product of the sugar processing industry. Maltodextrins, which are commonly employed in sugar free confectionery as bulking agents, also influence positively the *L. plantarum* strains.

In this chapter was also revisited the ability of some *L. plantarum* strains to produce exopolysaccharides, polyols, such as sorbitol and other sweeteners such as D-Tagatose, which could be of high interest in developing functionalized confectionery products. EPS were reported to possess some positive effects on human wellbeing, such as radical scavenging activity, anti-tumor, anti-bacteria, anti-mutagen effects or immune regulation. Some strains have the ability to consume fructose or lactose, alleviating some gastrointestinal disorders.

Strain of *L. plantarum* were also studied in their relationship with fermentation of the cocoa beans and the development of aroma in chocolate products. So far, *L. plantarum* was included in the formulation of dark and milk chocolates, also in their sugar free variant, in free or immobilized form, encapsulated, spray-dried or lyophilized form, these processing conditions having different effects on the cell's viability, depending on the presence of some protective agents. While too high or too low temperatures involved in the before mentioned processes might affect some strains of *L. plantarum,* other techniques such electro-hydrodynamic atomization could be an impediment for the up-scaling of the production processes and the transfer to industrial production. The usage of carbohydrates in designing protective layers for the microcapsules of the probiotic bacteria, can induce fat blooming, loss of shine and defects in chocolate products during storage, while the microcapsules can alter lipid crystallization during tempering of chocolate, leading to an altered texture of the chocolate and increased apparent viscosity of the chocolate mass. For this reason, even if chocolate may contain components that could potentially support the growth of *L. plantarum* such as sugar, proteins, cocoa and antioxidant compounds, is should not yet be targeted as an optimal host for the inclusion of probiotic bacteria, taking in regard its rich amount of fat and sugar and their combinations effects, the presence of theobromine and its implication on the central nervous system, which affects individuals differently based on factors such as body weight, tolerance, and overall sensitivity. Interestingly, none of the research conducted in chocolate, does not take in consideration the total cell count of *L.plantarum* per serving size, thus, as a further research topic, it would be of great importance to quantify if the effect of the probiotics outstands the negative effects which could arise from the higher consumption of chocolate, especially that containing sugar, which does not contain pure cocoa fat and high cocoa levels. Further research is encouraged in the relationship with food products consumption and nutritional or medical effects. *L. plantarum* is proved to reduce the blood glucose levels and the inflammatory responses, for which reason its inclusion in confectionery products is solving the problems related to hyperglycemia and insulin responses. The gut microbiota is proved to be involved in the etiology of diabetes, by influencing glucose homeostasis and insulin resistance, while probiotic bacteria, including *L. plantarum*, are successfully lowering blood glucose. It was revealed that positive effects on the consumers health depend also on the strain, the *L. plantarum* SCS2 strain may alleviate weight loss, correct insulin insufficiency, and minimize oxidative stress by enhancing antioxidant enzyme activity.

References

[1] Racolta E., Mureșan V., *Tehnologia amidonului-produse zaharoase Manual didactic ID, 2019,* EAP - Editura Academic Press, Cluj-Napoca, Romania, eISBN 978-973-744-729-6.

[2] World Health Organisation, Fact Sheet, Obesity and Overweight, 2023, Available online: https://www.who.int/news-room/fact-sheets/ (accessed on 10 MAY 2023).

[3] Konar, N., Gunes, R., Palabiyik, I., Toker, O. S., Health conscious consumers and sugar confectionery: Present aspects and projections. *Trends in Food Science & Technology,* 2022, *123*, 57-68.

[4] Pekdogan Goztok, S., Gunes, R., Toker, O. S., Palabiyik, I., Konar, N., Investigation of the use of various fruit juice concentrates instead of corn syrup in marshmallow type products: A preliminary study. *International Journal of Gastronomy and Food Science,* 2022, *30*:100616.

[5] Kasabova, K., Samokhvalova, O., Zagorulko, A., Zahorulko, A., Babaiev, S., Bereza, O., Ponomarenko, N., Tesliuk, H., Yukhno, V., Improvement of Turkish Delight Production Technology Using a Developed Multi-Component Fruit and Vegetable Paste, *Eastern-European Journal of Enterprise Technologies,* 2022, 6(11 (120), 51–59.

[6] Teixeira-Lemos, E., Almeida, A. R., Vouga, B., Morais, C., Correia, I., Pereira, P., Guiné, R. P., Development and characterization of healthy gummy jellies containing natural fruits, *Journal Open Agriculture,* 2021, *6* (1), 466-478.

[7] Delgado, P., Bañón, S., Effects of replacing starch by inulin on the physicochemical, texture and sensory characteristics of gummy jellies. *CyTA - Journal of Food,* 2018, *16* (1), 1-10.

[8] Čižauskaitė, U., Jakubaitytė, G., Žitkevičius, V., Kasparavičienė, G., Natural Ingredients-Based Gummy Bear Composition Designed According to Texture Analysis and Sensory Evaluation In Vivo, *Molecules*, 2019; 24 (7): 1442.

[9] Söderling, E., Pienihäkkinen, K., Gursoy, U. K. J, Effects of sugar-free polyol chewing gums on gingival inflammation: a systematic review, *Clinic Oral Investigations*, 2022, *26* (12), 6881-6891.

[10] Zumbe, A., Lee, A., Storey, D. J., Polyols in confectionery: the route to sugar-free, reduced sugar and reduced calorie confectionery. *The British Journal of nutrition*, 2001, *85* (S1), S31-S45.

[11] Homayouni Rad, A., Pirouzian, H. R., Toker, O. S., Konar, N., Application of simplex lattice mixture design for optimization of sucrose-free milk chocolate produced in a ball mill. *LWT* 2019, *115*, 108435.

[12] Belščak-Cvitanović, A.; Komes, D.; Dujmović, M.; Karlović, S.; Biškić, M.; Brnčić, M.; Ježek, D. J. F. c., Physical, bioactive and sensory quality parameters of reduced sugar chocolates formulated with natural sweeteners as sucrose alternatives, *Food Chemistry*, 2015, *167*, 61-70.

[13] Šeremet, D.; Mandura, A.; Vojvodić Cebin, A.; Oskomić, M.; Champion, E.; Martinić, A.; Komes, D.,Ruby chocolate–Bioactive potential and sensory quality characteristics compared with dark, milk and white chocolate, *Agricultural and Food Sciences,* 2019, *8* (2), 89-96.

[14] Weber, T., Solioz, M., Technology, Evaluation of chocolate as a source of dietary copper, *European Food Research and Technology*, 2014, *238*, 1063-1066.

[15] Gvozdjakova, A., Singh, R., Takahashi, T., Fedacko, J., Hristova, K., Wilczynska, A., Mojtová, M., Mojto, V., Chapter 19 - Cocoa Consumption and Prevention of Cardiometabolic Diseases and Other Chronic Diseases. In *The Role of Functional Food Security in Global Health*, 2019, Eds. Academic Press; pp 317-345, ISBN 9780128131480.

[16] Davani-Davari, D., Negahdaripour, M., Karimzadeh, I., Seifan, M., Mohkam, M., Masoumi, S. J., Berenjian, A., Ghasemi, Y., Prebiotics: definition, types, sources, mechanisms, and clinical applications. *Foods,* 2019, *8* (3), 92.

[17] Żyżelewicz, D., Motyl, I., Nebesny, E., Budryn, G., Krysiak, W., Rosicka-Kaczmarek, J., Libudzisz, Z. J. P., Probiotic Confectionery Products–Preparation and Properties. 2012, 261., IntechOpen, London.

[18] Şenöztop, E., Dokuzlu, T., Güngörmüşler, M., A comprehensive review on the development of probiotic supplemented confectioneries. *Zeitschrift fur Naturforschung,* 2022, *77* (1-2), 71-84.

[19] Lim, S.-M., Lee, N.-K.; Paik, H.-D., Antibacterial and anticavity activity of probiotic Lactobacillus plantarum 200661 isolated from fermented foods against Streptococcus mutans. *LWT* 2020, *118*, 108840.

[20] Zhang, Q., Qin, S., Huang, Y., Xu, X., Zhao, J., Zhang, H., Chen, W., Inhibitory and preventive effects of Lactobacillus plantarum FB-T9 on dental caries in rats. *Journal of Oral microbiology*, 2020, *12* (1), 1703883.

[21] Kaur, K., Nekkanti, S., Madiyal, M., Choudhary, P., Effect of chewing gums containing probiotics and xylitol on oral health in children: A randomized controlled trial. *Journal of Oral microbiology,* 2018, *10* (5), 237-243.

[22] Chundakkattumalayil, H. C., Kumar, S., Narayanan, R., Thalakattil Raghavan, K. T., Role of L. plantarum KX519413 as probiotic and Acacia gum as prebiotic in gastrointestinal tract strengthening. *Microorganism,* 2019, *7* (12), 659.

[23] Nart, J., Jiménez-Garrido, S., Ramírez-Sebastià, A., Buj, D., Huedo, P., Espadaler, J., Oral colonization by levilactobacillus brevis KABPTM-052 and Lactiplantibacillus plantarum KABPTM-051: a randomized, double-blinded, placebo-controlled trial (pilot study). *Journal of clinical and experimental dentistry,* 2021, *13* (5), e433.

[24] Karimi, N., Jabbari, V., Nazemi, A., Ganbarov, K., Karimi, N., Tanomand, A., Karimi, S., Abbasi, A., Yousefi, B., Khodadadi, E., Kafil, H. S., Thymol, cardamom and Lactobacillus plantarum nanoparticles as a functional candy with high protection against Streptococcus mutans and tooth decay. *Microbial Pathogenesis* 2020, *148*, 104481.

[25] Anurag, T., An over view on chemistry and applications of acacia gums. *Der Pharma Chemica,* 2010, 2(6):327-331,

[26] Wang, G., Chen, X., Wang, L., Zhao, L., Xia, Y., Ai, L. Diverse conditions contribute to the cholesterol-lowering ability of different Lactobacillus plantarum strains, *Food Function,*2021, *12* (3), 1079-1086.

[27] Kamil, R., Fadhila, F. H., Rachmasari, A. D., Murdiati, A., Juffrie, M., Rahayu, E., Development of probiotic gummy candy using the indigenous Lactobacillus plantarum Dad-13 strain; evaluation of its gastrointestinal resistance and shelflife prediction. *Food Research 2021*, *5*, 265-273.

[28] Feng, S., Wang, H., Lin, X., Liang, H., Zhang, S., Chen, Y.; Ji, C., Probiotic properties of Lactobacillus plantarum and application in prebiotic gummies. *LWT* 2023, *174*, 114357.

[29] Danesh, A., The Development of Nutraceuticals in Gummies Form, Based on Antimicrobial Lactic Acid Bacteria, Multifunctional Gels, and Berries/Fruits by-Products, Thesis, Lithuanian UNIVERSITY OF HEALTH SCIENCES VETERINARY ACADEMY 2022, available online at https://portalcris.lsmuni.lt/server/api/core/bitstreams/5ef256d5-624a-4d27-a76e-21ded2fcaaff/content, (accessed on 10 MAY 2023).

[30] Singh, P., Medronho, B., Miguel, M. G., Esquena, J. J. F. H., On the encapsulation and viability of probiotic bacteria in edible carboxymethyl cellulose-gelatin water-in-water emulsions, *Food Hydrocolloids,* 2018, *75*, 41-50.

[31] Devarajan, A., Mudgil, P., Aldhaheri, F., Hamed, F., Dhital, S., Maqsood, S., Camel milk-derived probiotic strains encapsulated in camel casein and gelatin complex microcapsules: Stability against thermal challenge and simulated gastrointestinal digestion conditions, *Journal of Dairy Science*, 2022, *105* (3), 1862-1877.

[32] Hadidi, M., Majidiyan, N., Jelyani, A. Z., Moreno, A., Hadian, Z.; Mousavi Khanegah, A., Alginate/fish gelatin-encapsulated Lactobacillus acidophilus: A study on viability and technological quality of bread during baking and storage, *Foods*, 2021, *10* (9), 2215, https://doi.org/10.3390/foods10092215.

[33] Juodeikiene, G., Zadeike, D., Bartkiene, E., Lėlė, V., Bernatoniene, J., Jakštas, V. , A new delivery system based on apple pomace–pectin gels to encourage the viability of antimicrobial strains, *Food Science and Technology International*, 2020, *26* (3), 242-253, https://doi.org/10.1177/1082013219881585.

[34] Foong, Y. J.; Lee, S. T.; Ramli, N.; Tan, Y. N.; Ayob, M. K. J. J. o. F. Q., Incorporation of Potential Probiotic L actobacillus plantarum Isolated from Fermented Cocoa Beans into Dark Chocolate: Bacterial Viability and Physicochemical Properties Analysis. *Journal of Food Quality,* 2013, *36* (3), 164-171.

[35] Gómez-Fernández, A. R., Faccinetto-Beltrán, P., Orozco-Sánchez, N. E., Pérez-Carrillo, E., Marín-Obispo, L. M., Hernández-Brenes, C., Santacruz, A., Jacobo-

Velázquez, D. A., Sugar-free milk chocolate as a carrier of omega-3 polyunsaturated fatty acids and probiotics: A potential functional food for the diabetic population. *Foods*, 2021, *10* (8), 1866.

[36] da Silva, M. N.; Tagliapietra, B. L.; do Amaral Flores, V.; dos Santos Richards, N. S. P. J., In vitro test to evaluate survival in the gastrointestinal tract of commercial probiotics., Current *research in food science*, 2021, *4*, 320-325.

[37] Kamil, R. Z.; Murdiati, A.; Juffrie, M.; Rahayu, E. S. J. N., Gut microbiota modulation of moderate undernutrition in infants through gummy Lactobacillus plantarum Dad-13 consumption: A randomized double-blind controlled trial. *Nutrients*, 2022, *14* (5), 1049.

[38] Han, Q., Kong, B., Chen, Q., Sun, F., Zhang, H., In vitro comparison of probiotic properties of lactic acid bacteria isolated from Harbin dry sausages and selected probiotics, *Journal of Functional Foods*, 2017, *32*, 391-400.

[39] Pavlovic, A., Mrmosanin, J., Krstic, J., Mitic, S., Tosic, S., Mitić, M., Arsic, B., Micic, R. J., Effect of storage temperature on the decay of catechins and procyanidins in dark chocolate. *Czech Journal of Food Science,* 2017, *35* (4), 360-366.

[40] Succi, M., Tremonte, P., Pannella, G., Tipaldi, L., Cozzolino, A., Coppola, R., Sorrentino, E., Survival of commercial probiotic strains in dark chocolate with high cocoa and phenols content during the storage and in a static in vitro digestion model. *Journal of Functional Foods* 2017, *35*, 60-67.

[41] Zoldan, J., De Marco, I., Verruck, S., Gomide, A. I., Cartabiano, C. E. L., de Melo Pereira, G. V., Lindner, Evaluation of viability to simulated gastrointestinal tract passage of probiotic strains and pioneer bioaccessibility analyses of antioxidants in chocolate. *Food Bioscience*, 2023, *52*, 102494.

[42] Lim, J. h., Yoon, S. m., Tan, P. L., Yang, S., Kim, S. h., Park, H., Probiotic properties of Lactobacillus plantarum LRCC5193, a plant-origin lactic acid bacterium isolated from kimchi and its use in chocolates. *Journal of Food Science,* 2018, *83* (11), 2802-2811.

[43] Mirković, M., Seratlić, S., Kilcawley, K., Mannion, D., Mirković, N., Radulović, Z. The Sensory Quality and Volatile Profile of Dark Chocolate Enriched with Encapsulated Probiotic Lactobacillus plantarum Bacteria, *Sensors*, 2018, 6;18(8):2570.

[44] Radulović, Z., Miočinović, J., Mirković, N., Mirković, M., Paunović, D., Ivanović, M., Seratlić, S. J. Survival of spray-dried and free-cells of potential probiotic Lactobacillus plantarum 564 in soft goat cheese, *Animal Science Journal*, 2017, *88* (11), 1849-1854.

[45] Konar, N., Palabiyik, I., Toker, O. S., Polat, D. G., Kelleci, E., Pirouzian, H. R., Akcicek, A.; Sagdic, O., Conventional and sugar-free probiotic white chocolate: Effect of inulin DP on various quality properties and viability of probiotics. *Journal of Functional Foods,* 2018, *43*, 206-213.

[46] Mulyaningsih, R., Nurhidayat, N., Mangunwardoyo, W. In Viability microcapsules Lactobacillus plantarum Mar 8 and KMar C2 in chocolate (Theobroma cacao L) for probiotic purposes, *Journal of Physics: Conference Series,* IOP Publishing: 2020; p 042073.

[47] Goranov, B., Teneva, D., Denkova-Kostova, R., Shopska, V., Oulahal, N., Denkova, Z., Kostov, G., Degraeve, P., Pagan, R. J. M., Biopreservation of Chocolate Mousse with Lactobacillus helveticus 2/20: Microbial Challenge Test. *Molecules*, 2022, *27* (17), 5631.

[48] Denkova-Kostova, R. S., Goranov, B. G., Teneva, D. G., Tomova, T. G., Denkova, Z. R., Shopska, V., Mihaylova-Ivanova, Y. J. A. S. P. T. A., Bio-preservation of chocolate mousse with free and immobilized cells of Lactobacillus plantarum D2 and lemon (Citrus lemon L.) or grapefruit (Citrus paradisi L.) zest essential oils. *Acta scientiarum Polonorum Technologia Alimentaria,* 2021, *20* (1), 5-16.

[49] Food Safety and Standards Authority of India, Indian snacks and sweets. 2021, *File No.1(13), Codex/FSSAI-2021.*

[50] Lasta, E. L.; da Silva Pereira Ronning, E., Dekker, R. F., da Cunha, M. A. A., Encapsulation and dispersion of Lactobacillus acidophilus in a chocolate coating as a strategy for maintaining cell viability in cereal bars. *Scientific Reports*, 2021, *11* (1), 20550.

[51] Champagne, C. P., Guertin, N., Raymond, Y., Strategies to improve the survival of probiotic Lacticaseibacillus rhamnosus R0011 during the production and storage of granola bars. *Canadian Journal of Microbiology,* 2022, *68* (3), 147-156.

[52] ElDeeb, G. S., Mokhtar, S. M., Control of Biogenic Amines in Peanut Butter by Incorporation of Some Probiotic Bacteria. *Egyptian Journal of Food Science*, 2020, *48* (2), 259-270.

[53] Fuso, A., Bancalari, E., Castellone, V., Caligiani, A., Gatti, M., Bottari, B. Feeding Lactic Acid Bacteria with Different Sugars: Effect on Exopolysaccharides (EPS) Production and Their Molecular Characteristics, *Foods*, 2023. *12*(1), 215.

[54] Suryawanshi, N., Naik, S., Jujjawarapu, S. E. A., Exopolysaccharides and their Applications in Food Processing Industries, *Food Science and Applied Biotechnology*, 2022, *5* (1), 22-44.

[55] KB, R., Radha, K., Sathian, C., Chinnu, M., Exopolysaccharide production potential of different strains of Lactobacillus plantarum. *Indian Journal of Dairy Science*, 2020, Vol. 73 No. 4.

[56] Desai, K., Akolkar, S., Badhe, Y., Tambe, S., Lele, S. J. P. B., Optimization of fermentation media for exopolysaccharide production from Lactobacillus plantarum using artificial intelligence-based techniques. *Process Biochemistry,* 2006, *41* (8), 1842-1848.

[57] Zhang, J., Zhao, W., Guo, X., Guo, T., Zheng, Y., Wang, Y., Hao, Y., Yang, Z. J. Survival and effect of exopolysaccharide-producing Lactobacillus plantarum YW11 on the physicochemical properties of ice cream. *Polish Journal of Food and Nutrition Sciences,* 2017, *67* (3).

[58] Zhang, M.; Lai, T.; Yao, M.; Zhang, M.; Yang, Z. Interaction of the Exopolysaccharide from Lactobacillus plantarum YW11 with Casein and Bioactivities of the Polymer Complex , *Foods*, 2021, 10(6): 1153.

[59] Siti, R. O., Effect of microencapsulated Lactobacillus plantarum on the rheological and sensorial properties of synbiotic ice cream. *International Journal of Current Research*, 2018, *19* (3), 506-514.

[60] Hanafi, F. N. A., Kamaruding, N. A., Shaharuddin, S., Influence of coconut residue dietary fiber on physicochemical, probiotic (Lactobacillus plantarum ATCC 8014) survivability and sensory attributes of probiotic ice cream. *LWT* 2022, *154*, 112725.
[61] Cinar, A., Altuntas, S., Altuntas, V., The addition of royal jelly to dairy probiotic dessert produced with predictive microbiology: Influence on physicochemical, rheological, microbial and sensorial properties. *LWT*, 2021, *146*, 111444.
[62] Ladero, V., Ramos, A., Wiersma, A., Goffin, P., Schanck, A., Kleerebezem, M., Hugenholtz, J. Smid, E. J.; Hols, P. J. A.; microbiology, e., High-level production of the low-calorie sugar sorbitol by Lactobacillus plantarum through metabolic engineering. *Applied and Environmental Microbiology,* 2007, *73* (6), 1864-1872.
[63] Nadiya Jan, K., Tripathi, A. D., Singh, S., Surya, D., Singh, S. P., Enhanced Sorbitol Production under Submerged Fermentation using Lactobacillus plantarum. *Applied Food Biotechnology* 2017, *4* (2), pp. 85-92.
[64] Zumbé, A.; Lee, A.; Storey, D., Polyols in confectionery: the route to sugar-free, reduced sugar and reduced calorie confectionery. *British Journal of Nutrition* 2001, *85* (S1), S31-S45.
[65] COMMISSION, T. E., REGULATION (EU) 2017/2470. *Official Journal of the European Union* 2017.
[66] Sun, Z., Miao, T., Yin, A., Qiu, H., Xiao, Y., Li, Y., Hai, J., Xu, B., Optimization of fermentation conditions for production of l-arabinose isomerase of Lactobacillus plantarum WU14. *Food Science & Nutrition* 2021, *9* (1), 230-243.
[67] Saavedra, S., Alejandro-Paredes, L., Flores-Santos, J. C., Flores-Fernández, C. N., Arellano-García, H.; Zavaleta, A. I., Optimization of lactic acid production by Lactobacillus plantarum strain Hui1 in a medium containing sugar cane molasses. *Agronomia Colombiana*, 2021, *39* (1), 98-107.
[68] Coelho, L.; De Lima, C.; Rodovalho, C.; Bernardo, M.; Contiero, J. J. B. J. o. C. E., Lactic acid production by new Lactobacillus plantarum LMISM6 grown in molasses: optimization of medium composition. *Brazilian Journal of Chemical Engineering*, 2011, *28*, 27-36.
[69] Alves de Oliveira, R., Filho, R., Rossell, C., High Lactic Acid Production from Molasses and Hydrolysed Sugarcane Bagasse. *Chemical Engineering Transactions,* 2016, *50*, 307-312.
[70] De Vuyst, L., Weckx, S. J. J. o. A. M., The cocoa bean fermentation process: from ecosystem analysis to starter culture development, *Journal of applied microbiology*, 2016, *121* (1), 5-17.
[71] Illeghems, K., Weckx, S., De Vuyst, L., Applying meta-pathway analyses through metagenomics to identify the functional properties of the major bacterial communities of a single spontaneous cocoa bean fermentation process sample. *Food Microbiology* 2015, *50*, 54-63.
[72] Djaafar, T. F., Monika, D. C., Marwati, T., Triwitono, P., Rahayu, E. S., Microbiology, Chemical, and Sensory Characteristics of Cocoa Powder: The Effect of Lactobacillus plantarum HL-15 as Culture Starter and Fermentation Box Variation. *Digital Press Life Sciences, 2020*, 2, 00008.
[73] Amanda, E.; Choo, W. S., Effect of refrigerated storage on the physicochemical characteristics and viability of Lactobacillus plantarum in fermented watermelon

juice with or without supplementation with inulin or fructooligosaccharide, *Journal of Food Processing and Preservation*, 2018, *42* (12), e13831.

[74] İspirli, H., Demirbaş, F., Dertli, E. J., Glucan type exopolysaccharide (EPS) shows prebiotic effect and reduces syneresis in chocolate pudding, *Journal of Food Science and Technology,* 2018, *55*, 3821-3826.

[75] Rodríguez-Rodríguez, R., Barajas-Álvarez, P., Morales-Hernández, N., Camacho-Ruíz, R. M., Espinosa-Andrews, H., Physical Properties and Prebiotic Activities (Lactobacillus spp.) of Gelatine-Based Gels Formulated with Agave Fructans and Agave Syrups as Sucrose and Glucose Substitutes, *Molecules,* 2022, *27* (15), 4902.

[76] García-Villalba, W. G.; Rodríguez-Herrera, R.; Ochoa-Martínez, L. A.; Rutiaga-Quiñones, O. M.; Gallegos-Infante, J. A.; González-Herrera, S. M. J. J. o. F. S.; Technology, Agave fructans: a review of their technological functionality and extraction processes, *Journal of Food Science and Technology,* 2022, 1-9.

[77] Espinosa-Andrews, H., Urías-Silvas, J. E., Morales-Hernández, N., The role of agave fructans in health and food applications: A review. *Trends in Food Science & Technology,* 2021, *114*, 585-598.

[78] Franz, M. J., Medical nutrition therapy for diabetes mellitus and hypoglycemia of nondiabetic origin, in *Krause's Food & Nutrition Therapy.* Canada: Saunders Elsevier, 2008.

[79] Aw, W.; Fukuda, S. J., Understanding the role of the gut ecosystem in diabetes mellitus, *Journal of diabetes investigation*, 2018, *9* (1), 5-12.

[80] Gurung, M., Li, Z., You, H., Rodrigues, R., Jump, D. B., Morgun, A., Shulzhenko, N. J. E., Role of gut microbiota in type 2 diabetes pathophysiology. *EbioMedicine*, 2020, *51*, 102590.

[81] Angelin J., Kavitha, M., Exopolysaccharides from probiotic bacteria and their health potential., *International Journal of Biological Macromolecules,* 2020, 162: 853–865.

[82] Huang, Z.; Lin, F.; Zhu, X.; Zhang, C.; Jiang, M.; Lu, Z. J. I. j. o. b. m., An exopolysaccharide from Lactobacillus plantarum H31 in pickled cabbage inhibits pancreas α-amylase and regulating metabolic markers in HepG2 cells by AMPK/PI3K/Akt pathway. *International Journal of Biological Macromolecules,* 2020, *143*, 775-784.

[83] Youn, H. S., Kim, J.-H., Lee, J. S., Yoon, Y. Y., Choi, S. J., Lee, J. Y., Kim, W., Hwang, K. W., Lactobacillus plantarum reduces low-grade inflammation and glucose levels in a mouse model of chronic stress and diabetes. *Infection and immunity*, 2021, *89* (8), e00615-20.

[84] Wu, L. j.; Long, L.; Sun, J. y.; Bu, L. l.; Cao, J. l.; Luo, Y.; Liu, H. j.; Wu, Y.; Meng, X., Exploring the antioxidant effect of Lactobacillus plantarum SCS2 on mice with type 2 diabetes, *Journal of food biochemistry,* 2021, *45* (8), e13781.

[85] Naruszewicz, M.; Johansson, M.-L.; Zapolska-Downar, D.; Bukowska, H., Effect of Lactobacillus plantarum 299v on cardiovascular disease risk factors in smokers. *The American Journal of Clinical Nutrition* 2002, *76* (6), 1249-1255.

[86] Nguyen, T. D.; Kang, J. H.; Lee, M. S., Characterization of Lactobacillus plantarum PH04, a potential probiotic bacterium with cholesterol-lowering effects. *International journal of food microbiology,* 2007, *113* (3), 358-61.

[87] Šeme, H., Bogovič Matijašić, B., Švigelj, K., Langerholc, T., Fujs, Š.; Horvat, J., Zlatić, E., Gjuračić, K., Petković, H., Štempelj, M., Kos, B., Šušković, J., Kosec, G., Generation of Lactobacillus plantarum strains with improved potential to target gastrointestinal disorders related to sugar malabsorption. *Food research international,* 2017, *94*, 45-53.

Index

A

acidification, 118, 122, 133, 140, 142, 178, 189, 192, 196
adverse effects, 77, 89, 95, 113
American Food and Drug Administration (FDA), 2, 87, 197, 206
ancient wheat species, 116, 120, 121, 122, 145, 153
antimicrobial activity, 85, 86, 106, 109, 116, 138, 142, 145, 157, 158, 190, 197, 200, 213, 216, 217, 218, 220, 222, 232, 238

B

Bacilli, 5, 24
bakery, v, vii, 115, 116, 120, 125, 126, 135, 139, 144, 147, 149, 152
beverages, 15, 16, 79, 80, 106, 204, 207, 208, 210, 215, 219, 221, 223, 224

C

cardiovascular disease, 29, 36, 41, 89, 94, 174, 198, 234, 254, 263
cereal-based beverages, 221
cereals, vi, vii, 78, 92, 120, 136, 139, 148, 207, 208, 210, 211, 220, 221, 222, 223, 224, 226, 230, 231, 248
cheese, 8, 11, 162, 163, 164, 168, 169, 170, 171, 173, 174, 175, 176, 177, 178, 179, 180, 181, 186, 187, 204, 216, 246, 260
chocolate, vi, vii, 237, 238, 239, 240, 244, 245, 246, 247, 248, 252, 255, 256, 258, 259, 260, 261, 263
chocolate-based products, vi, vii, 237, 238, 240, 244
cider, 213, 226
clinical application, 23, 24, 25, 37, 77, 258
cognition, 26, 37, 41
colonization, 25, 28, 31, 32, 39, 45, 47, 55, 90, 95, 100, 105, 113, 187, 258
controlled release, vii, 45, 46, 47, 59, 60, 63, 64, 65, 68, 73, 76, 79, 83
cooked meat products (cooked meat), 186, 188, 189, 191, 194, 195
COVID, 208, 209

D

dairy, vi, 2, 3, 8, 9, 10, 14, 17, 18, 21, 24, 39, 42, 47, 69, 70, 71, 78, 80, 92, 105, 106, 107, 109, 157, 158, 159, 160, 161, 163, 164, 167, 168, 169, 170, 171, 173, 175, 176, 177, 178, 179, 180, 181, 182, 183, 186, 202, 203, 204, 225, 229, 232, 237, 238, 240, 243, 259, 261, 262
dairy industry, 109, 159, 164, 167, 168, 170, 243
dairy products, vi, 8, 9, 24, 78, 80, 92, 157, 158, 159, 161, 164, 169, 170, 171, 173, 175, 178, 181, 186
diabetes, 33, 34, 40, 43, 45, 94, 98, 99, 104, 108, 111, 198, 238, 239, 253, 257, 263
durum wheat, 120, 121, 123, 124, 208

E

electrospinning, 50, 62, 63, 66, 71
emulsion, 48, 50, 53, 54, 55, 56, 67, 71, 72, 80, 82, 196, 199
encapsulating agents, 46
encapsulation, vii, 45, 46, 47, 48, 49, 50, 51, 52, 53, 54, 55, 57, 59, 60, 62, 63, 64, 65, 66, 67, 68, 69, 70, 71, 72, 73, 76, 77, 78, 79, 80, 81, 82, 83, 104, 105, 107,

108, 144, 150, 165, 182, 186, 190, 191, 192, 195, 199, 200, 206, 233, 241, 243, 247, 259, 261
encapsulation efficiency (EE), 46, 52, 55, 57, 60, 62, 64, 70, 82
encapsulation techniques, 45, 46, 47, 71, 76, 104, 105, 108, 243
exopolysaccharide production, 140, 154, 261
exopolysaccharides (EPS), 13, 24, 31, 93, 110, 118, 119, 136, 140, 153, 168, 170, 171, 173, 181, 222, 233, 249, 255, 261, 263
extrusion, 46, 48, 49, 50, 51, 52, 54, 67, 76, 80

F

fermented cereals, 221, 222, 243, 255
fermented foods, 1, 2, 3, 14, 15, 16, 38, 46, 78, 95, 104, 106, 114, 116, 119, 120, 150, 158, 159, 161, 168, 176, 180, 186, 187, 196, 204, 208, 209, 210, 216, 218, 221, 223, 227, 229, 234, 258
fermented meat products, 186, 188, 190, 196, 197, 198, 200, 204
fermented milk, 3, 19, 23, 109, 159, 160, 161, 168, 174, 176, 177, 180, 187, 202
Firmicutes, 5, 24, 34, 92, 93
food supplements, v, vii, 75, 76, 77, 86, 87, 91, 103, 104, 107, 109
fresh meat products, 186
fruits, vi, vii, 15, 47, 85, 109, 207, 208, 210, 211, 212, 213, 215, 216, 222, 223, 224, 227, 231, 232, 233, 248, 251, 257, 259
functional meat products, 186, 200
functional products, 116, 159, 160

G

gastrointestinal viability, 46
generally recognized as safe (GRAS), 2, 63, 64, 80, 94, 96, 112, 164, 167, 170, 193
genomic diversity, 2, 10, 13, 21
glucose response, 238
gluten-free (GF), 116, 139, 140, 141, 142, 143, 144, 145, 146, 148, 150, 151, 152, 154, 155
gluten-free products, 139, 140, 155
gut microbiota, 14, 18, 20, 31, 34, 38, 39, 40, 42, 43, 76, 77, 78, 84, 88, 90, 91, 92, 102, 103, 109, 111, 117, 137, 158, 182, 205, 252, 253, 256, 263

H

human health, vii, 14, 15, 23, 24, 25, 31, 37, 78, 85, 91, 94, 104, 137, 147, 158, 164, 166, 173, 174, 177, 182, 187, 200, 208, 209, 223, 224, 227, 252

I

ice cream, 164, 165, 166, 167, 177, 178, 180, 181, 238, 250, 251, 261, 262
inflammatory bowel disease (IBD), 32, 33, 43, 45, 78, 108, 209
isolation, 1, 3, 8, 9, 19, 43, 106, 108, 207, 208, 209, 210, 223, 224, 229, 231, 233, 235, 237, 238, 251, 252

J

juices, 46, 80, 107, 207, 211, 212, 214, 215, 219, 227, 228, 233, 234, 239

L

L. plantarum food supplements, 76
L. plantarum history, 2
Lactobacilliaceae, 24
Lactobacillus spp., 7, 19, 46, 150, 186, 263
literature review, 158, 207, 208

M

malolactic fermentation (MLF), 4, 16, 94, 112, 230

meat products manufacturing, vi, 185
meat reformulation, 186
mental illness, 35
microecology, 25, 31, 32, 37
microencapsulation, 47, 48, 49, 55, 57, 64, 65, 67, 69, 70, 71, 72, 73, 76, 79, 80, 84, 114, 144, 165, 167, 176, 177, 180, 229, 247
milk, vi, vii, 9, 18, 20, 21, 42, 47, 49, 50, 52, 53, 58, 63, 64, 66, 73, 80, 89, 92, 107, 110, 157, 159, 160, 162, 166, 168, 169, 170, 171, 172, 173, 174, 175, 176, 177, 178, 179, 180, 181, 182, 186, 216, 222, 227, 237, 238, 239, 240, 242, 243, 245, 246, 247,249, 250, 256, 258, 259, 260

N

nanocrystals (SNCs), 65
nanoemulsion, 50, 61
nanoencapsulation, v, 45, 46, 47, 50, 58, 59, 61, 62, 64, 65, 67, 68, 69, 73, 76, 79, 83, 84, 104, 106, 108
nanoencapsulation-functional foods, 83
nanospray drying, 59, 69
nutraceuticals, 15, 69, 72, 76, 86, 89, 109, 165, 259

P

pastry, v, vii, 115, 116, 145, 146
pharmaceutical(s), ii, v, vii, 24, 75, 77, 78, 79, 104, 108, 109, 119, 175, 218
prebiotic, 21, 25, 39, 66, 81, 88, 90, 110, 111, 117, 170, 171, 179, 239, 241, 247, 248, 251, 252, 255, 258, 259, 263
products formulation, 238

R

raw meat products, 188, 190
regulation, 16, 25, 31, 32, 33, 34, 37, 43, 76, 109, 202, 231, 250, 251, 256
regulation of microecology, 32

S

silage production, 208, 220
skin diseases, 35
sourdough, 105, 108, 115, 116, 117, 118, 119, 121, 122, 124, 125, 126, 127, 128, 129, 130, 131, 132, 133, 134, 135, 136, 137, 138, 139, 140, 141, 143, 144, 146, 147, 148, 149, 150, 151, 152, 153, 154, 163, 208, 210, 231
sourdough fermentation, 105, 115, 117, 118, 120, 121, 122, 124, 125, 126, 127, 129, 130, 132, 134, 138, 142, 143, 145, 146, 147, 148, 151, 152, 208, 231
spray-drying, 48, 56, 57, 59, 68, 73, 99, 214, 246
starch nanoparticles (SNPs), 65, 88, 110
sugar confectionery, vi, 237, 238, 240, 257
sugar confectionery products, 240
supplements, 5, 14, 34, 46, 67, 76, 77, 79, 83, 84, 87, 89, 104, 106, 109, 110, 111, 165, 201
symbiotic formulations, 77, 89

T

taxonomy, 2, 5, 14, 17, 167
therapy, 34, 40, 76, 84, 91, 93, 97, 98, 102, 103, 104, 113, 114, 147, 263
tolerance, 6, 18, 25, 31, 32, 40, 43, 90, 132, 136, 163, 171, 187, 220, 240, 246, 256
Type 2 diabetes, 33, 224, 253

U

United States Food and Drug Administration (FDA), 87, 94, 96, 109, 197, 206

V

vegetables, vi, vii, 8, 14, 15, 24, 47, 78, 80, 106, 160, 207, 208, 210, 211, 215, 216, 217, 218, 219, 222, 223, 226, 227, 228, 229, 230, 231, 251

W

wall material, 46, 47, 48, 49, 51, 52, 53, 57, 60, 63, 64, 66, 67, 69, 72
weight, 29, 30, 34, 86, 91, 92, 95, 101, 119, 130, 134, 254, 256
wheat, 105, 116, 117, 118, 119, 120, 121, 122, 123, 125, 126, 127, 128, 129, 130, 131, 132, 133, 134, 135, 136, 137, 139, 145, 146, 147, 148, 149, 150, 151, 152, 153, 154, 177, 221, 226
wheat species, 120, 151, 153
wine, 4, 11, 12, 15, 16, 24, 78, 94, 112, 123, 163, 213, 228, 232, 243

Y

yoghurt, 46, 71, 105, 106, 160, 161, 162, 171, 173, 174, 175, 179, 182, 183, 186, 204
yoghurt fermentation, 160, 172, 182